CHOLERA, FEVER AND ENGLISH MEDICINE 1825-1865

by

MARGARET PELLING

OXFORD UNIVERSITY PRESS

1978

Oxford University Press, Walton Street, Oxford OX2 6DP

OXFORD LONDON GLASGOW NEW YORK
TORONTO MELBOURNE WELLINGTON CAPE TOWN
IBADAN NAIROBI DAR ES SALAAM LUSAKA
KUALA LUMPUR SINGAPORE JAKARTA HONG KONG TOKYO
DELHI BOMBAY CALCUTTA MADRAS KARACHI

British Library Cataloguing in Publication Data

Pelling, Margaret
    Cholera, fever and English medicine, 1825–1865.
    — (Oxford historical monographs).
    1. Public health — England — History
    I. Title   II. Series
    614′.0942   RA487   77-30646

    ISBN 0-19-821872-9

*Set by Hope Services, Wantage
and printed in Great Britain by
Billing & Sons Ltd., Guildford, London and Worcester*

To

William Alexander Osborne

(1873–1967)

PREFACE

This book is based on a B. Litt. thesis submitted at the University of Oxford in October 1971, entitled 'Some approaches to nineteenth century epidemiology, with particular reference to John Snow and William Budd'. A certain amount of new material has been added to each of the chapters; Chapters 1, 2, and the Conclusions have been considerably altered. The text and the footnotes have been revised to bring them up to date.

My greatest debt is to Charles Webster, who was my supervisor and has subsequently taken an active interest in the process of revision. The finished product is no adequate indication of his contribution. Dr. Richard Harper of Barnstaple, who is a great-grandson of Richard Budd, and Mr. A.E.S. Roberts, late Medical Librarian of the Bristol Medical Library, concerned themselves very much with my work and showed me every kindness. I was helped by many people in Bristol and in Devon, particularly at Barnstaple and North Tawton, and by many libraries; of the latter the Radcliffe Science Library, Oxford, and its staff should be singled out. Mrs. Irene Ashton of Sheffield typed my manuscript with great speed and accuracy.

I am also indebted to the Wellcome Trustees for their generous support of this work from an early stage.

Those who gave me encouragement, advice, and support during the writing of my thesis and afterwards know how much I owe to them; but I should like particularly to thank my parents; Miss Diana Dyason, of the Department of the History and Philosophy of Science, University of Melbourne; and Colin, Sue, David, Lucy, and Oliver Matthew, for a whole range of benefits.

MARGARET PELLING

ACKNOWLEDGEMENTS

I wish to thank the following for permission to quote from papers in their possession: the Director of the Wellcome Institute, London; the Bristol University Library; Bristol Central Library; the Harveian Librarian of the Royal College of Physicians, London; and the London School of Hygiene and Tropical Medicine.

CONTENTS

Abbreviations x

1. The Origins of Official Doctrine:
   Chadwick and Southwood Smith 1

2. Later Developments: the General Board of Health and
   the Medical Profession 34

3. Epidemiology as Medical Science: William Farr 81

4. Morbid Poisons and Process: Justus Liebig 113

5. The Cholera–Fungus Controversy of 1849 146

6. Exclusive and Inclusive: John Snow and
   the Committee for Scientific Enquiries 203

7. The Smallpox Analogy: William Budd 250

8. Conclusions 295

Select Bibliography 311

Index 329

ABBREVIATIONS

Biog. Lexicon	*Biographisches Lexicon*
Braithwaite	W. Braithwaite (ed.), *The Retrospect of Practical Medicine* (1840–5); then *The Retrospect of Medicine* (1846–87)
Bristol Gazette	*The Bristol Gazette and Public Advertiser*
Budd Letters	Wellcome Institute of the History of Medicine, London. Autograph Letter Collection: William Budd.
College Cholera MSS.	Royal College of Physicians, London Cholera Commission Correspondence etc., Boxes 1–3
DNB	*Dictionary of National Biography*
DSB	*Dictionary of Scientific Biography*
Farley's Bristol Journal	*Felix Farley's Bristol Journal*
Farr, *Appendix* [*date*]	William Farr's 'Letters' appended to the Annual Reports of the Registrar-General (PP)
Henle, *Miasms and Contagions.*	'On miasmata and contagia', *Bulletin of the Institute for the History of Medicine: Johns Hopkins University*, 6(1938), 907–83. Translated by G. Rosen from *Pathologische Untersuchungen* (1840)
Munk	*The Roll of the Royal College of Physicians of London*, 3 vols. (2nd edn., 1878); *Munk's Roll*, compiled by G.H. Brown (1955)
OED	*Oxford English Dictionary*
PP	Parliamentary Papers
Plarr	D'Arcy Power, *et al.* (eds.), *Plarr's Lives of the Fellows of the Royal College of Surgeons of England*, 2 vols. (Bristol and London, 1930)
School of Hygiene Papers.	London School of Hygiene and Tropical Medicine, Budd Papers
Surgeon-General's Catalogue.	*Index-Catalogue of the Library of the Surgeon-General's Office, United States Army* (Washington, D.C., 1880–95; 2nd series, Washington, D.C., 1896–1916)
Venn	J. and J.A. Venn, *Alumni Cantabrigienses*, Pts I and II (Cambridge, 1922–54)

1

THE ORIGINS OF OFFICIAL DOCTRINE: CHADWICK AND SOUTHWOOD SMITH

Western industrialized society has achieved a high standard of physical health for most of its members, and the reality of medical progress goes almost unquestioned. Most dramatic of all have been the achievements based on bacteriological explanations of the etiology of disease. Hence, the identification of living organisms as agents of disease is conventionally regarded as the triumph of scientific medicine in the nineteenth century. Yet Louis Pasteur's theories seemed at the time, according to scientific criteria, to be anomalous. His claim that disease in an animal or plant was caused by another independent species, by means unknown, was contrary not only to the established trend of chemical explanation, but also to mainstream germ theory, since this development was based on advances made earlier in the century in the understanding of structure, growth, and differentiation. It looked not to independent living organisms, but to abnormal products of normal growth processes, for the agents in disease. If the bacteriological discoveries of the 1870s and 1880s are to be regarded as 'scientific', then the complex biochemical and physiological explanations of disease characteristic of earlier decades can hardly be less so. The comparative lack of explanatory power of hypotheses involving living organisms is more objectively demonstrated in relation to a somewhat earlier period, and this will be attempted in this monograph. Similarly, the important work of John Snow and William Budd will be reconsidered, and placed in context as involving aspects of theory and method typical of the complex epidemiological discussions of the period.

Asiatic cholera, a highly fatal bacterial disease of the gut endemic in India, and transmitted chiefly through the medium of contaminated drinking water, first began to extend pandemically in 1817, and reached England from Europe for the first time in October 1831.[1] The mortality (there were no national records for morbidity, or cases of disease not ending in death, until after 1899)[2] caused during this epidemic has been estimated, for England and Wales, as over 23,000.[3] The disease spread 'capriciously', neither following the usual patterns of human intercourse nor regularly affected by climate and similar factors.[4] It was assumed, as a matter of course, that the worst-conditioned parts of the population would be most subject to the disease, and this, in general, proved to be the case; yet the working poor suffered as much as, if not more than, the incapable and the 'vicious', and persons from the upper classes died who could have had no contact with the more common subjects of the disease. Potentially, therefore, if not actually, cholera threatened the prosperous, to some extent directly, but more nearly through the possibility of its regularly occurring among the mobile poor of large cities.

In the first epidemic, London (and even more the over-grown industrial slum of Birmingham) enjoyed a surprising exemption; the second did not occur for twenty years, but was the most fatal over all, causing 53,000 deaths in England and Wales. The third outbreak, 1853 to 1854, was most savage in London, causing there 11,000 of the total of 23,000 deaths. The last cholera epidemic of any scale in England took place in 1866 (14,000 deaths, of which 5,500 occurred in London); knowledge was by then sufficient for crude control, but the increasing failure of the disease to establish itself in

[1] A. Hirsch, *Handbook of Geographical Pathology* (1883-6), i. 394, 399. On cholera, see R. Pollitzer, *Cholera*, WHO Monograph Ser. 43 (Geneva, 1959); D. Barua and W. Burrows (eds.), *Cholera* (Philadelphia etc., 1974). That Asia is the original and natural home of cholera is disputed by S.N. De, *Cholera: Its Pathology and Pathogenesis* (Edinburgh, 1961). See also N. Howard-Jones, 'Choleranomalies: the Unhistory of Medicine as Exemplified by Cholera', *Perspectives in Biology and Medicine* (Chicago University Press), 15 (1972), 422-33; idem, 'Cholera Therapy in the Nineteenth Century', *J. Hist. Med.* 27 (1972), 373-95.

[2] On morbidity statistics and the notification of disease see R. Lambert, *Sir John Simon 1816-1904 and English Social Administration* (1963), pp.114-16, 193-40, 419-20; G.M. Ayers, *England's First State Hospitals and the Metropolitan Asylums Board 1867-1930* (1971), pp. 90-1; W. Farr and H. Ratcliffe, *Mortality in Mid-19th-Century Britain*, ed. R. Wall (1974).

[3] E.A. Underwood, 'History of Cholera in Great Britain', *Proc. R. Soc. Med.* 41 (1948), 165-73: 168.

[4] 'Spasmodic Cholera', *Westminster Review*, 15 (1831), 468.

Britain was probably also a function of differences in the later pandemics.[1]

The discovery of the cholera bacillus (*Vibrio cholerae*) in 1884 was one prize awarded in the race that followed the first successes of Pasteur and Koch; the rival teams of investigators found their nearest material in Alexandria.[2] 'Koch's postulates' for proving the agency of a given micro-organism in disease, which specified the isolation of the agent from a diseased subject, the experimental induction of the disease (or a regular diseased state), the re-isolation of the agent from the experimental subject, and the induction of the disease using this material in a second experimental subject, were not fulfilled in the case of cholera, which has an ambiguous and very limited effect on lower animals in the natural state. The Alexandrian findings were eventually accepted on the basis of analogy with others more fully proven.[3] The unqualified credit still given to Koch is a further indication of the importance of context. Although Koch was responsible for necessary innovations in technique, the eponymous postulates had, as is hardly surprising, been formulated earlier, for example by Koch's teacher, Jacob Henle.[4] Moreover, the discovery of *Vibrio cholerae* is now accredited, by a recent judgement of the Judicial Commission of the International Committee on Bacteriological Nomenclature, not to Koch, but to Filippo Pacini (1812–83), who published his findings in 1854.[5]

As a cause of death and debility in mid-nineteenth-century England, cholera was surpassed among epidemic diseases by

---

[1] Underwood, 'Cholera in Britain', pp. 168–70; Pollitzer, *Cholera*, pp.17–48. Cholera touched England from Germany in 1893, causing in England and Wales 287 attacks and 135 deaths. The British epidemics were episodes in successive pandemics (approximately 1817–23 [no British epidemic], 1829–51, 1852–9, 1863–75, 1881–96, 1889–1923 [no British epidemic]). Except in this note the mortality statistics for each epidemic have been reduced to round figures. Given the many sources of fallacy it is misleading to present seemingly more exact totals.

[2] Cholera has since 1962 been defined as including the condition caused by the 'el Tor' vibrio, first isolated by Gotschlich in 1905. On this agent see Barua and Burrows, *Cholera*.

[3] See W. Bulloch, *The History of Bacteriology* (1960); Pollitzer, *Cholera*, pp.98–101. For Koch (1843–1910), see *DSB*; Howard-Jones, 'Choleranomalies'.

[4] On the limitations of the postulates, see L.S. King, 'Dr. Koch's Postulates', *J. Hist. Med.* 7 (1952), 350–61.

[5] Howard-Jones, 'Choleranomalies', pp.422-3. For Pacini, see *DSB*. Pacini's priority was recognised by the Berlin Cholera Commission to which Koch presented his findings.

'common continued fever' (chiefly typhoid, relapsing fever, and some typhus), scarlet fever, smallpox, and measles, and accounted for only a very small proportion of the area of highest mortality, which occurred among infants and young children. All the known epidemic diseases were exceeded in incidence and effect by the many forms of tuberculosis, the different appearances of which were regarded, until about the middle of the century, as distinct diseases and as being constitutional, not epidemic.[1] Cholera has, however, attracted some of the kind of attention from historians that other diseases, excepting plague, have conspicuously lacked.[2] There are many reasons for this: the shock value of cholera, abundantly recorded at the times of its appearance; its coincidence with other dramatic and disturbing forces, particularly the social and the political; its assumed relation to innovation in institutional and administrative structures; the comparative superiority of the records of its appearances; and the abundance of its literature. The *Surgeon-General's Catalogue* alone records 777 separate works on cholera published in London, including authors' contributions to journals (medical only), for the years 1845 to 1856. The *Medical Directory* of 1853 gives the names of 11,808 practitioners (all of these being qualified, but a small proportion of them as physicians) for

[1] See E.H. Greenhow, *Sanitary Papers* (1858; 1973), especially p.131.

[2] See e.g. (of published and completed work), L.A.J. Chevalier (ed.), *Le Choléra: la première épidémie du XIXe siècle*, Bibliothèque de la Révolution de 1848, Tom. XX (La Roche, 1958); C.E. Rosenberg, *The Cholera Years: The United States in 1832, 1849 and 1866* (Chicago, 1962); N. Longmate, *King Cholera* (1966); R.E. McGrew, *Russia and the Cholera 1823–1832* (Madison etc., 1965); A. Briggs, 'Cholera and Society in the Nineteenth Century', *Past and Present*, no.19 (1960–1), 79–96; C.E. Rosenberg, 'Cholera in Nineteenth Century Europe: A Tool for Social and Economic Analysis', *Comparative Studies in Society and History*, 8 (1966), 452–63; R.E. McGrew, 'The First Cholera Epidemic and Social History', *Bull. Hist. Med.* 34 (1960), 61–73. Some recent studies also exist of the effects of cholera in particular localities, e.g. M. Durey, *The First Spasmodic Cholera Epidemic in York, 1832*, Borthwick Papers no.46 (York, 1974); cf. M. Barnet, 'The 1832 Cholera Epidemic in York', *Med. Hist.* 16 (1972), 27–39. Theses on cholera include T. Jones, 'The Cholera in Manchester, 1832' (University of Manchester B.A. dissertation, 1948); A. Gatherer, 'A Socio-Medical Study of the First Cholera Epidemic in Great Britain, 1831–2' (University of Aberdeen D.M. dissertation, 1960); M. Durey, 'A Social History of the First Cholera Epidemic in Britain, 1831–3' (University of York Ph. D. dissertation, 1975). The questions first raised by C. Smyth, 'The Evangelical Movement in Perspective', *Camb. Hist. J.* 7 (1942), 160–160–74, may be answered in a forthcoming work by R.J. Morris, *Cholera 1832* (Croom Helm Ltd.).

London and the provinces. Both figures are, of course, very approximate, although each is an underestimate; they are intended merely to give some idea of output on this subject compared with the number of likely authors.[1]

Clearly, the volume of works produced represents more than the usual, optional reaction of a profession to a problem within its expertise. Cholera was not a constant social factor of the same proportions as fever, tuberculosis, or alcoholism; but the same features which have led to its being noticed by historians caused an extremity of reaction, albeit shortlived, in those whom it threatened. Not at first, but by the time of the second epidemic, the literature on cholera reflects the full range of scientific and human resources available at the time, and more or less applicable to a crisis of this type. In an emergency, even the least qualified will act, and in the case of cholera, a new and intractable disease, each practitioner or concerned layman felt justified in publishing the results of his experience. Not only individuals were involved. Cholera made demands on (or was seized on as an opportunity by) newspapers, journals, Parliament, the churches, professional and other societies, charitable and similar institutions, and the plural organs of local administration; it elicited remark, if not always activity.

It is often assumed that, although the incidence of other epidemic diseases may be taken to be a constant or incidental factor, cholera by the very abruptness of its appearances and its novelty, must necessarily have acted, if not casually, at least catalytically. It is sometimes further assumed that because its clinical signs and symptoms are characteristic, and hardly to be mistaken when well developed, cholera must have had much to do with establishing in the minds of the prosperous, the reality of their interrelationship with the poor. The threat

---

[1] The 1841 census gave 33,339 persons as practising one or more branches of medicine: E.M. Little, *History of the British Medical Association 1832–1932* (1932), p.5. The *Medical Directory* of before 1858 depended on the initiative of practitioners for its contents, and was not equivalent to the Registers which began after the Medical Act of 1858, although these were also imperfect. An analysis of the 10,220 practitioners listed in the *Medical Directory* of 1856 finds that 54·6 per cent were qualified as M.R.C.S. Eng. and L.S.A. Lond., and 18·5 per cent as M.R.C.S. Eng. only; 3·9 per cent were M.D. or M.B. Oxford, Cambridge, or London Universities, and Fellows, Licentiates, or extra-Licentiates of the Royal College of Physicians: C. Singer and S.W.F. Holloway, 'Early Medical Education in England in Relation to the Pre-history of London University', *Med. Hist.* 4 (1960), 1–17.

posed by cholera, and the extent of the reaction to it, cannot be doubted, although neither was, in England at least, of the proportions that were at first feared. It is, however, one conclusion of the present book that, probably on all levels, cholera was a distraction rather than an impetus to reform, and that strenuous efforts had to be made at the time by reformers hoping to modify the reaction to it for their own ends. This is most clearly exemplified in the present context by the relation between interest in cholera, and concern over fever, of the greater importance of which as a perennial cause of death and debility, nineteenth-century public-health reformers were definitively aware. As far as persons with this interest were concerned, the necessity of making capital out of cholera was very obvious. Some effort was expended during the first epidemic, and a great deal more invested just before the second, some twenty years later, not to base the sanitary cause on the threat of cholera, but to force cholera, with respect to both theory and practice, into the same category as what was called 'the ordinary fever of the country'. It is partly as a result of these efforts that we are encouraged to assume that sanitary reform began with the first cholera epidemic.

'Official doctrine', in its theoretical aspect, was a minority view. The centralization of doctrine in epidemic disease may be said to have begun with Neil Arnott, James Kay, and Southwood Smith's reports (1838-9) for the Poor Law Commissioners on fever in the metropolis. Even less than the results of other official investigations were the findings of these and later reports on the public health based on a real consensus.[1] Chadwick and Southwood Smith, immediately upon their early involvement in the public-health question, exercised a monopoly of the official sources; Smith consequently emerges as the 'chief medical theorist of the sanitary reformers'.[2] Moreover, although official doctrine became more dogmatic, it did not materially alter over a period of twenty years. Southwood Smith's views on the nature of

---

[1] On the Benthamite manipulation of public enquiries, see S.E. Finer, 'The Transmission of Benthamite Ideas, 1820–50', in G. Sutherland (ed.), *Studies in the Growth of Nineteenth Century Government* (1972), pp.11–12.

[2] R.A. Lewis, *Edwin Chadwick and the Public Health Movement 1832–1854* (1952), p.35.

epidemic diseases were fixed by 1830, before the first cholera epidemic; large sections of his articles in the *Westminster Review* of 1825, and of his larger work on fever of 1830, were reproduced, or rather incorporated, into the Reports of the Metropolitan Sanitary Commission and of the General Board of Health, just as they were into the *Examiner* in 1831–2. Smith committed himself not to the evolution of principles, but to the campaign for their acceptance and use. The promulgation of his views at the later date had two consequences. Firstly, a false appearance was given of a climate of non- or anti-contagionism; secondly, their statement in theoretical terms in the late 1840s caused the united opposition of the medical profession to be added to the forces of resistance to the General Board of Health. Little hostility had been aroused previously, because the energies of all sanitary reformers were then devoted to establishing, on a national scale, the simple correlation between insanitary conditions and disease, and its practical connotations; and this activity was not felt to usurp professional prerogatives. The official retreat into dogmatism was chiefly the result of the need to deal with the renewed threat of cholera, which involved justifying a categorical stand on whether or not cholera was contagious.

Southwood Smith and Chadwick, who was twelve years Smith's junior, were both members of the last group of Benthamite disciples, serving as much the person of Bentham as his principles.[1] Both were interested in a range of reforms, including educational, legal, and penal; both were promoted by Place's Parliamentary Candidate Society of 1831.[2] Smith had been a widower, and was deeply religious. He was especially concerned to resolve the problem of pain by a belief in the possibility of spiritual and physical amelioration, and in later life was inclined to take measures of a self-protective

---

[1] Smith and Chadwick are both given credit for important assistance with the *Constitutional Code*, and for attending Bentham in his last illness. On the former point see [Chadwick], *University of London Election Address* (1867). On Chadwick as a Benthamite, compare Finer, 'Transmission of Benthamite Ideas', and J. Hamburger, *Intellectuals in Politics: J.S. Mill and the Philosophic Radicals* (New Haven and London, 1965).

[2] Ibid., p. 115, n.

kind.[1] His most radical public utterances were the incitements he offered to a (literate) working-class audience in 1847, not to violence or a disregard of Parliament, but to orderly agitation against vested interests. More characteristic activities were his involvement in model dwellings, the Health of Towns Association, and convalescent homes for unfortunate or isolated members of the middle classes.[2]

Although a medical man, Smith had adopted this profession as his second choice and from motives connected with earning a living for a young family. There is some evidence that he never built up much of a practice in London, except among his friends, and that, public health apart (which in any case comprehended a range of his closest concerns), he was interested in the physical aspects of life as they related to the mental and the moral.[3] Most of his medical views and activities can be seen as serving a sustained interest in the physiological and neurological bases of mental phenomena. His only appointments to institutions, the regular route to self-establishment, were atypical and unlikely to contribute towards the usual professional ends of advancement or varied experience. Smith's artificially exposed position as Chadwick's only medical colleague should not be taken as definitive.

It is not yet entirely clear why, or when, Smith developed extreme views with respect to medical theory. Little is known about his life and practice before he moved to London at the age of thirty-two. The period of his medical and philosophical education in Edinburgh appears to have been dominated by the activities consequent upon his conversion to Unitarianism.

[1] Thomas Southwood Smith (1788–1861), M.D. (*de mente morbis laesa*) Edinburgh 1816, L.R.C.P. 1821, F.R.C.P. 1847, F. Stats. Soc. 1841; educated Bristol Baptist College; co-founder and first secretary of Scottish Unitarian Association, 1813. His first public employment was as a Commissioner on the Royal Commission on the State of Children in Factories (1833). Founder member of the Health of Towns Association and of the Metropolitan Society for Improving the Dwellings of the Industrious Classes. For biography, see *DNB*; *Munk*; C.L. Lewes, *Southwood Smith, A Retrospect* (1898); F.N.L. Poynter, 'Southwood Smith – the Man (1788–1861)', *Proc. R. Soc. Med.* 55 (1962), 381–92.

[2] Smith, *An Address to the Working Classes*, published January 1847; idem, *Results of Sanitary Improvement* (1854); R.G. Paterson, 'The Health of Towns Association in Great Britain 1844–1849', *Bull. Hist. Med.* 22 (1948), 373–402; Lewes, *Southwood Smith, A Retrospect*, pp.93–4, 98, 107–11, 80–5.

[3] Poynter, 'Southwood Smith – the Man', pp.384–5; Bentham, *Works* (1843), xi. 35; Smith, *Philosophy of Health* (1865), Preface by G.H., and Introduction to 1st edn.

His rejection of Calvinist beliefs may have been, as different events were in other lives, the basis of his active commitment to the ideal of improvement; but neither this, nor his somewhat indefinite political outlook, is sufficient to explain the comparative particularity of his scientific ideas. His interest in fever is said to have dated only from his appointment to the London Fever Hospital, and the *Westminster Review* articles of 1825 largely paraphrase Charles Maclean. These articles were later described by a partial relative as 'the result of a *rapid glance* which had gone to the very root of things'.[1] However, his own experience (which apparently included no knowledge of the 'doubtful' diseases other than fever) and certainly his medical practice, resemble far more closely those of John Armstrong.

After qualifying at Edinburgh, where he was supported by the Unitarian Fund, Smith practised for three years in the provinces as both minister and physician, roles which later found combined expression in his services to public health. He moved reluctantly to London in 1820, and took what was still a common first step by becoming physician to a dispensary (the Eastern, in Whitechapel).[2] Metropolitan dispensaries were often at that time also teaching establishments; they offered clinical experience, and involved some exposure to the condition of the poor. Smith's only other substantial appointments were to the Jews' Hospital or asylum, of Mile End, Old Town, and, in 1824, the London Fever Hospital. His association with the Fever Hospital, still at that time the only institution of its kind in London, lasted for nearly forty years and constitutes his chief claim to be considered an expert on epidemic disease.[3] The policy, and even more the practice, of this hospital varied considerably from that of the

---

[1] Poynter, 'Southwood Smith — the Man', p.384; cf. pp.384-5. Lewes, *Southwood Smith, A Retrospect*, p.25. My italics.

[2] Poynter, 'Southwood Smith — the Man', pp.384-6.

[3] On the London Fever Hospital (L.F.H.), founded by the Society for Bettering the Condition of the Poor, and the Public or Carey Street (London) dispensary and medical school, see *Reports* of the parent Society, ed. T. Bernard (1798-1817); works by its physicians, especially Thomas Bateman, Southwood Smith, Alexander Tweedie, William Jenner, and Charles Murchison; published annual reports; T.A. Murray, *Remarks on the Situation of the Poor* (1801); *Report of Committee on Petition Respecting the Fever Institution*, PP, 1804, IV, Pt. 2; A. Highmore, *Pietas Londinensis* (1810), i. 111-23.

general hospitals. Here it can be noted, firstly, that elaborate case records were kept from the earliest years and post-mortems carried out as a matter of course, and secondly, that its governorship imposed what was virtually a research and publication requirement on its physicians, in the interests of the diffusion of useful knowledge.[1] The fund of data so provided, still unrivalled in 1864, supplied the basis for Smith's *Treatise on Fever*, which was almost his sole contribution to medical literature.[2] As we shall see, Charles Murchison's 'pythogenic' theory, the last and most sophisticated of 'sanitary' explanations of fever, was also based on London Fever Hospital records.

In the *Examiner*, and even more so in the later official reports, Chadwick and Smith are indistinguishable on all subjects. Smith's early writings are quoted from or paraphrased in all instances, but to what degree of collaboration this was owing may be indeterminable.[3]

Edwin Chadwick's character was evidently well marked, and his biographers have not found it difficult to describe.[4] He was no more than typical of the Benthamites, and of middle-class reformers in general, in having limited popular sympathies and no egalitarianism, except that which might lie in the assumption that all groups had a natural capacity for happiness (roughly equivalent to earning and learning power) and a natural life-cycle which ought not to be cut off or disrupted at the point of greatest skill and productivity. Pauperism and disease were alike gratuitous and preventable, and there was no such thing as the inevitable pressure of a

---

[1] Ibid. i. 121; Smith, *Treatise on Fever* (1830), Preface; *Edinb. Med. Surg. J.* 33 (1830), 337.

[2] J.S. Bristowe and T. Holmes, *Report on the Hospitals of the United Kingdom*, PP, 1864, XXVII. 725.

[3] For an attempt to arrogate to Smith from Chadwick, credit in areas besides the purely medical, see Poynter, 'Southwood Smith — the Man'. Contemporary admirers were inclined to make Smith responsible for the General Board of Health's cholera and quarantine reports: T. Baker, preface to Smith, *The Common Nature of Epidemics* (1866). Smith and Chadwick's colleague, Richard Owen, merely confirms their collaboration: R. Owen, *The Life of Richard Owen*, 2 vols (1894), i. 305–6.

[4] S.E. Finer, *The Life and Times of Sir Edwin Chadwick* (1952), and Lewis, *Chadwick and Public Health*, have not been superseded as biographies of Chadwick. See also Chadwick, *Sanitary Report*, ed. Flinn (1965); B.W. Richardson in *The Health of Nations* (1887; 1973).

willing and capable working population on the means of subsistence.[1] It is possible that Chadwick intended sanitary reform and the New Poor Law to have a relation far more intimate than was finally achieved. The rigid moral imperative of the new law would have been balanced by action taken upon the concession that the poor were subject to debilitating physical conditions which were outside their control and responsibility. The function of sanitary reform was to give the poor free use of their natural capacities; the provisions of the New Poor Law were intended for a population more or less healthy. Only an unbalanced half of Chadwick's poor-law programme was represented in the final report.[2]

Although reference is frequently made to Chadwick's earliest published articles, and to his contact in the 1820s with medical men, institutions, and events, it is none the less usually assumed that 'there is little evidence that his interest in public-health questions was anything other than minimal before 1838'.[3] The degree to which public-health questions were related to, and typical of, other aspects of reform, particularly in Benthamite ideology, might of itself give grounds for doubting this judgement. More direct evidence, however, is supplied by the enthusiasm for medical aspects of the 'condition of the people' question shown by the *Examiner* during Chadwick's subeditorship. It is possible that the *Examiner*, unlike the *Westminster Review* which carried little more than its quota of articles on medical and related subjects, was a regular vehicle for interests of this kind, but Chadwick's personal involvement in the trends shown during 1831-2 is demonstrated by the consistency between the *Examiner* and the later official reports.[4]

Most accounts of Chadwick's role in the development of public health on a national basis arrive at conclusions about

---

[1] See e.g. Chadwick, *Comparative Results of Poor Law Administration* (1864).

[2] Ibid., pp.8 ff., 15 ff.; J.R. Poynter, *Society and Pauperism: English Ideas on Poor Relief, 1795-1834* (1969), pp.318-19; Finer, *Life of Chadwick*, pp.69 ff.; Lewis, *Chadwick and Public Health*, pp.18-19.

[3] Chadwick, *Sanitary Report*, ed. Flinn, p.35.

[4] See Finer, *Life of Chadwick*, pp.33-4. Cf. Gatherer, 'Sociomedical Study of the First Cholera Epidemic', pp.254-60. For James Mill and his awareness of 'news' as part of the weaponry of politics, see J. Hamburger, *James Mill and the Art of Revolution* (New Haven and London, 1963); and see e.g. (on cholera), *Examiner*, 25 Mar. 1832, p.194.

his relations with medical men that require correction in the present context.[1] Chadwick's attitude to the profession was ultimately impersonal. It was formed at a time when he was benefiting from close contact with the physicians Arnott, Kay, and Smith, and was based on the entirely justifiable conclusion that the methods, content, and style of evaluation of English medical education were inadequate, unsystematic, antiquated, and corrupt, and compared unfavourably with those of France, even in cases, such as clinical teaching, where the English supposed themselves to be most advantaged. It followed, as a corollary, that eminence within the profession was regularly determined not by merit, but by influence and privilege. Chadwick therefore felt entitled not only to ignore but to despise the colleges and other institutions which most epitomized and guarded these defects; and further, to doubt the power of the average medical man, who was the product of this system and who, moreover, shared the delusions of other 'practical' men, to reason correctly in his own sphere. Chadwick's attitude to the higher echelons should be contrasted with his respect for the poor-law medical officers and for the system obtaining in the medical branches of the armed services, which he found in many ways admirable. He also showed a sympathetic awareness of the 'horrors and degradation' suffered by medical men in the competition for private practice, and acted consistently upon a conviction of the 'unreasonableness of expecting private practitioners to compromise their own interests by conflicts for the public protection with persons on whom they are dependant [*sic*] '.[2]

Chadwick's view of the medical profession was only proportionately more severe than his conclusions respecting other professions, which were based on a similar analysis of the defects in their educational and professional institutions. The chief effect of existing forms of professional education, he thought, was to destroy 'objectivity'.[3] The positive aspects

---

[1] But see Chadwick, *Sanitary Report*, ed. Flinn, pp.60-1.

[2] Chadwick, 'Centralization', *Lond. Rev.* 2 (1829), 536-65; *Examiner*, 17 Oct. 1830, pp.658-60; Chadwick, *On Local Medical Appointments* (1872); idem, *Sanitary Report*, ed. Flinn, p.404.

[3] On practical and professional qualifications see e.g. Chadwick, 'Life Assurances', *Westminster Review*, 9 (1828), 390-3.

of this critique were later illustrated by his recommendations
with respect to the civil service, which were also based on
the guiding principle of public accountability.[1] It must further
be conceded to Chadwick that he made a correct estimate, at
an early stage, of the limited extent to which the leaders of
the medical profession, its writers, and its institutions would
feel themselves engaged by public-health and epidemiological
questions. He took a realistic view, not only of the chief
occupations of practitioners and medical politicians, but also
of the limits of one man's experience and of the lack of contact with the circumstances of disease entailed in the hospital
and dispensary system of teaching and practice. Southwood
Smith's *Treatise* of 1830 might well have appealed to Chadwick
(as it did not to the profession) because of its philosophical
or methodological bias, and because the London Fever
Hospital, like the French hospitals, fulfilled some of the
criteria for a 'scientific' institution.[2]

Chadwick's views were not, of course, unique. They were
compatible not only with the attitude of the radicals to other
establishment institutions and forms of education, especially
the scientific, but also with the position taken by an important and growing minority in the medical profession itself.[3]
A minority which included William Lawrence and Thomas
Wakley was particularly active at the time when Chadwick's
views were formed.[4] Even his dismissal of medical therapeutics
was characteristic of the context of the 1820s and 1830s.

[1] Chadwick, *Health of Nations*, i. 324 ff.; Finer, *Life of Chadwick*, pp.477-82.

[2] The *Treatise on Fever* is described as 'one of the most able of the philosophical works that have aided the advancement of the science of medicine in the last
half-century' in the *Examiner*, 5 June 1831, p.355. For Smith's criticisms of the
structure and education of the profession, see his *Westminster Review* articles of
1825, and his contributions to the campaign for an Anatomy Act.

[3] See *Report of Select Committee on Medical Education*, PP, 1834, XIII. See
also G.N. Clark, *A History of the Royal College of Physicians of London*, 2 vols.
(Oxford, 1964-6), ii. 685n.; PP, 1833, XXXIV. 99-124; PP, 1835, XXXVII.
597-600. C. Newman, *The Evolution of Medical Education in the Nineteenth
Century* (1957), pp.150-2; S.W.F. Holloway, 'Medical Education in England,
1830-1858: A Sociological Analysis', *History*, 49 (1964), 299-324. On the whole
subject of medical reform, see J. Simon, *Public Health Reports* (1887), i. 491 ff.;
and the unsatisfactory W.H. McMenemey, *The Life and Times of Sir Charles
Hastings* (Edinburgh and London, 1959).

[4] See the early numbers of *The Lancet*, founded in 1823 by Wakley in association with Lawrence, William Cobbett, and James Wardrop; and C. Brook, *Battling
Surgeon* [Wakley] (Glasgow, 1945).

The average practitioner working in this context was likely in his reading to come across a variety of assertions of the rejection of systems, in favour of a new, cautious, 'scientific' character for medicine as well as other branches of knowledge, but his own practice would still have been dependent on largely eighteenth-century formulations.[1] Probably the most important of the older sources which were still able to dominate the regular medical education were contained in the teaching and textbooks of William Cullen.[2] Cullen's 'nosology' provided not so much a system as a set of histories or descriptions of diseases, made as complete as possible with respect to 'common and inseparable' or 'pathognomic' characteristics, for the positive guidance of the young physician. Attempts wholly to displace the Cullenian definitions were negligible until they were made as one reflection of the early nineteenth-century development of the pathologico-anatomical school of medicine.

Fever and inflammation were two generic disease states the discussion of the nature of which, during the late eighteenth and early nineteenth centuries, may be seen as epitomizing contemporary concepts of disease process.[3] Fever appeared as the fundamental phenomenon in a large number of diseased conditions where the whole body was affected; its explanation had, therefore, to be in terms of those fluids or organic systems (the circulatory, the nervous) which were capable of determining the state of the whole constitution. Equally, to arrive at a satisfactory account of fever was in some degree to determine the mode of operation and combination of bodily

[1] On this period in general, see C. Daremberg, *Histoire des sciences médicales* (1870); P.J.G. Cabanis, *Sketch of the Revolutions of Medical Science* (1806); J.H. Baas, *Outlines of Medical History* (1889; 1971).

[2] Cullen (1710–90), M.D. Glasgow 1740, F.R.S. 1777, professor of the 'institutes of medicine' at Edinburgh University from 1766, professor of physic 1773, began teaching chemistry and medicine in 1744 in Glasgow. See *DNB*; J. Thomson's *Life* (1859); and Daremberg, *Histoire des sciences médicales*, ii. 1102 ff. Seventeen British edns. of Cullen's *Nosology* appeared between 1769 and 1831; nine British full edns. of the supplementary *First Lines*, between 1785 and 1829.

[3] The best discussion of these complicated issues is in Daremberg, *Histoire des sciences médicales*, on which Baas's account of the eighteenth-century schools appears to have been based. C. Creighton, *Epidemics* (1965), ii, and C. Murchison, *Treatise on Continued Fevers* (1884), give epidemiological, bibliographical, and other information. See also M. Foucault, *Naissance de la clinique* (Paris, 1972), Ch. 10.

mechanisms. Inflammation was also a common factor in diseases, but was definitively local rather than general, and referable to the condition of the solids rather than to the fluids of the body. This period saw a protracted debate on the question of the nature of primary disease, or the body's first reaction to abnormal stimuli. Cullen's category of *Pyrexiae*, or febrile diseases, included most of the conditions now thought of as distinct, infectious diseases, and which then exemplified the various kinds of relationship between inflammation and fever. The subgroup *continuae* contained the most ambiguous and controversial febrile conditions; here Cullen perpetuated for the nineteenth century the very old terminology of 'synocha' and 'synochus', with 'typhus' (low fever), a term of eighteenth-century derivation. The continued fevers had as their exciting causes the so-called 'common' contagions, which, unlike the specific contagions, arose not from the body alone, but according to prevailing conditions. Cullen's definition of the character of febrile diseases in general, demonstrates the pragmatism of his approach, but was none the less a reflection of current developments in the physiology of the nervous system.

After Cullen's death, the pathologico-anatomical and clinical schools of France and elsewhere introduced a 'localizing' tendency which was opposed to the concept of essential disease. An interest in morbid processes or physiology as well as structure was restored by the aggressive Broussais, in whose monistic system all fevers were stages in a single organic process deriving from an irritability, and consequent inflammation, of the gastro-intestinal canal.[1] English medical men, however, tended to absorb the results of such developments rather than their significance. Partly because of the indigenous clinical and epidemiological emphasis, the doctrine of essential or idiopathic fever, that is, a generalized febrile state capable of arising independently of any other condition in the body,

---

[1] See Ackerknecht, *Medicine at the Paris Hospital 1794–1848* (Baltimore, 1967); Foucault, *Naissance de la clinique*; Daremberg, *Histoire des sciences médicales*; I. Waddington, 'The Role of the Hospital in the Development of Modern Medicine: A Sociological Analysis', *Sociology*, 7 (1973), 211–24. Broussais's character as a progressive has been stressed by E.H. Ackerknecht, 'Broussais: Or a Forgotten Medical Revolution', *Bull. Hist. Med.* 27 (1953), 320–43, and Foucault, *Naissance de la clinique*, Ch. 10.

was modified rather than at any time abandoned. Pathological findings, in particular those on which Broussais, Bretonneau, and Louis depended, were allowed as defining 'secondary affections', or complications that were readily attributable to ancillary factors in the constitution of the individual, his particular circumstances, or the prevailing epidemic tendency.[1] It will be seen from this that English medicine in this important area remained peculiarly liable to admit the influence on the body of factors in its environment, an inclination which, at the least, would allow the growth of interest in sanitary questions.

The renewed physiological emphasis most dogmatically expressed by Broussais, the chemical and physical analyses and experiments conducted by the later, 'eclectic' French school, and the progress being made in animal or organic chemistry, were all represented in a 'new humoralism' which was evident by the time of the first cholera epidemic in England (1831), and still prevalent at the time of the second (1849). William Stevens exemplifies the early, and Edmund Parkes the later period. As will be seen, the theories of epidemic disease prevailing between about 1830 and 1860 depended most heavily on a hypothetical or realized pathology of the fluids, and in particular of the blood.[2]

The dangers of moving out of context are obvious, but it is none the less possible to schematize the range of epidemic diseases of most concern in the nineteenth century, in order to define the areas of least knowledge. During the period under discussion it was generally agreed that there were two

---

[1] See e.g. R. Christison, 'Fevers', in *Library of Medicine*, ed. A. Tweedie, I (1840), especially p.121. On the history of the distinction between typhus and typhoid, see C. Murchison, 'Typhus and Typhoid Fever', *Med. Times Gaz.* 1857, ii. 642–3; idem, *Treatise on Continued Fevers;* E.W. Goodall, *William Budd* (Bristol, 1936), pp.44 ff.; A.L. Goodall, 'Glasgow's Place in the Distinction between Typhoid and Typhus Fevers', *Bull. Hist. Med.* 28 (1954), 140–53. All historical questions relating to the continued fevers are highly complex; pronounced but ill-defined changes in the incidence of typhoid occurred over the period under discussion. Here it should be noted that British writers saw the French discussions primarily as one aspect of the localist-essentialist debate.

[2] For 'neohumoralism' in France, see Ackerknecht, *The Paris Hospital*, pp.106ff. As one reflection of British studies, see Thomson, *Life of Cullen*, ii. 129, 158–9. See also J. Simon, Lectures II–VI and XI, *Lancet*, 1850, i. 709, 743, 769; 1850, ii. 1, 35,193, and especially p.194. For Stevens (1786–1868) and others see Christison, 'Fevers', pp.117–18; Howard-Jones, 'Cholera Therapy', pp.386–93.

types of disease having substantial causes which were in some
way external to the body, even though both types were necessarily defined in terms of effects. The diseases most definitive
of these types, smallpox and intermittent fever (malaria),
may be regarded as lying with some constancy at opposite
ends of a spectrum of contagiousness. Both could be thought
of as fevers, with or without additions; both were indigenous,
and endemic in England in the eighteenth and nineteenth
centuries. Intermittent fever or marsh ague, however, never
propagated from person to person by contact or extended
beyond certain areas, and seemed to be caused by the airborne
products of vegetable putrefaction as it occurred in marshes
and other low-lying regions.[1] Smallpox, unlike ague, was
thought to have a constant character independent of variations in the environment or in the constitution of the individual.[2] It affected each person only once; its usual course
consisted of a general constitutional reaction or fever, followed by a local cutaneous reaction including a crop of pustules. The pustules appeared to represent physical proof of
an increase in morbid matter since (as the practice of inoculation, not replaced by that of vaccination with cowpox until
after the end of the eighteenth century, had shown), the
smallest portion of their contents was capable of producing
the disease in another subject. Because the disease was
normally transmitted by human contact, it could be assumed
that a material substance passed between subjects, although
nothing peculiar could be extracted either from the pustules
or from supposedly tainted air. Of these two types, it will be
seen that smallpox, because it could be manipulated, was

[1] Unlike smallpox, malaria declined drastically through the eighteenth and
nineteenth centuries: see George Whitley, *Report as to the Quantity of Ague in
England*: Appendix to *6th Rep. of Med. Officer of Privy Council*, PP, 1864,
XXVIII. 430-54. The new writing on agues in the early nineteenth century was
based on observations made abroad: see F. Boott, *Inquiry into those Forms of
Fever Attributed to Malaria*, in vol. ii of his *Memoir of Armstrong* (1833-4). Most
'agues' were not true malaria: see Creighton, *Epidemics*, ii. Ch. 3.

[2] On smallpox, see C.W. Dixon, *Smallpox* (1962); J.D. Rolleston, *The History
of the Acute Exanthemata* (1937); G. Miller, *The Adoption of Inoculation for
Smallpox in England and France* (Philadelphia, 1957); Simon, *Public Health
Reports*, i. 169-407; R.J. Lambert, 'A Victorian National Health Service: State
Vaccination 1855-71', *Hist. J.* 5 (1962), 1-18; R.M. MacLeod, 'Law, Medicine
and Public Opinion: the Reaction to Compulsory Health Legislation, 1870-1907',
Public Law, 1967, pp.107-28, 189-211.

better understood than intermittent fever, although intermittent and remittent fevers were the subject of considerable interest in the early nineteenth century. It was consequently smallpox which was, whether consciously or unconsciously, most often used analogously, or as a standard against which to construct definitions of epidemic diseases.

Between the two fixed poles of smallpox and intermittent fever there can be seen to lie, even for Cullen, an increasing number of maladies the nature of which was ambivalent or undetermined, and it is these 'doubtful' diseases which dominate discussion throughout the period in question. Although the group also included yellow fever, 'typhus' and the other continued fevers and Asiatic cholera became its most important members, with typhus gradually becoming of less account. The intermittent and continued fevers were known from the eighteenth century to be pre-eminently dependent upon, or associated with, conditions such as putrefaction, overcrowding, famine, and uncleanness, and the group also included, often without distinction, such diseases as diarrhoea, scurvy, dysentery, and relapsing fever which was peculiarly associated with famine.

Thomas Southwood Smith's views on epidemic diseases and fever were, if not wholly derivative, at least not original. He associated himself with the minority rather than the majority principally in redefining 'epidemic' and 'contagious' to describe two absolutely distinct classes of disease. His approach bears many resemblances to that of Budd, although Budd's reference to the smallpox standard was natural and deliberate, and his concept of cause, although less acceptable to his contemporaries, gave far more support to his conviction that a non-contagious disease could never become contagious, or a contagious disease, non-contagious. It is significant, however, that Smith's contemporaries were as critical of his formulations in general as were Budd's, and on similar grounds; both periods favoured 'contingent-contagionist' solutions in respect of the 'doubtful' diseases, although the membership of this latter class differed with period.

It is clear from Cullen's classifications that there was nothing to prohibit a view of typhus and plague as entirely analogous diseases arising from similar conditions in different countries, regardless of whether they were contagious or not.[1] Yellow fever was already classified as a variety of typhus.[2] The first quarter of the nineteenth century introduced an element of disharmony. Plague remained an unknown, exotic, and potentially importable disease, while opinion on 'typhus' became subject to fluctuations. These arose in part from the lessening incidence of severe forms of typhus and the increasing incidence of typhoid, and were inevitable in the period immediately preceding firm demonstrations of the difference between these two diseases. Reports were, however, increasingly received of the behaviour of epidemic diseases in other countries or in their countries of origin. Some writers were prepared to merge the intermittent and continued fevers into a single class whose members owed their peculiarities to factors in the different climates in which they arose. The most important of these factors in each case was a form of animal or vegetable putrefaction, which was more or less encouraged by a variety of local conditions, including temperature and degree of humidity.[3] The prevalent notion of febrile disease as comprising a common, essential reaction and variable local phenomena would give scope to this simplification. John Armstrong held views of this kind, as well as the much travelled Maclean; Smith could have been influenced by either, or both. William Grant (d.1786), the follower of Sydenham, had suggested an absolute distinction between 'contagious' and 'epidemic' as early as 1775.[4] However, most English writers were not unnaturally oblivious to generalizations based on diseases outside their experience (which could include common fever), and persisted in their view of the mixed character of continued fevers.

Smith, in his *Treatise* of 1830, criticized both localist and essentialist schools alike for a tendency to mistake secondary for primary phenomena, and to postulate the existence of events and states for which there was no objective evidence.

[1] For a post-bacteriological inquiry into the history of the assumed relation between typhus and plague, see R. Crawfurd, 'Historical Contributions from the History of Medicine to the Problem of the Transmission of Typhus', *Proc. R. Soc. Med.* (Section Med. Hist.), 6 (1913), 6–17. See also Creighton, *Epidemics*, ii. 16–17.

[2] Thomson, *Life of Cullen*, ii. 143–4.

[3] See e.g. Boott, *Memoir of Armstrong*, ii; Thomson, *Life of Cullen*, ii. 136 ff.

[4] Daremberg, *Histoire des sciences médicales*, ii. 1198n. For Grant, see *Munk*.

His own was a 'wholly practical' work, in which the limits of current knowledge would be well defined. He based his conclusions on statistics and correlated clinical and pathological (or 'necrotomic') findings, which was beginning to be acceptable, but these data were dominated by a rigidly methodological argument consistent with his assertion that medical men received no training in the inductive methods proper to their science.[1] He placed most stress upon his having established, from observation, the invariable events in fever, and the fixed order of these events, using an approach calculated to avoid speculation as to causes which Cullen had also employed, deriving it directly from Hume; Smith had absorbed it indirectly, through Thomas Brown.[2] Smith stated that the nervous functions were first deranged; then the circulatory function; and lastly, the secreting and excreting functions. Differences in the degree to which each of these systems was affected produced the variety of appearances observed. However, in spite of his assertion that 'fever is not an entity, not a being possessing a peculiar nature ... but ... a series of events', which may be taken as a criticism of the 'natural history' approach to disease, Smith can be detected (and was by his contemporaries) as cherishing a unitary view of fever.[3] His one major distinction, between 'typhus' and 'synochus', was introduced for custom's sake and was based only on differences in intensity; and, although he admitted the peculiar signs of the exanthemata, he thought that the true character of these diseases was that of a varying degree of fever. He acknowledged diversity on the clinical, but not on the specific level; as we shall see, the tendency of Smith's views to cast doubt on the specificity of epidemic diseases ran, from the outset, counter to the trend in professional opinion, which was towards defining these diseases as clinically and pathologically distinct.

Smith's criticism of systems in general reflected current views and he arrived at a compromise between the two systematic extremes of opinion on fever, which had been put

---

[1] Smith, *Treatise on Fever*, p.30; Preface.

[2] Smith, 'Lectures on Forensic Medicine', *Lond. Med. Gaz.* 1837-8, i. 305-6; Thomson, *Life of Cullen*, ii. 131-2 and *passim*. For Brown (1778-1820), a pupil and colleague of Dugald Stewart at Edinburgh, see *DNB*.

[3] Smith, *Treatise on Fever*, p.46; *Lancet*, 1830-1, i. 586-7.

forward by Pinel and later by a number of British clinicians. He maintained that fever was a primary disease, but agreed with the localists in thinking that the solids rather than the fluids of the body were first affected. Where he abandoned compromise was in opposition to Cullen. Although claiming with Cullen that the nervous and sensorial functions were invariably the first to be involved, he was insistent that the primary phenomena were inflammatory rather than debilitating in character. From this it followed that the cardinal remedy in fever was 'moderate' bleeding at the earliest possible moment.[1]

This account of fever, Smith thought, held good for all forms, regardless of their causes. His remarks on causation very plainly provide a basis for sanitary activity, but they were not in themselves novel. The exciting or immediate cause of a fever he thought was a poison, not because there was any direct evidence of the existence of such an agent, but because the effects on the nervous system were analogous to those produced by poisons whose nature was to some extent understood. All that was known of this poison was that it could be formed by the putrefaction of animal and vegetable matter. Here Smith praised John Pringle's work on the putrefaction of animal substances, and further criticized Cullen for obscuring the importance of 'animal malaria' by his emphasis on the vegetable effluvia of marshes.[2] Plague, which was merely typhus in another environment, was caused by animal malaria — 'an old truth but forgotten'. Smith's conception of the predisposing cause conformed to the classical and traditional notion of the 'non-naturals': that is, 'whatever diminishes the vigorous action of the organs, impairs their functions, and so weakens the general strength of the system'. Such factors would include those of diet, regimen, and climate.[3] However, Smith also stated that 'of all predisposing causes, the most powerful is the continued presence and slow operation

---

[1] *Treatise on Fever*, pp.333–43. Cf. idem, 'Use of the Dead to the Living', *Westminster Review*, 2 (1824), 79.

[2] *Treatise on Fever*, pp.337, 348 ff., 361 ff. Thomson, *Life of Cullen*, ii. 136 ff., 147. For Sir John Pringle (1707-82), see *DNB*; Partington, *History of Chemistry*, iii. 249; D. Singer, 'Sir John Pringle and his Circle', *Ann. Sci.* 6(1948–50), 127–80, 229-61.

[3] Smith, *Treatise on Fever*, p.369.

of the immediate or exciting cause'.[1] This assertion of the pre-eminence of one among the range of environmental causes, and of the identity of different types of cause, is characteristic of dogmatic sanitary theory.

As was usual, Smith admitted the existence of diseases or states caused by a 'peculiar and specific' poison. These constituted no challenge to his conception of exciting cause, but appeared within it merely as a special case. Such diseases, smallpox for example, were caused by another form of animal matter, secreted only in the body, and capable of producing a series of specific symptoms. The body produced other poisons, for it had the power 'even when in sound health, much more when in disease, and above all when that disease is fever, to produce a poison capable of generating fever'.[2] This remark, which could be taken to represent the difference between the 'common' and the 'specific' contagions, aptly illustrates how naturally contemporary opinion would tend towards contingent contagionism in the explanation of the doubtful diseases, and how precarious was Smith's own categorical distinction between 'contagious' and 'epidemic'.

The two categories of contagious and epidemic Smith regarded as being defined by different behaviour, and by peculiar features: the epidemic type tended to decline when the number of those attacked was at its height, a fact inexplicable by contagion; a contagious disease, once the morbid matter was secreted, could be propagated at any time and amongst any number of persons, but usually to one person only once. In the case of epidemic diseases, Smith took into consideration the concept of 'epidemic atmosphere', since the hypothesis that these diseases were caused by a state of the air seemed to be the only possible explanation of the phenomena. He thought that certain conditions of the atmosphere, like heat and moisture, had an effect, but was critical of mysterious versions of the concept, and even of the term 'epidemic atmosphere', since 'to give a non-entity a name, is at once to convert it, in most men's imagination, into a sub-

---

[1] Here Smith cited examinations by Nathaniel Potter (1770–1843) of the blood in yellow fever: see *Treatise on Fever*, pp.371–4, also *Examiner*, 16 Sept. 1832, p.596. For Potter, see *Surgeon-General's Catalogue*.

[2] *Treatise on Fever*, p.365.

stance'. Smith preferred to rely on what was known, that is, that the air could be contaminated by putrid exhalations. It could be assumed, if only on *a priori* grounds, that these were material.[1] From these arguments it can be seen that a reasonable philosophical scepticism could also lead to a concentration on a single known cause.

Smith's notion of contagious disease was one Budd would have welcomed: in particular, he described as an 'absurdity' the notion that a disease like smallpox could generate spontaneously, or that a disease which was not contagious could under any circumstances develop that property.[2] Although Smith himself plainly thought otherwise, his account of epidemic and contagious disease depended for its definition on the positive characteristics of contagious diseases as they appeared to affect the individual.[3] No comparison was made with the very much less decisive picture presented by a variety of contagious diseases as they actually appeared in the field. Smith was therefore able to say that evidence for the contagious nature of a disease could only be either negligible, or overwhelming. Thus, the inevitable result of considering the behaviour in the field of a 'doubtful' disease like 'typhus', or yellow fever, or cholera (all of which are now known to travel indirectly from one to another subject), was its inclusion in the epidemic, non-contagious category. Smith was seeking to establish the contagious character as the exception rather than the rule; to put the onus of proof on the 'contagionists'; and to eradicate a supposed habit of mind which saw a contagionist explanation of two consecutive events in the field as 'intuitively obvious', regardless of the absence of evidence for the relation's being one of cause and effect. Similarly, he held up as absurdly *improbable* earlier accounts ascribing the introduction of plague to such means as a piece of silk imported by a Frenchman in 1665.[4]

[1] Smith, 'Contagion and Sanitary Laws', *Westminster Review*, 3 (1825), 145-6, 134 ff., 142. Compare, on the laws of epidemic diseases, Charles Maclean, e.g. 'Summary of Facts and Inferences Respecting Plague', *Pamphleteer*, 16 (1820), 154-6, 172-82; *Results of an Investigation* (1817-18), i, especially Books I and III.

[2] Smith, 'Contagion and Sanitary Laws', pp.139-41.

[3] As detected by *The Lancet*, 6 (1825), 337.

[4] Smith, 'Contagion and Sanitary Laws', pp.145-6. Cf. Maclean, *Results of an Investigation*, i. Smith, 'Plague, Typhus Fever, Quarantine', *Westminster Review*, 3 (1825), 503.

Smith recognized that very little separated the 'contagionist' and the 'anticontagionist' positions. With respect to more confined spaces, the two kinds of disease, even as he defined them, could be said to share a mode of propagation. The special matter of a contagious disease could be carried from person to person in the air; matter generated by a patient with typhus or yellow fever could also contaminate the air and produce fever in a healthy person. Smith suggested that there would be no dispute at all if the term 'contagious' were restricted to diseases which arose from a specific contagion, and if 'infectious' were used to describe those diseases which arose from every other such poison. In 1825 he proposed that all fevers that were not contagious should be called 'con-taminative'.[1] However, no clarification which was dependent upon little-known causes, regardless of epidemiological be-haviour, was acceptable at this time or later.

As an 'anticontagionist', Smith took an interest in plague which was scarcely shared by his contemporaries, even during the earlier debates over quarantine. He naturally asserted that cases of alleged importation should instead be given a 'con-taminative' interpretation, but his dependence was rather upon observations made by persons working in countries like Egypt and India in which epidemic diseases were said to originate. Observations of this kind made at earlier periods and according to different preconceptions did not have to be discarded, since even a contagionist was obliged to give an account of the origin of any disease.[2] As Smith saw it, all the evidence pointed to those local conditions which could be assumed to produce particularly rich putrid effluvia. Since a disease thus generated could not then become contagious or travel contagiously, it followed that a corresponding disease arising in England was caused by corresponding conditions. Thus typhus was a form of plague; and the overcrowded lodgings of the poor in London corresponded to the appalling living conditions of the fellahin. Smith thought that efficient ventilation (that is, a practical preventive measure) provided an acid test of the distinction between epidemic and con-

---

[1] Smith, *Treatise on Fever*, p.366; idem, 'Plague, Typhus Fever, Quarantine', pp.520–1.

[2] As *The Lancet* was quick to notice, Smith himself avoided this obligation with respect to diseases he regarded as contagious: ibid. 6 (1825), 340–2.

tagious diseases: 'No fever produced by contamination of the air can be communicated to others in a pure air'.[1] His contemporaries were, of course, unlikely to admit his distinction on this ground, since ventilation had been used to control all diseases capable of propagating through the air. Smith also stressed the disproportionate incidence of fever suffered in particular localities, especially in London.

The reviews of Smith's work provide much evidence of the state of controversy as to the nature of disease and show, in general, a resistance to polarization on all questions.[2] Some weariness with the subject of fever is expressed, which is attributable to the academic nature of many of the issues involved, the difficulty experienced in resolving any of them, and to the quantity of works produced on the subject since the epidemics of 1818-19.[3] The chief reaction to Smith's book was none the less not of this generic nature. Far from being 'hailed enthusiastically' by the medical journals, the *Treatise* was criticized as categorical, philosophically affected, and redolent of a lack of both sobriety and experience.[4] Its dogmatism as to the relationship between inflammation and fever and consequently as to therapeutics, was regarded as likely dangerously to mislead the beginner, and as a 'practical work' it was invariably contrasted with Alexander Tweedie's work on fever, which appeared simultaneously. This shorter and more modest study was also based on London Fever Hospital records (Tweedie being Smith's colleague in that institution), and was favourably reviewed.[5] Tweedie's account,

<hr>

[1] Smith, 'Plague, Typhus Fever, Quarantine', pp.514-20; idem, *Treatise on Fever*, pp.360 ff.

[2] The following will be used here: *Med. Chir. Rev.* 12 (1830), 337-61, 385-400; *Edinb. Med. Surg. J.* 33 (1830), 337-54; *Lond. Med. Gaz.* 6 (1830), 232-40, 306-10, 337-45, 1012-15; *Lancet*, 1830-1, i. 582 ff., 584-9, 641-5, 705-9.

[3] See e.g. *Lond. Med. Gaz.* 6 (1830), 232; and Murchison's bibliography of British and foreign works consulted for his *Treatise on Continued Fevers*, pp.699-718.

[4] Cf. Poynter, 'Southwood Smith — the Man', p.387; see also Lewes, *Southwood Smith, A Retrospect*, pp.24-5. The least critical of the journals was in effect claiming priority for the similar views of its editor, James Johnson: *Med. Chir. Rev.* 12 (1830), especially pp.342-3.

[5] Tweedie, *Clinical Illustrations of Fever* (1830). For reviews, see above, note 2. For Tweedie (1794-1884), M.D. Edinburgh 1815, F.R.S. 1838, see *Munk*; *DNB*; *Correspondence and Editorial Comments on the Points at Issue between Dr. Tweedie and Dr. Murchison* (1863).

according to the *Edinburgh Medical and Surgical Journal* (which was not entirely without some bias in favour of a disciple of William Alison), was 'more consonant with nature' or the natural history of fever.[1] Smith's claim to have reached a definition subordinating the whole range of febrile epidemic diseases was scarcely taken seriously; regardless of its title, his work was treated as dealing only with the 'common continued fever' of England, or rather of London.[2] The reviewers, referring to the 'recent fashion for strict pathological researches in this disease [fever]', criticized Smith for his minuteness, and for a *naïveté* in regarding all the pathological and postmortem appearances in his class of patient as attributable to fever alone.[3] Smith, although 'labouring for originality', was chastised for being extreme rather than original. The *London Medical Gazette*, repeating a charge levelled by *The Lancet* in 1825, accused the author of the *Treatise* of tacitly deriving his views from those of the late notorious John Armstrong, who preceded Smith at the London Fever Hospital and at Grainger's Webb Street medical school.[4] Most of the reviewers found Smith's condemnation of Cullen (a further imitation of Armstrong) the more ill judged as they detected Smith's share in the common dependence on a modifiedly Cullenian view of fever.[5] Smith had achieved only a novelty of manner, not of matter.[6]

The reviewers clearly also had in their minds as they wrote, Smith's earlier and more polemical articles on epidemic diseases in the first numbers of the *Westminster Review*.[7] General references in 1830 to an 'unbelief in contagion' as a factor in disease described the ill effects of a publicly conducted controversy over quarantine, which had come to a head in 1824–5, and been resolved in favour of a less anomalous practice by a

---

[1] *Edinb. Med. Surg. J.* 33 (1830), 343. But see also *Lancet*, 1830–1, i. 707.

[2] See e.g. *Lond. Med. Gaz.* 6 (1830), 232; *Edinb. Med. Surg. J.* 33 (1830), 343.

[3] *Lancet*, 1830–1, i. 703; *Edinb. Med. Surg. J.* 33 (1830), 348–9; *Lond. Med. Gaz.* 6 (1830), 306–9.

[4] *Lond. Med. Gaz.* 6 (1830), especially pp.233, 235 ff., 339, 341, 342, 344–5. The *Gazette* refers to the earlier charge, p.345. See *Lancet*, 7 (1825), 192; for Smith's (anonymous) denial, and further comment, see ibid., pp.280–1.

[5] See e.g. *Lond. Med. Gaz.* 6 (1830), 233, 235; *Edinb. Med. Surg. J.* 33 (1830), 339–41. See also Thomson, *Life of Cullen*, ii. 119.

[6] *Lond. Med. Gaz.* 6 (1830), 233; *Edinb. Med. Surg. J.* 33 (1830), 339; *Med. Chir. Rev.* 12 (1830), 343–4.

[7] Smith, 'Contagion and Sanitary Laws'; 'Plague, Typhus Fever, Quarantine'.

committee on the maintenance and improvement of foreign trade. The old and obviously fatuous quarantine law had been condemned as 'injurious to commerce' from before 1800, and the conflict between interested parties which took place between 1815 and 1825 did so in the absence of any immediate threat of disease.[1] The establishment reaction was predictably defended in the quarterlies by such medical writers as Robert Gooch and William MacMichael, but since the diseases concerned were not indigenous but exotic, the witnesses consulted during the official inquiries exhibited not a developed 'contagionist' position but rather an often entire ignorance. On the question of principle, the establishment, including the Royal College of Physicians and the major figure of Sir Gilbert Blane, merely came down on what it considered to be the side of economic, social, and actual safety. In this it was joined by less conformable arbiters, including *The Lancet.*[2] The initiative in medical terms lay instead with a very small number of activists who were attempting to force an anticontagionist position with respect to plague, yellow fever, and other quarantinable diseases. The chief of these was Charles Maclean,[3] a wandering servant of the East India and Levant Companies and enemy of the Holy Alliance, who held the idiosyncratic view that the 'doctrine of contagion' was a pious fraud, first perpetrated by the legates of Paul III at the Council of Trent, and preserved as the basis of the instrument of quarantine by the Venetian Republic and other

[1] Some details on quarantine may be obtained from the otherwise limited J.C. Macdonald, 'History of Quarantine in Britain during the Nineteenth Century', *Bull. Hist. Med.* 25 (1951), 23–44; C.F. Mullett, 'A Century of English Quarantine (1709–1825)', ibid. 23 (1949), 527–45. See also the works of Gavin Milroy (1805–86), listed in *DNB*.

[2] [R. Gooch], 'Plague, a Contagious Disease', *Quarterly Review*, 33 (1826), 218–57; cf. J. Bowring, *Observations on the Oriental Plague* (1838). *Report of Select Committee on the Doctrine of Contagion in Plague*, PP, 1819, II; (*Second*) *Report of Select Committee on Foreign Trade: Quarantine*, PP, 1824, VI. *Lancet*, 6 (1825), 342.

[3] Maclean (c. 1766–1825), M.D., ship's surgeon with East India Co. 1788; expelled from India by Wellesley in 1798 for refusing to retract a published criticism of the local justiciary: P.E. Roberts, *India under Wellesley* (1929), pp.176–7; Maclean, *To the British Inhabitants of India* [1798]. None of Maclean's publications on this occasion can fairly be called a 'radical political pamphlet': cf. E.H. Ackerknecht, 'Anticontagionism Between 1821 and 1867', *Bull. Hist. Med.* 22 (1948), 562–93: 583. For biography see ibid., pp. 582–4; *DNB* (an unfair account).

trading or tyrannical nations who found that instrument pol-
itically and commercially useful. An energetic campaign was
conducted by Maclean and his supporters on the strength of
his undeniably first-hand experience of plague, Asiatic cholera
and yellow fever in their natural habitats. His views were
pressed in the House of Commons by his friend the Liberal
John Smith and also by the then radical John Cam Hobhouse.[1]
Maclean's own political views are perhaps best described as
anti-authoritarian, but he seems to have formed a loose connection with the Benthamites and their Liberal fellow-travellers
which led to Southwood Smith's articles in the *Review* and
to Southwood Smith's being described in the House as the
'most zealous of the doctor's [Maclean's] medical coadjutors'.[2]

Maclean's notoriety affected public opinion and so did
that of Armstrong, whose influence had led, again according
to the reviewers of 1830, to a deplorable 'extra-professional
belief' in the omnipotence of malaria or bad air. Armstrong,
whose Benthamite connections are slightly more definite
than Maclean's, was described by John Smith as being 'more
conversant with cases of fever than any other physician in the
metropolis'. He had written and lectured extensively and
with great éclat on 'typhus fever' and had further made out a
parallel between typhus and the plague. Praised by *The Lancet*
as a 'reformer' to the last, 'ever a lover and ardent admirer of
liberal principles and open institutions', Armstrong also
shared Maclean's antischolasticism.[3]

Southwood Smith's articles were congruent in tone with
Review rhetoric in general, the Royal College of Physicians
being a natural object for attack. Some of the strongest
passages, such as those alleging the obfuscating effect of the
current forms of medical education, and the superior judge-

---

[1] Maclean, *Results of an Investigation*, i. 184 ff. See also *Examiner*, 29 May
1831, p.344; 18 Sept. 1831, p.600. *Hansard*, 2nd series, XII and XIII (1825),
especially cols. 1315–23.

[2] Smith was so described by Mr. Hudson Gurney, a member of the Select
Committee of 1819 on the plague: *Hansard*, 2nd series, XII (1825), col. 1321.

[3] *Edinb. Med. Surg. J.* 33 (1830), 343, 344; *Hansard*, 2nd series, XII (1825),
col. 1319. Armstrong had first asserted the analogy between typhus and plague *c.*
1816, on pathological grounds — at which time he thought both diseases contagious: Boott, *Memoir of Armstrong*, i. 23–4. *Lancet*, 1830–1, ii. 401. For
Armstrong (1784–1829), b. Durham, M.D. Edinburgh 1807, L.R.C.P. 1820, see
Boott, *Memoir*; *Munk*; *Br. For. Med. Rev.* 1 (1836), 34–70.

ment on the question of quarantine displayed by the commercial classes, are reproduced almost unchanged over twenty
years later in the General Board of Health's First Report on
Quarantine.[1] Many of the illustrations given in the *Westminster
Review* and in the *Treatise* are repeated more than once in
later official reports.[2] With respect to quarantine, the articles,
like the Reports of 1849 and 1852, dwelt on the system's
injustices and its failure to succeed in its own terms. On contagion, 'a question of science, to be decided by facts which
every one can understand', Smith stressed points which later
became rebarbative in the debate over cholera: the evidence
of persons familar with the countries of origin; outbreaks on
board ship; the apparently 'crucial' experiment of importation;
the susceptibility or otherwise of attendants on the sick; and
the nature, relevance, and obstinacy of popular conviction on
the subject.[3] That quarantine and contagion could, in spite of
their supposed status as matters for professional expertise, be
regarded in the same light as other reform questions is illus-
strated in the works of both Smith and Maclean by their use
of the argument that the application of quarantine, and the
popular belief in contagion, led to social, moral, political, and
even medical evils. The distinction between scientific and
professional expertise represented not merely an attack on
groundless professional privilege but also the characteristic
radical belief in scientific knowledge as pre-eminently, if not
definitively, available to all.[4]

Smith's articles, according to *The Lancet*, were 'powerfully
instrumental in influencing' the public mind, but professional
opinion remained convinced that contagion existed as one
cause of epidemic diseases, that plague and yellow fever (very
little was said of cholera) were specific and very likely con-

[1] Smith, 'Contagion and Sanitary Laws', pp.135 ff.; cf. *Report on Quarantine*,
PP, 1849, XXIV. 19 ff. [137 ff.].

[2] Cf. Smith, 'Contagion and Sanitary Laws', pp.148, 150, 157; idem, *Treatise
on Fever*, pp.350–64; idem, *Report on Removable Physical Causes of Mortality*,
PP, 1837–8, XXVIII. 233, 240–2; *Report on Quarantine*, pp.37, 44. Smith
similarly repeated himself in evidence to Commissions: M. Greenwood, *Some
Pioneers of Social Medicine* (1948), p.44.

[3] Smith, 'Contagion and Sanitary Laws', p.135. For popular reaction interpreted
as a result of 'taxes on knowledge', see *Examiner*, 31 July 1831, p.482.

[4] According to the pronouncement attributed to Bentham, after Bacon: 'let
experience be fertile and custom be barren': Bowring, *Autobiographical Recollections* (1877), p.337.

tagious, and that common fever had a separate status which was a matter for debate. *The Lancet* chose to defend the profession in an impertinent review which none the less conveyed serious criticism not only of Smith's anticontagionism and concept of epidemic disease but also of the rigidity of his notion of contagion.[1] 'This author', it stated, in the same vein as the reviewers of 1830, 'defines, divides, deduces and dogmatizes . . . the trinity of epithets, contagious, epidemic and sporadic, being all applicable to the same disease, cannot serve as the basis of nosological distinction . . . [he has] dressed up contagion in an armour best suited to fight his battle . . . Are contagious diseases really independent of atmospheric influence, unmodified by place, climate and constitution?' In addition, 'daily experience must convince every man of the spontaneous generation [in the human body] of specific animal poisons'. *The Lancet* concluded that the public were misguided in assuming that the late discussions had thrown new light upon the laws of contagion, and that something more commercial than mere philanthropy or a love of truth had actuated the participants in the dispute.

It appears to be the case that the word 'sanitary', in any of its nineteenth-century spellings, and regardless of a difference in the Latin roots which might imply a distinction between 'health' and 'healing', was first used by Maclean in his *Evils of Quarantine Laws* (1824), and directly transferred from there to Smith's *Review* articles of 1825.[2] Maclean used the term in entirely pejorative contexts to refer to quarantine laws and institutions, presumably as an adaptation of the French expression for a state health regulation, *cordon sanitaire*.[3] 'Sanitary' and 'sanative' were used indiscriminately in official documents during the first cholera epidemic in headings over quarantine and other precautionary regulations that included measures directed towards improvement in

---

[1] *Lancet*, 7 (1825), 114–20; 6 (1825), 336–42.

[2] Maclean, *Evils of Quarantine Laws*, p.xxvi and *passim*; Smith, 'Contagion and Sanitary Laws', pp.134 (heading) and 137; *Lancet*, 6 (1825), 336, 342. Cf. *OED*. I have since found usages for 1779 and 1796 in J. Knyveton, *Man Midwife*, ed. E. Gray (1946), but these may be mistranscriptions.

[3] The French adjective and its equivalents must have been common in the late eighteenth and early-nineteenth-century literature on State medicine and medical police. See e.g. M. Ryan, *A Manual of Medical Jurisprudence* (1836), p.xxxiii.

comfort and cleanliness. At the same time, 'sanitary' was applied by Bentham and by the *Examiner* both to quarantine regulations and to what might be regarded as standard sanitary procedures, aimed at reducing the incidence of fever.[1] Although the Benthamite sanitarians did not introduce the term, it would seem that they gave it the positive, environmental connotations which it has today. It was still something of a novelty when it appeared in the titles of Arnott, Kay, and Southwood Smith's reports on fever of 1838 and Chadwick's Report of 1842.[2] It is perhaps significant that one of the few others to employ it between 1832 and 1837 was William Farr.[3]

The *Examiner's* reaction to the first cholera epidemic represents the first and most decipherable combination of the resources of Chadwick and Southwood Smith. Lengthy sections of Smith's *Treatise* were reproduced by Chadwick in his capacity of subeditor to the *Examiner*, an employment which coincided in duration almost exactly with the period of the first epidemic. Before this, Chadwick had shown a constructive interest in medical education and the advancement of medical knowledge in his articles on French medical charities (hospitals etc.) and preventive police. He had perceived a parallel between crime and disease, and may have been led to an independent awareness of the existence of 'fever nests' — 'ghettoes' occupied only by the poor, in which there was a constant incidence of fever — through his analysis of police reports.[4] Before cholera first emerged as a threat to Britain, the *Examiner* was carrying bulletins on the regular incidence

[1] C.F. Brockington, *Public Health in the Nineteenth Century* (Edinburgh and London, 1965), pp.118, 120, 123, 124; spelling regularized. Bentham, Appendix II to *Constitutional Code*, *Works*, xi. 648-9; *Examiner*, 5 June 1831, p.355; 13 Nov 1831, p.723.

[2] Gibson records a use of 'sanatory' reported of Robert Slaney in *The Times* of 1840, and a debate in *The Times* of 1847 over the current spelling of the term: 'The Public Health Agitation in England, 1838-1848 — A Newspaper and Parliamentary History' (University of North Carolina Ph.D. dissertation, 1955), p.47 and note.

[3] Farr at this time tended to use the term in the sense of 'health-giving', or 'with respect to health', as did James Clark slightly later. Farr also used the word 'sanability'. Farr, 'Lecture on Hygeine [*sic*] and Public Health', *Lancet*, 1835-6, i. 240; idem, 'Vital Statistics' in J.R. McCulloch (ed.), *Statistical Account of the British Empire* (1837), ii. 567, 583.

[4] Finer, *Life of Chadwick*, pp.34-5; Chadwick, 'Centralization'; idem, 'Preventive Police', *Lond. Rev.* 1 (1829), 252-308; idem, 'Progress of Sanitation', *Trans. Natn. Ass. Soc. Sci.* 25 (1881), 646.

of fever in London, and was pointing out that the rich knew nothing of the moral and physical condition of the poor unless this was accidentally exposed, whereupon it was assumed that some set of extraordinary circumstances was at work. The *Examiner* further criticized the Government's continued lack of responsibility for the preservation of the public health, as well as the circumstance that it was not possible, as it was in France, to co-ordinate the activities of medical institutions to meet cholera or any other such emergency. It was not suggested that emergency Boards of Health were useless, but that there should be, in addition, a special board of two to four persons combining expert knowledge of the regular fever of the country and of the conditions and usages of parishes. This special board would, probably with the help of the new police, locate and remove the most powerful and general predisposing causes in the living conditions of the poor. This sanitary work was to be carried out in conjunction with other measures, for example, the removal of the sick into a pure air. Later, when the cholera had reached Sunderland, it was proposed that the City of London's Board of Health could best direct its energies by making maps of fever incidence and removing local causes where fever was found to be most prevalent. A suggestion to the same effect was recorded at the same time by Bentham in a note to his 'Constitutional Code', and it was of course this sort of inquiry which was finally conducted on an official level in 1837.[1] The *Examiner* provides no evidence that Chadwick had at this stage evolved his full circle of sewerage, continuous water supply, and agricultural improvement, or realized the whole extent and economic importance of the ordinary incidence of fever, presumably because he had not yet investigated these matters for himself.[2] But the option of attacking 'the most powerful and general' causes of disease, in the shape of drains, stagnant water, and accumulated organic filth, was clearly reasonable from every point of view. It could be justified on traditional grounds as well as on the

---

[1] See e.g. *Examiner*, 5 June 1831, p.355; 3 July 1831, pp.425–6; 7 Nov. 1831, p.760; see also 11 Dec. 1831, p.793; 4 Mar. 1832, pp.154–5. Bentham, *Works*, ix. 648–9.

[2] Credit for allocating to Chadwick the questions of arterial drainage and water supply was claimed by James Kay-Shuttleworth: *Autobiography* (1964), p.18.

basis of more modern theories, and it had already been proved effective on a small scale. It was, as well, both preventive and economical of effort, and it was practicable: sanitary practice as opposed to sanitary administration was very much an art of the possible, it being obvious to all sectors of opinion that most causes of epidemic diseases, especially remote causes, were outside current knowledge or control.[1]

[1] This course of action conformed in a literal manner to the methodology for 'interference in a social wrong' formulated by Chadwick in 1829. See [D. Masson], 'Edwin Chadwick', *N. Br. Rev.* 13 (1850), 49.

2

LATER DEVELOPMENTS: THE GENERAL BOARD OF HEALTH AND THE MEDICAL PROFESSION

The background of this chapter is the best-known period in the campaign for the public health, that from 1838 to 1850. Effective legislation was long delayed, but the pressure was kept up by a series of commissions and their reports, and by the Health of Towns Association. Chadwick's Report of 1842 was followed by that of the confirmatory 'Commission for Inquiring into the State of Large Towns and Populous Districts', or 'Health of Towns' Commission (First Report, 1844; Second Report, 1845). This commission, although dominated by Chadwick in the public-health interest, was also a continuation of the inquiry into municipal government begun in 1833. London was a special problem and had to be taken separately.[1] Three reports were produced by the 'Commission Appointed to Inquire whether any and what Special Means may be Requisite for the Improvement of the Health of the Metropolis' in 1847 and 1848. The 'Metropolitan Sanitary Commission' was handed to Chadwick by Lord John Russell; Southwood Smith was also a member, with Richard Owen, Richard Lambert Jones (for the City interest), and Lord Robert Grosvenor. The first Public Health Act (which excluded London) was passed in 1848 and Chadwick's General Board (Chadwick, Southwood Smith, and Lord Ashley) was gazetted in September of that year. Meanwhile, other important inquiries were carried out and legislation proposed on intramural interment, building regulations, wash-houses, and sewage manure.[2] Until the end of this period, the relevant views of Chadwick and Smith

---

[1] Finer, *Life of Chadwick*, stresses the peculiar difficulties and importance of London's administration.

[2] Ibid., pp.290–1, 314–15, 338–9. On building regulations, interment, and wash-houses see Gibson, 'The Public Health Agitation, A Newspaper and Parliamentary History', or idem, 'Baths and Wash-houses in the Public Health Agitation 1839–48', *J. Hist. Med.* 9 (1954), 391–406.

remained more or less static. Others, however, joined the campaign and published a variety of opinions on sanitary subjects; those who will be considered include Arnott, John Sutherland, William Alison, and Edmund Parkes. The present discussion examines how far 'a growth of anticontagionism to the middle of the century' can be regarded as an accurate and sufficiently comprehensive description of developments in medical opinion in relevant areas between 1835 and 1850.

The fever investigations of 1837, conducted along pre-ordained lines under the umbrella of the Poor Law Commission, are said to have constituted 'an entirely new sort of Government action . . . a first step in the modern utilisation of Medicine by the State'.[1] Even as a retrospective judgement, and assuming the word 'modern' is intended to exclude such precedents as the deliberate employment of Richard Mead in 1719, as well as other cases, which could perhaps be described as consultative, this statement requires considerable qualification.[2] Firstly, the investigations of 1837-8 are equally regarded as representing the first (presumably public) involvement of members of the profession in social questions. Arnott and Kay's contemporaries would have found this a meaningless distinction, and certainly it seems to limit the lives of medically qualified persons in the eighteenth and nineteenth centuries to professional matters in a way that is anachronistic. Secondly, a growing body of medical men, especially in the provinces, was already concerned about the liability of the lower ranks of the profession to be exploited in the public service, and saw this as a dangerous tendency of many reform proposals.[3] Both of the statements in question therefore suffer from an over-concentration on central government administration. Thirdly, if it is necessary to conclude that the medical profession made no greater contribution in the first half of the century than its part in furthering the sanitary

---

[1] J. Simon, *Sanitary Institutions* (1897), p.185.

[2] G. Newman, *The Rise of Preventive Medicine* (Oxford, 1932), p.157. The early vaccination establishments constitute another kind of precedent: see Simon, *Public Health Reports*, i.

[3] See e.g. N. Rumsey *et al.*, 'Observations on Medical Relief for Sick Paupers', *Trans. Prov. Med. Surg. Ass.* 5 (1837), 441-55; J. Yelloly, 'Observations on the Relief of the Sick Poor', ibid., pp.456-88.

movement, then it should also be said that medicine as a science had little to do with this. Furthermore, in this first phase as distinct from the second under John Simon, medical men were not engaged without being also somewhat detached from the profession, and especially from that part which was most self-consciously professional (Wakley undoubtedly being a special case).[1] One cannot make simple statements as to the involvement of medicine with government on the basis of taking Arnott, Smith, Kay, and even William Farr as representative. This tends to be borne out also on the theoretical level. Similar points may be made about the obscure poor-law and services medical officers whom Chadwick used so exclusively as witnesses.[2]

John Simon rightly said of the results of the fever investigations that they 'did not pretend to reveal anything medically new; but . . . showed . . . for the information of Parliament, that, under parliamentary sufferance, masses of population in this chief city of the world [London] were in physical circumstances which made healthy life impossible to them'. The titles of the Reports are of course indicative.[3] The Union medical officers were asked to describe the places where fever was most prevalent, and where sanitary defects were persistent. The argument required only that there be such places; an officer might find it difficult to assign causes precisely, but the range of possible factors was almost infinite. No special definition of terms was offered or required. The term 'contagion' is used casually; it was often employed for the aerial poison, however produced. Poisons thought to cause a great variety of fevers were evolved into the air by organic decomposition; even if not directly responsible for a disease, such poisons could cause it to become more virulent, or increase the incidence of such sporadic conditions as scrofula.

---

[1] Cf. Chadwick, *Sanitary Report*, ed. Flinn, pp.21–2.

[2] Munk observed that very few of his subjects had published works concerned with public health.

[3] Simon, *Sanitary Institutions*, p.182. Southwood Smith, *Report on Removable Physical Causes of Mortality*; idem, *On the Prevalence of Fever in 20 Metropolitan Unions*: Appendix to *5th Ann. Rep. of Poor Law Commissioners*, PP, 1839, XX. 100–6 [112–18]. N. Arnott and J.P. Kay, *Report on Prevalence of Removable Physical Causes of Fever*: Appendix to *4th Ann. Rep. of Poor Law Commissioners*, PP, 1837–8, XXVIII. 67–83.

Once a disease was induced, overcrowding alone could lead to fatal results, since the bodies of affected persons could give out a 'contagious malaria' which acted more quickly than the original cause. The medical officers spoke of 'typhus' as showing various degrees of contagiousness. The districts inspected were chosen on the basis of the long record they held at the London Fever Hospital as fever sites.

Smith drew together in the minds of his readers familiar but scattered facts, items, and stories — items in newspapers, noting the deaths of workmen from sewer gas; older stories of the decimation of armies and ships' crews, of the fatality of marshes and the destruction caused by foreign climates, and vaguer notions about bad airs and unhealthy places. The common and justifying factor in all such accounts, Smith asserted, was the influence of an aerial poison, produced by the putrefaction of animal and vegetable matter — or so it had been 'induced' from the fact that 'its virulence is always in proportion to the quantity of animal and vegetable matters present, and to the perfect combination of the circumstances favourable to their decomposition'. As in 1830, Smith recalled earlier writers, Pringle on the British Army in Flanders (1751), Mead on the generation of plague in Cairo (1720); respected observers, who now had the added merit of having inferred the existence of the poison of decomposition while knowing nothing of it directly. These independent findings had been based only on what was observed, and constituted, Smith thought, the most unimpeachable support for the modern explanation.[1]

In spite of their language, there was no quantitative basis for Smith's statements. However, Smith did think that he could offer something better than inductive evidence, however sound: the poison 'now ... may be procured in such a palpable and concrete form as to enable us actually to experiment with it'.[2] Examination of the residuum obtained by

---

[1] Smith, *Report on Removable Physical Causes of Mortality*, pp.83, 92-3, 94.

[2] Ibid., p92. Smith appears to have had some interest in chemistry, especially chemical or humoral pathology: see *Treatise on Fever*, pp.328-30. For his experiments on the febrile poison, see ibid., pp.367-8. He is later described as having found an organic substance (or possible fever poison) in London streets: R.A Smith, *On the Air and Water of Towns*, PP, 1850, XXII. 83. For other (physiological) experimentation by Southwood Smith, see *Report on Quarantine*, p.56.

condensing the 'vapour' in contaminated air had shown the poison to be putrefying animal and vegetable matter. Its virulence had been proved by injecting drops of the condensed fluid into the veins of dogs.[1] All the symptoms of yellow fever, including the black vomit, had been reproduced; and 'by varying the intensity and the dose of the poison . . . it is possible to produce fever of almost any type, endowed with almost any degree of mortal power'. It had also been proved by physiological experiment that, when inspired, the poison entered the blood; and that the fever produced varied further according to whether animal or vegetable matter predominated in the poison. The vegetable exhalations of bogs and marshes tended to produce intermittent and remittent fever; the predominantly animal wastes of crowded cities in temperate climates led to 'continued fever of the typhoid character'.

It would appear that, although his proofs of existence were hardly adequate, Smith was still averse to hypothetical entities or substances. However, his notion of the agent is no better defined because of this. He does not appear to have had in mind a spectrum of poisons; effects ranging from instant death to yellow fever to a non-specific weakening of the system could be produced merely by differences in the concentration of 'the poison'; and yet it produced ague or continued fever according to differences in composition.[2]

Smith did not, in his reports for the Poor Law Commission, take up a combative position with respect to contagion. Rather, he simply stated that in really bad conditions, once a fever had broken out, it could acquire a virulence which might extend to the whole of the household and to attendants on the sick. Like Arnott and Kay, he stressed instances in which fever, long present in a certain locality, had ceased to occur after sanitary work had been carried out.

---

[1] *Report on Removable Physical Causes of Mortality*, p.83. The experiments referred to here are probably those of Marie H. Bernard Gaspard, 'Mémoires sur les maladies purulentes', *J. Physiol. Expér.* 2 (1822), and F. Magendie, ibid. 3 (1823). Baas, *Outlines of Medical History*, ii. 899, 1004.

[2] *Report on Removable Physical Causes of Mortality*, pp.83–4. 'Typhoid' is of course used adjectivally. On the history of views on absorption, see M.P. Earles, 'Early Theories of the Mode of Action of Drugs and Poisons', *Ann. Sci.* 17 (1961), 97–110; J.M.D. Olmsted, *François Magendie* (1944), pp.33–44. Relevant here were the experiments of Potter of Baltimore.

It is clear that Arnott, Kay, and Smith functioned in these inquiries, and were presented to the public, not as expert witnesses in the modern mode, ostensibly silent on all subjects save one, but rather as men entitled to speak from their profound first-hand knowledge of the areas in question.[1] Smith found scope within the terms of the inquiry to develop the theme of the high economic cost of disease.

R.A. Lewis divides the activity of the years after 1838 and before the Public Health Bill of 1848 into three phases: revelation, recommendation, and legislation. The work of these years demanded no greater complexity of medical doctrine than that provided by Southwood Smith in the reports of 1838 and 1839. Evidence for the functional elements of the doctrine was, of course, greatly amplified. Using the new statistical information provided by the Registrar-General's Department, the sanitarians expressed their commitment to group prevention rather than individual cure. Farr established a 'norm of mortality' based on the average mortalities of 'healthy areas'.[2] Chadwick supported with maps, tables, and eye-witness accounts his contention that an Englishman's expectation of life varied directly with his social class, and that the reasons for this were not economic but physical: so many factors brought about the deaths of the few starving, but a high mortality among wage-earners living in squalor explained itself. The most satisfactory feature of this diagnosis was the existence of a remedy which was feasible, violated no other principle, and could be used on a scale commensurate with that of the problem itself: sanitary improvement. These conclusions and the weight of data supporting them are set out in Chadwick's famous Report of 1842.[3] This Report contains the equally famous statement as

[1] For Kay, later Sir James Kay-Shuttleworth (1804–77), M.D. Edinburgh 1827, see *DNB*; the *Life* by F. Smith (1923); the *Autobiography*.

[2] Lewis, *Chadwick and Public Health*, p.105. Farr, *Appendix 1840*, p.11; idem, *Appendix 1841*, pp.20 ff. For Farr's several attempts at a norm, or ideal, of healthiness, see J.M. Eyler, 'William Farr 1807–1883: An Intellectual Biography of a Social Pathologist' (University of Wisconsin Ph.D. dissertation, 1971), pp.132–3, 229–39.

[3] The *Sanitary Report* was also issued as a House of Lords paper from the Poor Law Commission. Two volumes of *Local Reports* were similarly issued, I: England and Wales; II: Scotland.

to the respective roles of the physician and the civil engineer; but even in the report itself, as Flinn has pointed out, this apparent dismissal must be seen in the context of Chadwick's employment of medical testimony and of his plans for the involvement of the profession in the public service.[1]

The Report of 1842 interested itself in the incidence of a range of diseases and diseased conditions. Chadwick's remarks were less specific than Smith's had been in 1838, and he had, of necessity, adopted the single 'epidemic, endemic and contagious' grouping introduced by Farr in 1839. The cholera of 1831–2 was noticed chiefly for having produced no lasting and useful result, although a spot-and-shade map of Leeds was included which showed (rather approximately) the identity of the tracks of cholera and fever. Some awareness is shown of conflicting views on fever, from which Chadwick affected to dissociate the Report:

The medical controversy as to the causes of fever; as to whether it is caused by filth and vitiated atmosphere, or whether the state of the atmosphere is a predisposing cause to the reception of the fever, or the means of propagating that disease, which has really some other superior, independent, or specific cause, does not appear to be one that for practical purposes need be considered, except that its effect is prejudicial in diverting attention from the practical means of prevention . . . the decision upon [the controversy] will not alter the practical value of cleanliness, or of its protective effects in prevention, whether it remove an original or only a predisposing cause.[2]

Most spokesmen for the profession, such as Benjamin Brodie in the *British and Foreign Medical Review*, were willing enough also to confine themselves to 'matters of practical value', and to admire the Report as 'the most valuable and complete treatise on certain departments of medical police ever published, either in this or any other country', not because it contained 'anything wonderfully new, either in principle or detail', but because of the 'authenticity and number of the facts'. The relation of the Report to larger issues did not go unnoticed; the reviewer was an adherent of Archibald Alison's doctrines of population, and regarded the

---

[1] Chadwick, *Sanitary Report*, ed. Flinn, pp.396, 60–1.

[2] Ibid., pp.111, 397, 50–1, 214. See also Chadwick to the Select Committee on Metropolitan Sewage Manure, PP, 1846, X. 654.

Report as supplying the proof of these. Yet as a medical reformer Brodie's recognition of the 'great and solemn' duty incumbent upon the medical profession, to work 'a greater and more beneficial revolution in England, than ever it has passed through', is clearly outweighed in real terms by his concern that 'the desire for medical knowledge and skill exhibited by government and public bodies has always been accompanied by a desire to get it for nothing — or less'. This remark was made with particular reference to the employment of surgeons by factory-owners.[1]

As long as they were taken literally, there was little possibility (or need) of refuting Chadwick's statements of correlation. The danger lay in their hardening into a positive and final view of the causality of disease. This was not detected of the 1842 Report; but Chadwick and Smith's certainty that the causes of fever were physical, and that fever was the cause, not the result, of destitution, had already aroused an adverse reaction among Scottish medical men, principally William Pulteney Alison. Chadwick's calculated disqualification of theory had a particular rather than a general reference. William Alison, brother of Archibald Alison, was a teacher of great influence and moral authority in the Edinburgh medical school. A pupil of Dugald Stewart, whom Stewart might have considered as his successor, Alison retained a markedly religious and philosophical bent and a particular interest in the doctrine of vital affinity.[2] Alison worked consistently among the very poor of Edinburgh, and introduced others to this level of existence; one of these was Kay, who did not relish the experience, and wondered how Alison could persist in it.[3]

Alison was chiefly responsible for the reform of the Scottish poor law, and his objections to the 'London writers' should be seen in the context of the distinction maintained between Scottish and English poor-law ideology and practice, as well

---

[1] [B. Brodie], 'Mr. Chadwick's Report', *Br. For. Med. Rev.* 15 (1843), 329, 333, 338–9: i.e. Sir Benjamin Collins Brodie (1783–1862).

[2] Chadwick, *Sanitary Report*, ed. Flinn, pp.214 ff.; Brodie, 'Mr Chadwick's Report', p.336. For Alison (1790–1859), M.D. Edinburgh 1811, D.C.L. Oxon. 1850, see *DNB*; W.T. Gairdner, 'Dr. Alison', in *The Physician as Naturalist* (1889), pp.388–430. On Alison's physiology, see ibid., pp.403 ff.

[3] Kay, *Autobiography*, pp.4 ff.

as in relation to the differences that delayed a Public Health Act (Scotland) until 1867.[1] The Scottish reformer's refusal to separate poverty from indigence threatened the Benthamite principle of less eligibility. Chadwick's reaction to this adds colour to the suggestion that he thought of poor-law and sanitary reform as integrally related. Southwood Smith and Chadwick maintained on all occasions that fever was a disease of the temperate and able-bodied, not of the destitute; it chiefly affected not immigrants to the towns, or even children, but rather established, mature members of the workforce.[2] No excess of mortality *necessarily* attached to the period of childhood; like the adult population, children suffered proportionately to the conditions in which they lived. Poverty ('the state of one, who, in order to obtain a mere subsistence, is forced to have recourse to labour') was not the object of attack, but rather those circumstances in their environment that turned the poor into the indigent (to whom the principle of less eligibility was not intended to apply); those circumstances, that is, that denied to the poor the life-span enjoyed by the rich. Similarly, high wages were no guarantee or measure of health.[3]

Alison had earlier objected to the tenor of the reports by Arnott, Kay, and Smith; his views (not in a very lucid form) were included in the Appendices to the Report of 1842, together with a reply by Arnott, who had investigated fever in the two major Scottish cities for Chadwick.[4] Alison, Arnott, and Southwood Smith were all much of an age, that is (in 1840), about fifty; the views of all three on medical questions,

---

[1] Chadwick, *Sanitary Report*, ed. Flinn, pp.62, 72–3. On the reform of the Scottish Poor Law, see Alison's own works, and G. Nicholls, *A History of the Scotch Poor Law* (1858); J.E. Graham, *The History of the Poor Law of Scotland Previous to 1845* (Cupar and St. Andrews, 1924). For Alison's role see Gairdner, 'Dr. Alison', pp.406 ff.

[2] This was an observation of Robert Willan: Creighton, *Epidemics*, ii. 140. For a later contradiction, see Greenhow, *Sanitary Papers*, p.104.

[3] Chadwick, *Comparative Results of Poor Law Administration*; idem, 'On Representing the Duration of Life', *J. Stats. Soc.* 7 (1844), 1–40; Smith, *Results of Sanitary Improvement*, pp.4, 12; Poynter, *Society and Pauperism*, pp.319–20; Chadwick, *Sanitary Report*, ed. Flinn, e.g. p.215.

[4] Arnott, *Report on Fevers in Edinburgh and Glasgow, Local Reports: Scotland*, PP (Lords), 1842, XXVIII. 1–13; W.P. Alison, *Observations on the Generation of Fever*, ibid. 13–33; Arnott, *Remarks on Dr. Alison's 'Observations'*, ibid. 34–9.

and especially the nature of fever, had been formed well before the controversies of the 1840s. Alison's association with the Edinburgh New Town dispensary had begun with its establishment in 1815, at the beginning of a punctuated but progressive real decline in economic conditions in Scotland.[1] He had lectured on medical police in 1820, and an article of 1827 on fever, which mentioned Armstrong, Percival, and Bateman, expressed a typical moderate, clinically oriented response to the medical controversies of that decade. This article pressed the epidemiological argument for the contagiousness of the fever prevalent in Scotland, gave it a mixed pathological character, distinguished it from the form prevalent in France, in which diarrhoea and ulceration of the bowel were common incidents, and suggested that in its most epidemical form it appeared as the link between exanthematous, and other continued fevers.[2] Again on clinical grounds, Alison ventured, as he put it, to question the benefit of ventilation, where this involved a removal to hospital and cold, pure air as an unaccustomed stimulus. There is some difference in purpose, but little in doctrine, between this article and Alison's position on fever after 1840.[3] The idea of a close connection between epidemic fever and destitution had occurred to him early, but 'developed itself into a practical shape more gradually, as his ideas of social economy became more matured'. Alison further ascribed scrofula, from before 1822, to the influence not of climatic factors but of the deprivations suffered most obviously by the inhabitants of towns.

In 1843 occurred an epidemic of what Alison at first thought of as a 'nova febris' (Sydenham), and which Christison asserted to be a specific form, later recognized as relapsing fever, and as a feature of earlier Scottish epidemics and of the epidemic of 1818–19. Alison subsequently revised his view of the unity of the fever poison, and worked out publicly and to

---

[1] Gairdner, 'Dr. Alison', pp.393–4. J.H.F. Brotherston, *Observations on the Early Public Health Movement in Scotland* (1952), pp.42 ff.

[2] Alison, 'Observations on the Epidemic Fever Now Prevalent in Edinburgh', *Edinb. Med. Surg. J.* 28 (1827), 233–63. For an experience of Edinburgh fevers similar to Alison's see T. Watson, *Principles and Practice of Physic* (1843), ii. 689.

[3] See L. King, 'The Blood-Letting Controversy — A Study in the Scientific Method', *Bull. Hist. Med.* 35 (1961), 1–13.

his own satisfaction that there were two, coexistent types of continued fever.[1]

Neil Arnott, who had become an expert on the scientific principles and practice of ventilation, appears to have shared Smith's views on the variable, but single, nature of the fever poison, but he cannot be regarded as an anticontagionist; instead, he exemplifies the way in which standard views could be modified by a strong practical commitment. He described as a 'great impediment' to correct thinking among medical men the opinion

that diseases might proceed from contagion alone, or else from certain combinations of such circumstances . . . occurring in the ordinary course of nature, but that the same could not proceed indifferently from both one source and the other. Yet no truth in medicine is now better ascertained than that diseases proceeding from the influence of an accidental combination of ordinary circumstances do become contagious . . .

In the particular context of the dispute with Alison, he stressed the lack of grounds for disagreement between them. In 1840 Alison limited himself to asserting the capability of contagion irrespective of other modes of communication. Arnott, as if accepting for the purposes of the argument a stress on the origin rather than the extension of fevers, returned that 'to hold contagion to be the sole cause of any disease, is in effect to assert that the first person who had the disease got it from somebody who had it before him, or that the disease was created in him as a separate and distinct existence, neither of which opinions has ever been deliberately maintained'. Arnott went on to detect the influence of 'malaria' as the common denominator among the conditions alleged by Scottish writers to be the cause of misery and disease: destitution (Alison), lack of education, lack of religious or moral training (Chalmers), and alcoholism. These other conclusions, Arnott stressed, did not contradict the 'London answer', or suggest any obstacle to its being carried out and *at once*; merely, they did not answer precisely the question of the immediate cause of fever. A good poor law might remove most of the conditions inhibiting an application of other remedies, but it would not reduce the inci-

---

[1] Gairdner, 'Dr. Alison', pp.395, 402, 396–7. Christison himself called the 'nova febris' 'synocha'.

dence of disease.[1] Southwood Smith, as well as Chadwick, also stressed this precedence of the physical over the moral. No form of education or spiritual enlightenment could usefully or fairly be applied to a fluctuating and debilitated population.[2] Arnott's remark that the best of governments might be unable to guarantee the material necessaries of life to all its people, but that any government could, by simple legislation, drain and ventilate, might be merely pragmatic, or indicative of an agreement with Chadwick's views on the feasibility and necessity of the labouring man's providing for himself.[3]

Alison on his side drew heavily, but inconclusively, on the recent Irish experience of fever and destitution (especially starvation). He could not, he said, answer the questions specifically framed by the Commissioners, because in Edinburgh destitution was not seen in the absence of filth. Sanitary reform in Edinburgh had not been followed by a similar improvement in medical terms. He admitted the influence of malaria, but denied that it was a sufficient or necessary cause in the origin of fever, and expressed surprise that this 'old doctrine of fevers in this climate' should issue from so respectable a source. The causes which led directly to the generation of fever were unknown; miasma was merely a predisposing cause, and of predisposing causes destitution was by far the more important, since it was known (as filth, in his view, was not) to promote the diffusion of contagious as well as other fevers. The Commissioners' case against filth ignored the incidence of such destructive diseases as smallpox.[4] Behind all Alison's objections however lay the concern that persons believing in the London writers' view of fever would consider nothing incumbent upon them with respect to direct intervention in the conditions of life of the inhabitants of towns, other than the removal of substances likely to become pu-

---

[1] Arnott, *Report on Fevers in Edinburgh and Glasgow*, pp.6–8; see also *Remarks on Dr. Alison's 'Observations'*, p.39. For Arnott (1788–1874), M.A. 1805, M.R.C.S. 1813, M.D. (by creation) Aberdeen 1814, L.R.C.P. 1817, F.R.S. 1838, surgeon to East India Co., inventor and popular scientific writer, see *DNB*.
[2] See e.g. Southwood Smith, *Results of Sanitary Improvement*, p.22.
[3] Arnott, *Report on Fevers in Edinburgh and Glasgow*, pp.5–6.
[4] Alison, *Observations on the Generation of Fever*.

trescent. Alison remained a severe critic of London-based public-health reform and poor-law theory; he later appears also as a critic of Farr's nosology, and as a sponsor of William Budd. Attempts were made in the English official reports to cancel his authority by reference to the views on poisons and fevers of his 'brother professor', Robert Christison.

By November 1847 cholera had reached Russia, and there seemed no reason why it should not for the second time spread to the rest of Europe, and eventually to Britain. Chadwick and Southwood Smith must have realized that if a General Board of Health were created during the next session of Parliament, cholera would be the first, and to the public mind, the most important, of its problems; and that, if they could in the current state of unease convince the public of their grasp of this particular problem, the chances of the Bill's passing would be so much the greater. With such considerations in mind, Smith, Chadwick, and Richard Owen formed themselves into a subcommittee of the Metropolitan Sanitary Commission, specifically to deal with the cholera.[1]

Chadwick and Smith at least among the sanitarians were aware that the threat of cholera would not necessarily serve the interests of their cause. The disease had still to be regarded as a 'foreign' epidemic, or exotic; it attracted, in proportion to the mortality it occasioned, more than its share of popular attention; and the people, fearfully watching its approach, or (as seemed more generally to be the case) surprised by its sudden arrival in their midst, were prone to lapse into the 'instinctive' belief that it was imported and spread among them by contagion. Secondly, for more educated persons, whatever their views, there was nothing in the history of the first epidemic to encourage them in the belief that they might control the second. The debate over fever in relation to the public health had acquainted Smith and Chadwick with the inconclusiveness of contemporary epidemiology. As evidence

---

[1] Lewis, *Chadwick and Public Health*, p.154. (Sir) Richard Owen (1804–92), M.R.C.S. 1826, F.R.S. 1834, may have met Chadwick while engaged in private practice in Lincoln's Inn Fields in the late 1820s; first served as a Commissioner on the Health of Towns Commission (1843). He early achieved a social standing and was no doubt shrewdly chosen as a 'name that carried weight': Finer, *Life of Chadwick*, p.232. For Owen on his Commission work, cf. ibid., p.233, and Owen, *Life of Owen*, i. 305–6, 329, 364–5.

from the field multiplied, it appeared to present a more, rather than less, equivocal picture, and yet the debate over cholera was continually being forced into oversimplification. The details of the progress of the doubtful diseases (which by this time included influenza) were constantly being arranged into abortive confrontations, at a time when the pressure for open, categorical decisions was also increasing.[1] Only the more advanced writers saw that it was first necessary to decide what content terms like 'contagious' had, and what they meant in relation to the body.

For the sanitarians, the obvious danger was that cholera would again be regarded as a problem different in kind from that of the familiar homebred diseases on which their case for the virtue of sanitary measures had, since 1831, publicly been built. The threat of cholera could easily blot out the new awareness of the true problem, which was the mortality suffered *constantly* by the labouring population because of the prevalence (which had been, it was alleged, of epidemic proportions since 1838) of 'fever'. Above all, Chadwick wished to prevent any reversion to quarantine procedures. Therefore, he and Smith set about systematically to compress cholera into the existing class of preventable diseases — a move 'purely practical' in intention, but leading inevitably to theoretical responsibilities. In their Second Report they went on to do the same for influenza.[2]

In the present instance the Commissioners published in some respects prematurely, in order 'to submit early the first clear practical conclusions which they [our inquiries] presented for executive action, namely, the conclusions at which we had arrived in relation to the identity of the tracks of cholera and typhus, and to measures preventive of both'.[3]

---

[1] In both 1831 and 1849 one finds medical gatherings 'deciding' the question of the contagiousness of cholera by majority decision: Ackerknecht, 'Anti-contagionism 1821-1867', p.577; *The Times*, 31 Aug. 1849.

[2] *First Report of Metropolitan Sanitary Commission*, PP, 1847-8, XXXII. 16 [20] (signed November 1847); *Second Report of Metropolitan Sanitary Commission*, PP, 1847-8, XXXII (signed February 1848). On influenza, see T. Thompson (ed.), *Annals of Influenza* (1852); F.A. Dixey, *Epidemic Influenza* (1892); Creighton, *Epidemics*, ii, Ch. 3. For later references see L. Ovenall's bibliography in Creighton, *Epidemics*, i. 155-7.

[3] *2nd Rep. Metrop. Sanitary Commission*, p.1.

The Second Report of the Commissioners analysed and stressed the causes of death already rampant in London (influenza, diarrhoea, and typhus), and discussed means for preventing cholera, including disinfection. Apart from the chemical and engineering experts, the witnesses examined were most frequently surgeons practising in poor areas who had experienced the cholera of 1832. They were asked, primarily, what the state of their districts had then been, and whether conditions had improved since: questions which could hardly fail of answers supporting the cause.

The argument now published was similar to that put by Smith in 1825 in relation to plague and by the *Examiner* in 1831-2 in relation to cholera itself. Typhus fever, the Commissioners stated, was 'the type of the entire class of epidemic diseases that infest this country' and 'epidemic cholera is to be regarded in its essential circumstances, as an exemplar of epidemic disease in general'. No clear attempt was made at this time to prove that cholera was a form of typhus, although it was later asserted also to be an 'intense form of fever'. There was, furthermore, no attempt to define the differences between the two diseases, the concern being not with essences, but with proving dependence upon the same conditions regardless of their exact aetiological status. Frequent references were made to cholera in India since (as in 1825) it was assumed that the true relations of the disease were most clearly to be seen in the country of origin. Recognized features of cholera, such as its preference for water-courses, were explained in sanitary terms. In Britain, apart from the obvious fact that the poor were disposed to suffer disproportionately from any epidemic, it could be shown that the cholera of 1832 had prevailed in just those areas which had since suffered most severely from fever. Hence, it was concluded, 'cholera observes in its progress the laws of ordinary epidemics, being influenced by the same physical conditions, and attacking similar classes of persons'. Naturally, what had been proved of typhus applied to cholera as well: that the most powerful predisposing condition was not destitution or starvation, but the 'habitual respiration [*sic*] of impure air'. There was, of course, nothing in these remarks which had not been assumed impulsively (and in more pathological detail) by the *Examiner* during the first epidemic:

All epidemic diseases are fever ... The cholera is an epidemic fever, differing not more from other epidemic fevers than these differ from each other ... the fever consecutive of cholera is indistinguishable from the prevailing fever of the season ... Cholera takes up its abode in the haunts of fever; it has assumed the place of fever, because it has nearly banished it from the metropolis and has itself become the epidemic of the season ... the one is merely a modification of the other.

The *Examiner* did not fail to stress the practical importance of this conclusion, which brought the 'monster', unknown malady 'under the class of epidemic diseases, having analogous causes and requiring analogous remedies, both preventive and curative.'[1] The later official reports do not cite the Benthamite newspaper, either as an early authority, or to give priority to their position; this does not seem surprising. Chadwick's connection with the *Examiner* was abandoned in 1833 as being prejudicial to his public advancement.[2]

The problem of the communication of cholera from person to person was dealt with at length by the Commissioners, with the implication that this was a question that could be decided categorically more or less independently of other questions. Twin propositions were advanced: first, that no restrictions on the movement of men or goods had succeeded in confining the disease; second, that it frequently failed to spread when given every opportunity to do so. This second assertion, if not known to be an unreasonable requirement, is to suppose that the nature of a disease may be directly inferred from the sum of the circumstances of its operations in the field, a presumption under which other authorities were certainly labouring, and to which nineteenth-century methodology peculiarly conduced. The Commissioners were further assuming, in the case of contagion, that a cause is no cause unless it is seen to be followed by its effects under all observed conditions. This approach is, of course, consistent with Smith's earlier arguments. The mixed selection of facts

---

[1] *1st Rep. Metrop. Sanitary Commission*, pp.10, 14; *2nd Rep. Metrop. Sanitary Commission*, p.1; *Report on Quarantine*, p.43; *Examiner*, 19 Aug. 1832, p.531. The 'epidemic' classification referred to was of course that defined by Southwood Smith.

[2] Finer, *Life of Chadwick*, p.96.

offered by the Commissioners did include some direct evidence, in the shape of the negative results of several daring but unsystematic attempts at inducing the disease artificially.

By the time of their Second Report, the Commissioners were able to state that their views as to practice were confirmed by 'nearly all the most recent experience of the disease'.[1] They could not pretend, however, that all the facts recorded gave them positive support. A Swedish report on which they otherwise depended wondered aloud whether the spread of cholera from village to village might not be best explained by an infected person's travelling from one to the other. Recent incidents, and some case-histories recorded by the English local boards of 1832, also seemed inescapably to suggest something of the sort.[2] The comment of the Commissioners exemplifies the fate of even a 'proven' anomaly (or 'crucial experiment') in an established theoretical framework or context:

... after a careful examination of the cases cited ... we have to observe that these cases would indeed accord with the opinion, that one mode by which this disease is propagated is by communication from person to person, if that opinion were established by other and satisfactory evidence, but they are quite insufficient of themselves to prove its truth.[3]

These few cases all admitted of 'a different and more probable' interpretation, that is, as instances of the effects of contaminated air in confined spaces. It was cases such as these that had led to the old belief in contagion, and deceived such valuable observers as Sir John Pringle. Furthermore, no such mode of importation was suspected or known in India, where the disease was most 'intense and direct'.

In superseding cure with prevention, the Commissioners had in the case of cholera an advantage which amounted to a justification: all attempts at cure, whether empirically or deductively based, were widely regarded as having failed. As they themselves put it, 'it is one of the peculiar characteristics of this disease, that it sets at defiance, to a great degree, the resources of medical art and science'. But sanitary procedures

---

[1] See e.g. their account of the altered state of opinion in Russia: *2nd Rep. Metrop. Sanitary Commission*, pp.4 ff.

[2] For the English experience see C.F. Brockington, 'Public Health at the Privy Council, 1831–34', *J. Hist. Med.* 16 (1961), 161–87: 184.

[3] *2nd Rep. Metrop. Sanitary Commission*, p.8.

achieved their aim slowly and, many suspected, indirectly; the threat of cholera was immediate and personal. Here the Commissioners showed a surprising virtuosity. Their investigation of the last epidemic, they announced, had revealed that the definitive stage of collapse did not set in suddenly, without warning, but was preceded always by a stage of diarrhoea, lasting from a few hours to several days.[1] This was the 'most important practical lesson, especially with reference to individual safety, which our past experience of cholera has taught'. Diarrhoea could be cured and prevented by the simplest measures, measures which might be taken by the patients themselves; it only needed vigilance, and the intractable second stage could be averted altogether. This stress on the first stage was in 'perfect accordance with Indian opinion and practice', and with the recent Russian experience; indeed, the prevalence of diarrhoea in cholera towns had been notorious in 1832, but the real connection had not been clearly and generally made out. The existence of premonitory diarrhoea had been recognized, but not that it was the 'key to control'.[2]

During the epidemic of 1849 the Commissioners, as the General Board of Health, instituted a system of house-to-house visitation on the local level. The visitor inquired as to the incidence of diarrhoea, 'looseness', or uneasy sensations among the household and, if necessary, dispensed costive medicines, or directed those affected to the nearest dispensary. Those who remained healthy were, if possible, removed from the dangerous locality to a house of refuge.[3] After the epidemic the Board made strong claims for the success of this system, which were to some extent admitted, and it featured prominently in the campaign conducted by Chadwick after

[1] *1st Rep. Metrop. Sanitary Commission*, p.48. For current opinion on diarrhoea as a concomitant, precursor, and mild form of cholera, see P. Manson-Bahr (ed.), *Manson's Tropical Diseases* (1966), p.396.

[2] *2nd Rep. Metrop. Sanitary Commission*, pp.10 ff. The confidence of the Commissioners in this matter was ostensibly based on information given Chadwick by a surgeon friend, Joseph Hodgson, who had witnessed the severe outbreak at Bilston in 1832 and the apparently successful system instituted there by Dr. Francis MacCann, sent by the then Central Board of Health. See W. Leigh, *The Melancholy Occurrences at Bilston* (1833); Minutes of Evidence, pp.1, 6, *2nd Rep. Metrop. Sanitary Commission*. But see also *Examiner*, 15 Feb. 1832, p.122; Simon, *Sanitary Institutions*, pp.175–6. For a claim to priority made out against MacCann, see ibid., p.176.

[3] Finer, *Life of Chadwick*, pp.341–3; Lewis, *Chadwick and Public Health*, pp.190–2.

the fall of the Board, for the principles upon which the Board had acted. Chadwick asserted that he had been able to tell, from the returns, if the system had been interrupted; that 'some 50,000 lives' could be said to have been saved in Britain by the Board's precautions; and that the adoption of the English system by the Russian authorities in 1866 was avowed by them to have led to a drastic reduction in their mortality rate from that epidemic.[1]

Although 'preventive', this measure represents the closest approach of the sanitarians to the problem of the individual case. None the less, this encroachment does not seem to have been much resented by medical men, partly because they were themselves involved in it, and partly because their interest lay, as Chadwick had always assumed, in the second or developed stage of the disease, and in the needs or demands of a rather different sector of the population. These factors were illustrated at the local level by the difficulty of finding properly qualified visitors: 'at this time, when there was the greatest pressure for the public service, there was the conflict of the preponderant private interest in the greatest pressure upon the officer for his service to his private patients'.

The general acceptance of the reality of a modifiable 'first stage' in cholera allowed great force to Chadwick's arguments for the influence of locality. A large proportion of the population of Mevagissey, for instance, was saved from the epidemic of 1849 by being moved out of the town into tents. Chadwick stressed that whenever an inhabitant had left the tents and returned to the town, he had immediately become subject to diarrhoea; but that this premonitory symptom had always, and repeatedly, been arrested upon that person's removal from the dangerous vicinity of the town back to the tents.[2]

Although in some respects an isolated excursion, the Board's view of premonitory diarrhoea is a major example of an increasingly and consciously Sydenhamian approach to epi-

---

[1] *Report on Cholera*, PP, 1850, XXI. 88–124; see also Southwood Smith, *Results of Sanitary Improvement*, pp.18–21. Chadwick, *On the Prevention of Epidemics* (1882), pp.10–12.

[2] Chadwick, *On the Prevention of Epidemics*, pp.10, 7; Longmate, *King Cholera*, p.176 and facing p.148.

demiology adopted by Chadwick and Smith in the 1840s. It must not be supposed that the sanitarians were alone in their adoption of this author although, as a name known to laymen, he suited their particular purposes. Sydenham enjoyed a status similar to that of Bacon or Locke in the nineteenth century, but his works themselves were probably less well known than the works of either. The Sydenham Society was founded in 1843, and produced as one of its first publications a complete edition of Sydenham's writings, but it chose to do so in Latin, at a time when that language was no longer a medium of communication between medical men except with respect to prescription.[1] The experience of a medically qualified reviewer of nineteenth-century editions of Sydenham was probably typical. He had, he said, picked up 'at college' the 'current commonplaces', most of which were anecdotal and personal; his teachers had told him that, although born into the 'Dark Ages' of medicine, Sydenham had done a great deal for his profession, had managed cases of smallpox with great skill, and had known the nature of epidemics, dropsies, etc. More seriously, Sydenham had, like Cullen, provided many excellent rules for diagnosis, and was the origin of 'many of our most common and valuable therapeutic doctrines'.[2]

It was possible for nineteenth-century medical writers to call upon Sydenham in a range of different contexts; the reviewer just mentioned, John Brown, was appealing in a reactionary spirit for a respect for 'experientia' as well as 'experimenta' in 'this intensely scientific age'. Benjamin Richardson was later able to find in Sydenham elements of the most prominent modern doctrines: 'His diseases from bad air are our diseases from the same cause; his fermentative diseases are our zymotics; his diseases from the products of fermentation and putrefaction are our auto-toxaemias and blood poisonings'; all he had missed in his system or method was 'the influence of vibrations and the nervous reflexes'. The *Examiner* in 1831 gave an account of a pamphlet, by J. Rymer, on Sydenham's clinical description and experience

---

[1] *Thomae Sydenham, M.D., Opera omnia*, ed. G.A. Greenhill (London, 1844); R.G. Latham produced a translation, with a life, for the Sydenham Society in 1848–50. For previous collected editions, see *DNB*, art. 'Sydenham'.
[2] [J. Brown], 'Locke and Sydenham', *N. Br. Rev.* 12 (1849), 65–6.

of 'cholera'. It was, however, Sydenham's epidemiology that acquired a real authority. The frequency and variety of epidemics occurring on home ground in the 1830s and 1840s were such that medical writers inevitably turned to Sydenham for information on, if not always explanation of, the interaction of epidemics. Characteristically, they felt it was necessary that Sydenham's qualitative language be replaced by quantitative expressions, and various attempts were made in this direction. John Conolly proposed, just after the first cholera epidemic, that local 'Natural History' societies should be established, and should co-operate with local committees of the Society for the Diffusion of Useful Knowledge in collecting data to test or substantiate Sydenham's views on the sequence, mutual relations, and environmental associations of epidemics.[1] These views were, of course, noticeably multifactoral. It should be stressed that Sydenham's influence was not limited to those who put his name to the ideas they were discussing. His views were adopted and transmitted more or less anonymously by many eighteenth-century writers who were more familiar than Sydenham himself to those of the nineteenth.

The *Examiner* talked freely of cholera's 'assuming the place of fever' to become the 'epidemic of the season'. The self-taught John Armstrong was an unusually active admirer of Sydenham, but it is scarcely necessary to propose so specific an influence on Chadwick and Southwood Smith.[2] After the first cholera epidemic, Smith used a Sydenhamian explanation both to account for recent changes in the nature of London fever, and to reinforce his conception of a single epidemic class of fevers. 'Six months' before the first cholera cases, 'London fever', hitherto acute and inflammatory, changed its character to that of a disease of debility, very like the 'consecutive fever' of cholera.[3] That such a change had occurred between about 1820 and 1830 was generally accepted, but

---

[1] Ibid., p.81; B.W. Richardson, *Disciples of Aesculapius* (1900), ii. 666, 671–2; *Examiner*, 31 July 1831, p.490; see also 'Spasmodic Cholera', *Westminster Review*, pp.458–9. J. Conolly, 'County Natural History Societies', *Trans. Prov. Med. Surg. Ass.* 1 (1832–3), 180–218.

[2] See e.g. *Examiner*, 19 Aug. 1832, p.532.

[3] Southwood Smith, *Epidemics Considered* (1856), pp.6–7.

variously interpreted.[1] For Chadwick and Smith, the significance of the change was best put in Sydenhamian terms: warning of the approach of an epidemic was given by the 'sudden outbreak and spread of some milder epidemic' (like diarrhoea, or influenza) or the 'transformation of ordinary diseases into diseases of a new type, more or less resembling the character of the extraordinary disease at hand'. The latter phenomenon could include diseases of animals as well as of men. Thus, it was not the habit of epidemics to arrive so suddenly and 'capriciously' that nothing could be done about them; isolated cases occurring in any locality during the prevalence of a general epidemic constitution were a sign of an impending outbreak 'over that place'. On the other hand, it followed that an epidemic was present and in operation well before it assumed its distinct and proper form, so that it was foolish to take no steps until the disease declared itself characteristically. It could be concluded that quarantine was useless, and that the most effective measure was constant attention to local causes and to the ordinary, modifiable but preventable forms of disease.[2]

Other Sydenhamian pronouncements included an argument from pathology against the contagiousness of cholera, presented in the Sanitary Commission's Second Report. This excursion, which was more typical of the *Examiner* than of the later official reports, involved a humoral and eliminative explanation of contagious disease. It will be seen that Sydenham's views were as likely to form the justification as the inspiration of Smith and Chadwick's approach. This is most evident with respect to their increasingly positive assumption of the existence of some kind of travelling epidemic atmosphere or remote cause, an important element in the General Board's dogmatism which will be dealt with more fully below.

In their capacity of Metropolitan Sanitary Commissioners

[1] See e.g. C.W. Bell, 'On the Advance of Asiatic Cholera', *Lond. Med. Gaz.* 5 (1847), 801; Christison, 'Fevers', pp.121-2; Watson, *Principles and Practice of Physic*, ii. 691-3; Murchison, *Treatise on Continued Fevers*, p.7. John Armstrong changed his view of 'typhus' over the same period.

[2] Smith, *Epidemics Considered*, pp.4-7; *Report on Cholera*, pp.17-18; *Report on Quarantine*, pp.12 ff. See also *2nd Rep. Metrop. Sanitary Commission*, p.16.

therefore Chadwick and Smith made no attempt to distinguish ordinary from premonitory diarrhoea, because they saw, or claimed to see, its relation to cholera as Sydenham might have seen it. Diarrhoea was a basic condition, which occurred whenever the atmosphere was impure; thus it appeared as a concomitant, and perhaps precursor, of typhus. In the absence of cholera, it was a 'distinct species' of disease; but because it resembled cholera, it was readily 'assimilated' by that disease when it prevailed as an epidemic. In controlling diarrhoea, one was preventing possible deaths from cholera, typhus, and diarrhoea itself. Chadwick later suggested that plague and yellow fever as well as cholera might have a premonitory stage of the same kind and significance, which would facilitate a similar control of these diseases.[1]

This more specialized argument was used to give support to the familar and fundamental contention, that the application of simple and accustomed sanitary measures could not fail to be beneficial, even if the cholera stayed away altogether. It was indeed part of the Commissioners' case that an epidemic situation (demanded under the terms of the only relevant legislation, the Nuisances Removal and Contagious Diseases Prevention Act) already prevailed.[2] This was owing in part to influenza, another exotic disease, established by Sydenham as an omen of other epidemics, and placed in particular relation to Asiatic cholera by Thomas Hancock; but in greater part to an excess of common lung diseases brought on by cold, damp, and impurity. This situation constituted, in the opinion of the Commissioners, 'the state of evil contemplated by the Contagious Disease Prevention Act, which authorises the appointment of local Boards of Health, with powers for cleansing and the adoption of other preventive measures'.[3] The case put by the Commissioners with respect to this Act is a particularly interesting example of the continuous attempt to provide for 'ordinary' conditions

---

[1] *2nd Rep. Metrop. Sanitary Commission*, pp.8–9, 16; Chadwick, 'The Plague', *J. Soc. Arts*, 27 (1879), 329–30.

[2] *2nd Rep. Metrop. Sanitary Commission*, p.34. An equivalent claim had been made in 1831: *Examiner*, 5 June 1831, p.356.

[3] Conolly, 'County Natural History Societies', p.193. For Hancock (d. 1849), see *Munk. 2nd Rep. Metrop. Sanitary Commission*, p.34. For the Act (an amended version of one passed in 1846), see PP, 1847–8, IV. 9. [537].

in the context of sporadic provisions meant to apply only to extraordinary circumstances. The Act was not put into operation until October 1848, after the cholera reached England. By that time, both Chadwick and Smith were members of the new General Board of Health, which had been gazetted in September.

So far, the sanitarians had needed to pay only haphazard attention to theory. Though not an empiricist, Chadwick, provided his practical claims were admitted, was prepared to take little or no interest in medical doctrines. Most medical men were, for most of the time, subscribing to the same dichotomy. Virtually all agreed in principle with the crusade for better physical conditions, being as least as liable as other classes to approve of these means of dispelling unrest, and concurred in the sanitary generalization in one form or another. In relation to familiar diseases, it was possible for the sophisticated medical man to keep distinct the statistical language and concepts of prevention, and his personal world of the particular case. Pragmatically, he was able to accept Chadwick's claims with respect to familiar epidemic diseases. The case for cholera, however, was an extrapolation, not supported by massed correlative evidence concerning either the whole range of diseases or a confused entity such as fever, but by arguments which involved a certain amount of speculation about a disease readily recognized to be specific. To accept Chadwick's view of cholera was, most importantly, to believe that cholera was never imported and never contagious. The Commissioners had adopted a categorical position, based on Smith's earlier views but made mandatory by practical and administrative considerations. It was, perhaps, not in their power to admit that cholera was contagious under some circumstances, that is, contingently contagious. These were not the terms in which the public could be instructed. If such terms meant anything, it seemed, they meant that countries, towns, and households were not safe unless there was quarantine and isolation of the sick; and this even the contingent contagionists did not believe. The danger in this position was that it could at any time be recognized as contradicting contingent contagionism as such. The categorical position was also open to the objection that it assumed too much in assuming that, because cholera had been removed from one class (the strictly contagious) it necessarily belonged to another, the purely epidemic — which was not generally, of course, recognized as a class at all. In a similar way, the positive practical claim was being put more forcibly at the expense of the earlier reserve as to the exact relation of cause and effect. Sanitary arrangements, 'instead of being incidental and collateral to other measures, are paramount, and principal, and effective, not only against cholera, but also against other epidemics'.[1]

Some criticism has already been noted of the categorical position as asserted by Smith in a private capacity, before the first cholera epidemic. It is only towards the end of the active phase of the 1840s that his view began fully to emerge as 'official doctrine'. In the meantime, the fervour of the sanitary movement, and the increasing occurrence of its tenets as articles of popular faith, were beginning to breed the inevitable reaction against such oversimplification. There was, for instance, some criticism of 'sanitary quackery'. A quackery was any simple and universal (and usually commercially profitable) remedy which could be employed independently of the profession. In this case, the remedy was disinfection, and the quackery especially deplorable because members of the profession and other respectable persons were involved in it, primarily (it appeared) on the commercial level. The *London Medical Gazette* blamed 'some Parliamentary Reports' for encouraging the 'disinfecting mania' and inveighed against 'absurd experiments' in which Sir William Burnett's fluid was proved better than M. Ledoyen's by its superior deoderant effect on bowls of faeces.[2] It must be conceded that these commercial trials could not compare with eighteenth-century attempts at investigating the processes of putrefaction and disinfection.

---

[1] *1st Rep. Metrop. Sanitary Commission*, p.48.

[2] *Lond. Med. Gaz.* 5 (1847), 939. The Parliamentary reports referred to came out six months before those of the Metropolitan Sanitary Commission and involved Southwood Smith, Richard Grainger, and Henry Leeson: *Reports on Disinfection*, PP, 1847, LVII. 1. 'Official' experiments were carried out by Faraday and others in 1831, but Faraday at least was already investigating disinfection: Brockington, 'Public Health at the Privy Council, 1831–4', p.168; A.E. Jeffreys, *Michael Faraday. A List of His Lectures and Published Writings* (1966).

The modern, as well as the contemporary, reader is liable to read into such proceedings a commitment to the well-known generalization 'all smell is disease', or worse still, 'all disease is smell'.[1] For some modern historians and contemporary critics, sanitary theory, or 'the miasmatic theory', consisted of, or achieved no better than, these risible equations. But before concluding that sanitary theory was to this extent empiricism posing as or flying in the face of science, one should recall, in this connection in particular, the extent to which sanitarianism as a movement was directed at the laity and then at the people. One did not have definitively to believe in these equations in order to think that it was an excellent thing for the poor to believe them, for laymen and medical men alike to act as if they believed them, and for the clergy to state that man's sense of smell had been supplied by providence for the detection of unwholesome influences. 'All smell is disease' is a slogan, making good use of natural feelings and providing a reasonable rule of thumb for the citizen wishing to improve his own household or district. The busy practitioner or poor-law surgeon, less concerned with processes than with the sequence of events, thought his patients' accounts of sickness following exposure to some evil odour (an event unlikely to be missing from any patient's recent experience) a sound enough representation of sanitary science. Hence this question and answer in the evidence of the First Report of the Metropolitan Sanitary Commission:

Q. [anon.]: May it not be stated with confidence, as a *general* conclusion derived from your experience, that all offensive smells (the consequence of decomposing animal and vegetable matter)[2] are *eventually* disease?

A. (Mr. Bowie, surgeon): I have not the slightest doubt that in *certain constitutions* of the atmosphere there is nothing so likely to produce disease.[3]

Odours, good and bad, had long stood for otherwise intangible atmospheric influences, and in nineteenth-century science provided an analogue for the dissemination of gases

---

[1] Finer, *Life of Chadwick*, p.298.

[2] Possibly an insertion into the text.

[3] Minutes of Evidence, p.9, *1st Rep. Metrop. Sanitary Commission*. My italics. Robert Bowie was a favourite witness, and employee of the Board. He is referred to in the *Examiner*, 20 Nov. 1831, p.744.

or volatile substances.[1] For some years, odour was regarded as a sufficient indication of the presence of substances too subtle for the balance. It should be remembered that, even in the case of smallpox, where the *materies morbi* could be localized to the blade of a lancet, nineteenth-century epidemiologists were, nevertheless, having to deal with a material but 'invisible' substance, known only by its effects. The nature of odours, which are now more narrowly defined, is still largely unknown; no precise classification is possible, or any fixed relationship between odour and chemical structure. Many diseases are still admitted as being characterized by a peculiar odour, including the later stages of tuberculosis, as well as typhoid, measles, scarlet fever, and smallpox.[2]

That the correlation between smell and disease became an article of popular faith was a triumph of sanitary propaganda. On the other hand it is, of course, true that propaganda can rarely be kept distinct from theory. However, in the present case the reports of the Sanitary Commissioners qualified the question and answer quoted above. On the subject of disinfection, they took evidence from Lyon Playfair and his assistant Robert Angus Smith, Richard Grainger (of the Webb Street medical school and later of St. Thomas's Hospital) and Henry Leeson (also of St. Thomas's). This evidence, they concluded, was of scientific interest but to some extent conflicting. Nothing could be said conclusively.[3] Of course they had reason to distrust disinfection, as a palliative rather than preventive measure; but in addition they made it clear that smell was an inadequate index to the presence of noxious influences, and the elimination of odour by chemical means, no indication of the destruction of these influences. Chadwick was able to remark caustically that 'the capacity and condition of a local administration may confidently be tested by the nose', but he was at the same time aware that some of the most deadly gases emitted during putrefaction had a very faint odour or none at all. It is possible that Chadwick was

---

[1] See e.g. Farr quoting Thomas Graham, *Appendix 1843*, p.206.

[2] See C.P. MacCord and W.N. Witheridge, *Odours, Physiology and Control* (New York, 1949).

[3] *2nd Rep. Metrop. Sanitary Commission*, p.19. For Leeson (1803–72), F.R.C.P. 1847, F.R.S. 1849, see *Munk*.

more cautious in respect to disinfection than others, including Southwood Smith. Over all, however, the sanitarians did not encourage a dependence upon deodorants and disinfectants. This was a source of complaint to some, for example Henry Condy, who introduced 'Condy's fluid' in 1857.[1]

More specific early warning signs of resistance to the categorical position appeared in the *London Medical Gazette*, which piqued itself on having held a contingent contagionist position since 1831: 'Our own belief . . . is that it [cholera] is not a pure epidemic, nor a universally infectious malady; but that it can be decidedly propagated by human intercourse.' There might be a great many cases of outbreaks in which there was no evidence of communication by infection; but

. . . Our answer is, that the same observation has been repeatedly made regarding typhus fever [regarded by the *Gazette* as contagious] and that facts do not neutralise each other like acids and alkalies — hence one good affirmative instance, as in the simple transference of the cholera from this country to Canada in 1831–32, cannot be overturned by a hundred negative cases.[2]

Elsewhere there was apparent harmony. The *Monthly Journal of Medical Science* agreed with the Sanitary Commissioners as to the 'inherent fallacy' of the arguments for the contagiousness of cholera which always arose wherever the disease first appeared. These were 'popular delusions', contradicted by all those who witnessed the disease on a large scale, and by the Indian practitioners in particular. 'Of late years', commented the *Journal*, 'the different facts and arguments opposed to the contagious nature of cholera, have undoubtedly gained much in force and extension; and governments, in consequence, have begun to see the impolicy and inutility of quarantine regulations as preventive measures'. The *British and Foreign Medico-Chirurgical Review*, however, gave an account of the real position:

The conclusion arrived at [in 1831–2] by almost the whole medical press, was that the doctrine of contagion, in the strict sense of the word,

---

[1] Chadwick, 'Progress of Sanitation', p.637. See especially Chadwick's evidence in *Report of Committee on Sewage Manure*, pp. 106, 109 [648, 651], where he argues for dilution rather than 'chemical manipulations'. H.B. Condy, *Disinfection and the Prevention of Disease* (1862), p.1.

[2] *Lond. Med. Gaz.* 5 (1847), 983.

— that doctrine which supposes that there *must be* contact or proximity between man and man, in order that the morbid poison may pass from one to another, — cannot explain the phenomena of the diffusion of cholera . . . At the same time, it seemed to be generally admitted, that it would require further research . . . before we could venture decidedly to affirm that the poison of cholera *could not* multiply itself during its passage through the body; that it could not, like smallpox, find in the human organisation the materials for its growth and reproduction, but that its subtle principle was exhausted in the effect it produced, and annihilated in the system which bore evidence to its potent agency.[1]

This last point, the *Review* stressed, was undecided, but of 'little practical value' and certainly irrelevant to the activities of legislation and prevention. The *Review* then praised the reports of the Commission for their practical qualities, and the Commissioners for keeping to their own province.

It is clear that, so long as the profession felt that the sanitarians had done this, it was not alarmed by scattered statements on the causation of disease. Apart from their basis in Smith's writings, these may be seen in sum as a combination of the familiar facts of the attachment of certain diseases to particular localities, and of formulations, after the manner of Sydenham, about epidemic conditions and the reaction of one epidemic with another. Some epidemic influence was by implication responsible for the special characteristics of the epidemic. Cholera was defined as an 'ordinary epidemic' not by exploring this concept but by equating the path of this disease with that of typhus. Impure air and humidity were the most powerful predisposing causes. Cholera 'appeared to be caused' by a poison diffused in the atmosphere, but nothing further was said about the nature of this agent. It was not related to Smith's experimental claims of 1838 or to any work currently being done on the products of putrefaction (or indeed to any earlier research on this subject).

'Miasmatic theory' is a description which, like (for example) 'atomic theory', is only inappropriately applied without specification to signify a single theory, and is best used of a type of theory, or for a particular component of theories. It has often been written about as if it were the peculiar property of nineteenth-century epidemiology, but in that case it is most substantial in the eye of the beholder, and the observer

---

[1] *Mon. J. Med. Sci.* 8 (1847-8), 676; *Br. For. Med. Chir. Rev.* 2 (1848), 65-6.

is usually critical if not hostile. However, the formulations of 1848 did, through dogmatism, take on the appearance of a body of theory. An account has been given above of the resources which the sanitarians were likely to call upon during this process. These were, very largely, not current sources. This mattered less than that such a theory should never have been produced at all. Its appearance was owing not so much to misplaced ambition on the part of the sanitarians, as to external pressures, real and imagined. A parallel case is that of Edward Jenner and vaccination. Jenner's discovery was originally presented as a fact, verified by experiment and independent of any other kind of justification. (The phenomena of vaccination were, of course, more precise than those involved in sanitary reform.) When, however, difficulties and exceptions arose, Jenner resorted not to further practical data, but to theoretical and philosophical preconceptions, previously excluded, in order to justify his conclusions.[1] These additions, being idiosyncratic, weakened rather than strengthened the appeal of his discovery. It is characteristic of such situations, which naturally occur in the biological, and especially the medical, rather than the physical sciences, that demands are made for a total explanation; that is, the 'facts' which are brought forward to be explained, by well-wishers as well as opponents, are apparently placed in no order of importance. A minor inconsistency presents the same difficulties as a major anomaly. Hence, where the demand for solutions is very strong, there is a tendency towards comprehensiveness and multifactoral theories.

At the end of 1848, in the midst of a great many other activities, the new Board of Health drew up a Report on Quarantine. The quarantine authorities at the Privy Council were making moves to pre-empt the authority of the Board, and the Report was designed to be as final as possible. It stated, in sum, that the epidemic extension of *any* disease was not due to contagion; and that, even if it were, the quarantine system could in no way prevent it. With respect to 'official doctrine', this Report (which is not usually given much attention) was probably the most important of all; not

---

[1] E. Jenner, *An Inquiry into the Causes and Effects of the Variolae Vaccinae* (1798). Dixon, *Smallpox*, pp.265, 270, 273, and especially p.260.

by reason of its merits (which were few), but because it had the effect of arousing the latent opposition of the medical profession.[1] It was this report that led to all subsequent impressions of the Board's being 'wedded to a theory', which have accumulated to the present day.[2] This development was not necessitated by any real change in the views held by the Board, although, as we have seen, much had often been left unstated. The result may be described as ironic, since the profession in no way disagreed with the Board's recommendations, and therefore required no theoretical justification of them. It could be argued that the Report was not directed primarily at the profession, in which case one can only conclude that it was, at this time, the more ill judged. The most offensive passages are taken directly from Southwood Smith's less public and certainly unofficial writings of twenty years before. These passages may have been reproduced in an attempt both to flatter lay opinion and obviate the need for any professional pronouncement on the subject in question. In this case, it would appear that medical opinion was at this time much less anticontagionist than has been supposed and known by the Board to be so, and perhaps also that medical men declared themselves on the subject of contagion (however they themselves might talk about the 'climate of opinion') not absolutely, but in context, that is, with respect to a particular disease.[3]

The reproduced passages include not only the reflections on the profession itself, but also the statements as to the resemblances between epidemic diseases. The Report put it as a question whether typhus, plague, scarlatina, influenza, yellow fever, and cholera depended on peculiar and specific causes or on one common agent modified by circumstances; and then stated that, regardless of the answer to this, these diseases were all fevers, all dependent upon certain atmospheric conditions, all obedient to similar laws of diffusion, all infesting the same sorts of localities, all attacking the same

---

[1] Cf. Lewis, *Chadwick and Public Health*, p.346, and Chadwick, e.g. 'The Plague'.

[2] The phrase is *The Lancet*'s: 1849, ii. 97.

[3] See *Mon. J. Med. Sci.* 9, Pt.3 (1849), 911, 917.

classes and age groups, and all increased in severity by the same sanitary and social conditions.[1]

Typhus, of course, was not in their view contagious. Of exotic diseases, plauge was taken as the type, and the arguments now familiar advanced against its contagiousness. As in the reports of 1847, circumstances held by many to fulfil the criteria for proof of a disease's being contagious (in particular. an outbreak among healthy persons following the arrival of a sufferer from the disease) merely proved the infectiousness, not the contagiousness of that disease.[2] Here the Report was using the former term as Smith once wished to use either 'infectious' or 'contaminative', that is to signify a property of extension through the atmosphere, which came and went and varied in intensity according to prevailing conditions.[3] Once again the chemical composition of these local miasms was not considered, except in an elementary way.[4] To the modern reader, the Board's account seems perverse, since, following Southwood Smith, it admitted the danger of emanations from the body and the evacuations, but only when these were concentrated by lack of ventilation; or, the body itself might 'take in and concentrate' the poison, and then release it. The Report cited authors (Haygarth, Currie, Arnott, Christison) who thought that, while the products of animal and vegetable decomposition were capable of permanent suspension in air, exhalations from the body were not, and were neutralized and destroyed by a sufficiency of good air, although liable to become virulent and even permanent if pent up. This was 'providential', for men would otherwise have been unable to live together.[5] Moreover, though exhalations from the sick body were clearly worse, Robert Angus Smith's experiments with expired air had proved that the

[1] *Report on Quarantine*, p.5.

[2] For one version of these criteria see 'the dictum of Dr. Elliotson' cited by W. Davies, 'Fever in its Relations to Sanitary Reform', *Trans. Prov. Med. Surg. Ass.* 4 (1849), 76.

[3] Elsewhere, in the Board's Second Notification of Cholera, the no more fortunate term 'catching' is used: PP, 1849, XXIV. 109. This term was later suggested by Budd as a proper replacement for both 'infectious' and 'contagious'.

[4] e.g. by Arnott in connection with the ventilation of ships: Appendix, *Report on Quarantine*, p.144.

[5] *Report on Quarantine*, p.51. See also *Second Report on Quarantine: Yellow Fever*, PP, 1852, XX. 69–70.

wastes exhaled by healthy persons were dangerous enough, if concentrated.[1] These, if inhaled, accumulated in the blood and led to (putrid) fever. The Report adopted the view of the Board's 'inspector', John Sutherland, that the degree of infectiousness developed in a given situation depended on the intensity of the epidemic influence, but that this influence was inoperative in the absence of 'localising conditions'. It may be noted here that Sutherland's views, like those of Arnott, cannot be described as anticontagionist. Sutherland was quoted by the Board as declaring 'I look on the poison which propagates cholera in an epidemic atmosphere as being truly zymotic, but not contagious. Why may it not be the same with other pestilences?'[2] As already indicated, 'not contagious' does not mean 'epidemic' in Southwood Smith's exclusive sense. The significance of 'zymotic' will be explained in Chapter 4 below. Again, as in the case of Arnott, Sutherland's practice in no way differed from that of the Board.

Southwood Smith's old views on fever had appeared before, though not so plainly. More novel, in deployment if not in conception, was the notion of epidemic influence presented in the Report. As we have seen, the existence of such a remote cause had been implicit in Southwood Smith's contributions to official doctrine since the first cholera epidemic, but little stress had been placed upon it, and Smith had earlier registered a philosophical objection to the concept. Now it was inflated to supersede the function of contagion even in contagious diseases. As in the Metropolitan Sanitary Commission Reports, contagiousness was treated not as a property of particular diseases but as a concept, once prevalent but now discredited. In the absence of an epidemic atmosphere, stated the Report, no contagion, imported or native, could cause a disease to spread epidemically: 'Allowing, therefore, to contagion all the influence which anyone supposes it to possess, and to quarantine all the control over it which it claims, there remains the condition, the primary and essential condition, which confessedly it cannot reach, namely the epidemic

---

[1] See e.g. R.A. Smith, 'Remarks on the Air and Water of Towns', *Phil. Mag.* 30 (1847), 478.

[2] *Report on Quarantine*, p.55.

atmosphere'.[1] The Report's usages are not clear, and they are the less so because of the subservience of every statement to the single aim of abolishing quarantine. In 1825 Smith had, while admitting the liability of diseases like smallpox to sudden extension, thought it inadvisable to call such an extension an epidemic when this term had already (for him) a specialized use. This latter notion of 'epidemic' is also present in the Quarantine Report. No clear definitions are given. In 1849 Chadwick, for one, was determined that quarantine should not be employed even if it were decided that a disease was invariably or contingently contagious, and contagion is, therefore, subordinated to 'epidemic atmosphere'.

Since it might be assumed that, whatever its nature, such an atmosphere would be beyond the reach of quarantine, little substance was given to this concept beyond reference to the facts it was intended to explain. It replaced importation; covered, as contagion alone could not, the rapidity of advance shown by some epidemics and the occurrence of simultaneous rather than consecutive outbreaks; and provided a blank space in which might be written the reason for the periodicity in the rise and fall of epidemics. This periodicity appeared in some way to reflect that of the seasons; similarly, the epidemic influence was thought to be in some way represented by the 'physical disturbances in the condition of the atmosphere', which traditionally ushered in epidemic disease. As well as conventional meteorology there were the more subtle forces of electricity and magnetism, about which little was known. It was not made clear whether the epidemic atmosphere would consist of some material entity, or of a set of laws defining an unusual concurrence of familiar events. The Report suggested at one point that physical and meteorological agents might determine the direction and distribution of cloud-like miasms; or else generate a 'peculiar force' which would do this, at least in the cases of cholera and influenza.[2]

To justify their inflation of this concept, the Board had the undeniable fact that (because of the prevalence of the doubtful diseases) 'over the last fifty years more stress has been placed

---

[1] Ibid., p.6.
[2] Ibid., pp.6–10, 53.

on terrestro-aerial agents as causes of fever'; but they depended most heavily again on traditional authorities, who, as already pointed out, were rather more useful to them than their true contemporaries. The chief of these was, of course, 'the celebrated Sydenham'. The difference between this and earlier reports is one of stress amounting to a positive view where there was none made out before. It will be remembered that Smith first wrote about epidemic diseases at a time when no exotic had actually reached England for over 150 years, a factor which, in the formation of his views, outweighed any reference to yellow fever and plague as other than localized diseases. The sanitarians' public position was built upon indigenous fevers; it had to be adjusted to include indigenous diseases which 'travelled'. By 1849, Britain had been included in the pandemic cycles of at least two diseases which were, unlike the indigenous fever, highly characterized in their effects. This apparent specificity was attributed by the members of the General Board, as it might have been by Sydenham, to the influence of a particular epidemic atmosphere on diseases already prevailing (especially the 'common fever'), and on a heavily predisposed population.

Both 'localising conditions' and epidemic influence were treated as necessary to the production of a particular disease form, but this was not done with precision, and the different writers quoted by the Report seem to differ as to which cause might have been said to cause cholera rather than any other disease. Certainly it was assumed that some kind of fairly rampant disease could be caused merely with the aggravation of common fever by a 'deleteriously impregnated air'. The concept of epidemic atmosphere is made even less precise in that the term was also used for an atmosphere infected or corrupted by local conditions, particularly in the case of diseases allowed, or at one time allowed, to be contagious, and which became 'epidemic' when already specific.

Before dealing with the hostile reaction to this Report, it is of interest to note what appeals were made in it to current opinion. Such appeals were made chiefly with reference to the question of contagion, but authors were also cited simply for their support of the practical measures advocated by the Board. Sometimes, and especially in the case of Scottish authorities, this was done regardless of differences in the opinions behind such measures. On contagion, the Report referred correctly enough to a modification over the previous half-century (one might have said even longer) of the 'strict notion' of contagion, that is, the communicability of disease exclusively by contact, direct or indirect; but it went on unfairly to imply that, as a result of this change, a climate of anticontagionism was a *fait accompli*.[1] The Royal College of Physicians, for example, was treated as having changed its mind entirely from one categorical position to the other between the first and second cholera epidemics. This account misrepresents the difference between the cautious recommendations based on hearsay alone, and the predictable modification of view which took place in most quarters under the influence of an actual experience of the disease.[2] The reader's first impression of radical change is further modified by the curious admixture in the Report of statements taken from Smith's earlier works. These were numerous enough to amount to a rehearsal of the polemical anticontagionism of 1825. They made it appear that enlightenment had in reality extended only to countries other than England, principally France; to those who had actually observed the relevant diseases (medical officers in charge of fleets and armies, practitioners in large city hospitals or with experience of the cholera in India); or to those fortunate enough not to have received a standard medical education. As in 1825, it was claimed that the question was not technical, but simply one of evidence, so that any 'unprejudiced' observer was convinced of anticontagionism in proportion to his opportunities for direct observation. Moreover, the Board seemed to be aware that 'mere medical opinion' varied, or 'clashed', on some important points of science.[3] The latter remarks did not reflect real knowledge on the part of the Board as much as an interest in revealing a lack of authority within the profession. It can be concluded that the Board knew or cared little about

[1] See e.g. ibid., pp.18 ff.; Letter from General Board of Health to Lords of Privy Council, Appendix, ibid., p.131.
[2] The Board gave a different account of the College in the *Second Report on Quarantine*, pp.2–3. See below.
[3] *Report on Quarantine*, p.21.

current opinion, that it had taken few steps towards gauging it, and that it was concerned only that something diametrically opposite to the 'old contagionism' (which belonged, even on the Board's account, to the period before 1800) should be the basis for practical decisions. The haste with which the Report was prepared was also very evident.

As well as relying on 'authentic sources' (allegedly not 'our own medical staff', mere treatises, or the merely eminent), the Board undertook a kind of research on its own account.[1] It was always thought that a disease's mode of spread could most easily be determined from a study of the first cases to occur in a given locality, when the relevant circumstances were fewest.[2] Such situations are for towns the nearest approach to the epidemiology of villages, which again present the closest approximation possible in the field to the deliberately restricted conditions of laboratories. Accordingly, the Board asked Edmund Parkes, who had had three years' experience of cholera and dysentery in India, to investigate the circumstances of the first cases recorded in London in 1848.[3] Parkes was of the family which 'played a large part in the social history of the century'; he was first cousin once removed of Joseph Parkes the Birmingham politician, his grandfather was nephew and partner to Josiah Wedgwood, and his family had been prominent in the group of Unitarians in Warwick closely associated with Priestley in Birmingham.[4] Edmund Parkes was connected with University College London from 1834. The direct contact of both Chadwick and Southwood Smith with this institution had taken place rather earlier and been comparatively brief, but regardless of any linkage of this sort, Parkes's background determines him as a representative

---

[1] Chadwick, 'The Plague'.

[2] The absence of this type of investigation had been deplored by the *Examiner* in 1831: 18 Dec. 1831, p.809. An inquiry into the first cases in Manchester was carried out by Kay: *Autobiography*, pp.9 ff.

[3] Edmund Alexander Parkes (1819–76), M.R.C.S. 1840, M.B. 1841. Educated University College and Hospital, London. 1842–5, asst. surgeon to 84th Regiment in India. 1846, M.D. London. Later the associate of Nightingale and Herbert. Parkes is described, perhaps parochially, as 'the founder of the science of modern hygiene': *DNB*; and as the author of the system of medical instruction in the military services: H. Hale Bellot, *University College London, 1826–1926* (1929), p.274.

[4] Ibid., pp.273–4.

of the reforming class, his particular bias being towards public health questions. He may have been influenced in the direction of medicine by his uncle, Anthony Todd Thomson, for whom he lectured on medical jurisprudence in 1841.

In addition to his Indian experience, Parkes had to reccommend him the reputation earned by an extremely sound work on cholera published in 1847. This gave a well-reasoned discussion of the pathology and symptomology of cholera based on limited aims and a large number of post-mortems, and since it avoided speculation without also abandoning pathological hypothesis, it was greeted by reviewers with relief and approbation. The work included details of two Indian epidemics observed by Parkes in 1843 and 1845, and in it Parkes stated that he had 'never observed any indication of contagion. In common with the great majority of Indian writers my evidence is on the negative side.'[1] Parkes produced for the Board a detailed study of twenty-eight early cases which occurred in ten different districts in London between 28 September and 9 October 1848.[2] 'In not a single instance,' the Board announced, 'as far as could be traced, had the first person attacked in one locality been in contact or proximity with a person previously sick in another locality, and in some instances such contact or proximity was impossible.'[3] These latter cases occurred in convict hulks moored in the Thames at Greenwich and Woolwich. Far from advancing in succession, cases in general occurred nearly simultaneously, and were widely scattered. Parkes's investigation also showed that the first cases appeared in 'fever nests', for which such an event had been predicted.[4] Elsewhere, the Board quoted from Parkes's accounts of cholera in the field in India.

Parkes's origins and experience, his lack of prepossession,

---

[1] See e.g. *Prov. Med. Surg. J.* 12 (1848), 208. Parkes, *Algide Cholera* (1847), pp.190 ff.

[2] There was inevitably some controversy over whether Parkes had included all the first cases: *Lond. Med. Gaz.* 10 (1850), 127, 305. Snow criticized 'the documents furnished to Dr. Parkes by the General Board of Health': *On the Mode of Communication of Cholera* (1849), p.27 n.

[3] *Report on Quarantine*, p.26.

[4] See the Board's Second Notification of Cholera, PP, 1849, XXIV. 99, 101.

and many of his views on epidemic disease, might have been
expected to guarantee his compatibility with the Board. In
his professional capacity, he appeared to possess the same
neutral virtues as Frederick Brittan, who was also employed
by the Board at this time.[1] Yet, as in the case even of Arnott,
Parkes's over-all conception and his account of current opinion
differed significantly from those of the Board, and since he
developed his views with clarity and in detail, these constitute
an excellent illustration of the distinctions between the
official and the professional positions. No single writer of
this period may be taken as entirely representative of the
views of the profession, even if one considers only its more
thoughtful and articulate members, but Parkes's qualifications
for this role are probably the best possible; as good, that is,
but no better than, those attributes implying a proximity to
the approach of the Board. His position will, therefore, be
given in some detail.

Although preserving the appearance of approval, the Board
did not publish Parkes's report, and its general conclusion on
his results was temperate.[2] The report appeared instead in
the *British and Foreign Medico-Chirurgical Review*, of which
Parkes later (in 1852) became editor. As already indicated,
much of the report might be supposed to have been highly
acceptable to Chadwick and Smith. In addition, Parkes had
suggested that a 'peculiar force' might be responsible for the
capricious path pursued by cholera. He had also concluded
that cholera was best explained by allowing, firstly, that 'the
degree of the several local conditions (the state of the receiving bodies remaining constant) will determine the prevalence
of a disease in one locality rather than in another', and that
this was a sufficient basis for prediction; and secondly, that
'in countries where cholera is not indigenous, in addition to
these local conditions, a general atmospheric state (the nature
of which is as yet unrecognised) may be assumed'. Nevertheless,

---

[1] Parkes and three other physicians were employed on a day-to-day basis
during the cholera period, at a rate of 2 guineas a day. No detail is given of the
services performed by these physicians (and by a similar group of surgeons) but
at least two of them, F. Brittan and G. Milroy, engaged in inspection rather than
'research': PP, 1851, XLIII. 371.

[2] *Report on Quarantine*, p.26.

Parkes was neither an anticontagionist nor a non-contagionist, and (like Wakley in 1825, Arnott in 1838, and Simon in 1865) he denied the existence of a body of opinion which could rightly be given either of these denominations; except in the case of one particular disease, influenza. He maintained that current opinion could be comprised under two heads, strict contagionist and modified contagionist, and that these had in common the view that epidemic diseases were caused by 'specific and uninterchangeable poisons'. The modified contagionist view, which he himself thought the more valid, and which was capable of including the strict view, had arisen as a result of the better knowledge of the new or doubtful diseases like cholera and yellow fever. It allowed a lesser role to the body, and a greater to the environment; an origin, propagation, and multiplication of the morbid poison outside the body; and a variation in the degree to which such poisons multiplied in the body according to contingent circumstances.[1] Unlike the other, this view held that epidemic constitutions and local conditions could directly affect the capabilities of the disease virus (or poison) by acting on the virus itself. It could as well be called contingent as modified contagionism; and provides a counterpart, in generally chemical terms, of the conclusions reached in biological terms in the same circumstances by Jacob Henle.

In tracing the historical development of this view, and in discussing the influence of environmental conditions, Parkes covered much the same ground as Smith and Chadwick. The greater lucidity of his arguments stemmed from their having as centre an assumption of the existence of *special* agents which were material, and whose properties could therefore be discussed. Other factors could then become factors affecting distribution or development, and their nature could be decided upon by a reasoned discussion of probabilities, such as Parkes gave in accounting for his twenty-eight cholera cases. His assumption of specificity in epidemic disease, which was fundamental to his approach, and perhaps the most important shared item of belief among his contempories, was based ultimately on his awareness of clinical and

---

[1] Parkes, 'Inquiry', *Br. For. Med. Chir. Rev.* 4 (1849), 271, 253.

pathological differences. Recognition of uniformity in appearances led directly to the requirement of a single special cause (however this might be combined in operation with other causes), which was better satisfied by a special morbid poison than by any combination or variation of conditions or substances.[1]

Not surprisingly, there were from the outset explicit differences between Parkes and the Board. Parkes, for instance, stated of a particular case not only that the effluvia from a drain were incompetent to cause cholera, but also that (given the circumstances) the effluvia could not have had any accessory effect.[2]

It is not contended that the profession had at this time any consistent or single view of epidemic disease to be contradicted by the Board's Quarantine Report. The point is rather that they recognized, as if for the first time, that the Board had 'ventured into the depths of theoretical medicine' and constructed a view with which they could not agree, in spite of the disagreements in their own ranks. Some account has already been given of the largely benevolent reaction to earlier official reports. As the Board itself pointed out, there had been no criticism of the conclusions of the Metropolitan Sanitary Commissioners, and even some praise. The journals now discovered that the views of the sanitary reformers had been 'peculiar' from the beginning, and that, while they would have preferred to have left the Board to work out its own perdition, the slights cast upon the profession were such that they were obliged to defend themselves.[3] As others have noticed, interest tends to erect for itself a screen of ideas, and it is true that medical men were reacting to the Board in the same manner as other professional groups. Professional pique was all the sharper because the lay press had approved the Quarantine Report. However, although it is obvious that the attacks on this report gained much of their spirit from the aspersions it cast (which, though as valid as

---

[1] Parkes, *Algide Cholera*, pp.156 ff.

[2] 'Inquiry', p.263.

[3] C.W. Bell, 'Address in Medicine', *Trans. Prov. Med. Surg. Ass.* 5 (1850), 4; Appendix, *Report on Quarantine*, p.143; *Mon. J. Med. Sci.* 9, Pt. 3 (1849), 909; *Lancet*, 1849, ii. 97.

they had previously been, were now quite out of context), the difference in ideas was real. The outcry at there being only one medical man on the Board, and he responsible to no one, was not raised until the Board left off engineering and began to put out 'medical and erroneous' opinions.

The current dichotomy between practice and theory was further underlined by the care taken by reviewers not to dissociate themselves from most of the measures advocated by the Board. The profession did not wish to disagree with sanitary solutions, nor (just as important) did they wish to appear to do so. They did not want to be understood as supporting the quarantine system as then existing, or as disputing the fact of its inutility in the past. They could not, however, agree that it should be abolished entirely.

The counter-attacks designed to repel the Board's 'invasion of our peculiar province' covered three main areas: the specificity of disease, the nature of epidemic influence, and the question of contagion.[1] With respect to the first, the *Monthly Journal of Medical Science* stated that 'a growing distrust of the existence or efficacy of the specific causes of epidemic diseases, and a disposition to refer all, or at least the great number of these diseases, to similar local and general causes' was definitive of the views of the sanitary reformers. From its objections to the Board's list of the characteristics in common among epidemic diseases, it is clear that the notion of specificity current in the profession at this time did not necessarily depend on a definite idea of a specific agent. Edmund Parkes's emphasis on specificity was a typical result of the prolonged stress on chemical pathology and pathological anatomy in a strongly clinical context. The reaction of the *Journal* indicates a general acceptance of specificity as a principle; it was prepared to differentiate in a particular case simply on the basis of age groups or classes affected, or of mode of travel, or climatic area most favoured by the disease. This perhaps exemplifies the persistence in England of the 'natural history' concept of disease. Predictably, many objections were made to the Board's (or Smith's) grouping of the epidemic diseases, on the basis of views held about a particular

---

[1] Bell, 'Address in Medicine', p.4.

disease. For instance, typhus was regarded by most reviewers as a specific disease and at least contingently contagious. Again, Smith's view of scarlet fever as a form of continued fever, not an exanthem, and as most closely related to plague, had been regarded as eccentric when it was first published and was by now extremely out of date; the inclusion of this disease in the Board's epidemic category appeared to some also to demand the presence of smallpox, the typical contagious (and exanthematous) disease.[1] For many, apparently unaware of Smith's peculiar notions, the inclusion of scarlatina implied views on specific contagious disease which the Board perhaps did not hold.

With respect to epidemic influence, it will be remembered that Parkes used the term, and his case may be taken as an example of that in which most writers on epidemic disease found themselves. It appeared to be necessary to posit some cause or causes for the sudden extension of a disease over large areas, or to believe that atmospheric conditions had an effect on the distribution of disease. What was objectionable was the Board's elevation of this token cause, with or without invoking Sydenham, into a 'magnificent creation . . . the "primary and essential" condition of the diffusion of epidemic disease', especially if scarlatina and typhus were to be included as epidemic diseases.[2]

Most time and energy were devoted to the Board's views on contagion, to which its ideas on specificity and epidemic influence were recognized as being in practice subservient. In general, the objections take the form of an assertion of the possibility of contingent contagionism in epidemic diseases, which the Board had previously ruled out as a practical consideration, but was now ruling out absolutely. The *British and Foreign Medico-Chirurgical Review*, having applauded the first exercise, vigorously opposed the second:

The Board seem to be perfectly incapable of comprehending that contagion may be one agent in the spread of epidemic diseases, without being the sole or even the principal agent; or of admitting that while

---

[1] *Mon. J. Med. Sci.* 9, Pt. 3 (1849), 910, 913; *Lancet*, 6 (1825), 339; Smith, *On the Prevalence of Fever in 20 Metropolitan Unions*, p.100; *Lancet*, 1849, ii. 97.

[2] *Mon. J. Med. Sci.* 9, Pt. 3 (1849), 914–15; Bell, 'Address in Medicine', pp.23 ff.

noncontagion is the rule in some diseases, contagion may be the occasional exception, the possibility of which must be acknowledged . . . The rejection of the idea of contagion in regard to every epidemic disease because 'its communication from the sick to the healthy has not been proved, either by the inoculation of a tangible virus, or by a weight of evidence amounting almost to demonstration in favour of atmospheric contagion' was, said the *Monthly Journal of Medical Science*, a habit common enough among the 'so-called non-contagionists of France', but opinions tending to displace contagion as a sufficient cause 'have never had any very extensive influence on medical opinion in this country'. Contagiousness could be proved of any disease regardless of other modes of communication. As to the manner of this proof, the reviewers could not agree with the Board's contention that the bulk of the evidence was the best of the evidence, especially where it was intended to prove a negative. 'Exceptional' cases, commented the *Review*, must be considered because often these were positive evidence where all else was negative, and the former had a higher value.[1]

Furthermore, the Board's account of the properties of 'contagion in the strict sense' was a 'monstrous caricature, or rather misrepresentation' of the views actually held on the subject. Contagion signified the transmission of disease from person to person, regardless of the channel of communication, and the Board's distinction between contagion and infection was therefore unwarrantable. (On this point, all reviewers agreed, and with several it is made quite clear that their view depended on pathology rather than behaviour in the field.) Like *The Lancet* in 1825, the *London Medical Gazette* accused the Board of first inventing a concept of contagion and then triumphantly refuting it. The Board's arguments depended upon the infallibility of contagion, that is, the assumption that if the cause had been present, it must have acted.[2]

The reaction of the journals makes it quite plain, if it is necessary to talk in such terms, that there was by the middle

---

[1] *Br. For. Med. Chir. Rev.* 4 (1849), 213; *Mon. J. Med. Sci.* 9, Pt. 3 (1849), 910.
[2] *Mon. J. Med. Sci.* 9, Pt. 3 (1849), 918; *Lond. Med. Gaz.* 8 (1849), 986.

of the century not a peak of anticontagionism, but a general adherence to a newer concept of contagion; that the profession regarded the older view as outmoded, and much resented its being ascribed to them or brought into play out of its context. In this respect the history of this concept resembles that of spontaneous generation.

The Board went on to produce a Report on Cholera (1850) and a second Report on Quarantine (1852). The Cholera Report was concerned mainly to point out the way in which the progress of the epidemic had confirmed the predictions of the Metropolitan Sanitary Commissioners. The experience had 'extended no light on the primary or proximate causes' of the pestilence, or on the treatment of developed cases. However, it was amply confirmed that cholera was governed by the same laws as other epidemics, and could be prevented by attention to local conditions, including overcrowding, filth, malaria from putrescent mud, dampness, want of drains and bad drains, graveyards, unwholesome food and water.[1] As we shall see more clearly in later chapters, such catalogues should not be regarded as in any way absurd. A pathology could be suggested in which such agents had a direct effect, as well as an indirect influence acting towards the suppression of the normal processes (especially respiration and perspiration) of excretion. The result was a form of septicaemia:

If we could suppose that certain organic impurities, existing in the atmosphere of unhealthy neighbourhoods, passed into the blood through the lungs, so as to follow the circulation, and that similar impurities taken into the stomach with articles of food or drink are likewise absorbed into the blood; if we could moreover suppose that the epidemic influence possessed the power of assuming such organic matter to its own poisonous nature, we should be enabled to include a number of complex phenomena under a hypothesis which would indicate the requisite measures of prevention.

These remarks do not appear in the body of the Report, but in an Appendix by Sutherland.[2] They reflect, as the Report does not, the most common of current influences on epidemiology, Liebigian chemistry. Where Sutherland, Arnott, and other authors, agents and long-term associates of Smith and

---

[1] *Report on Cholera*, pp.143–4, 36–66. For the Board on the influence of impure water in producing fever and cholera, see ibid., pp.59–63.

[2] J. Sutherland, Appendix A, p.8, *Report on Cholera*, [p.198].

Chadwick together differ from their professional colleagues is not in their being anticontagionist, but in their lesser concern for the principle of specificity in epidemic disease.[1]

As did most other official reports on disease outbreaks, the Board's Cholera Report contained extensive tabulated data on cholera mortality in relation to such factors as barometric pressure, temperature, dewpoint, rainfall, free electricity, and 'magnetic force'. As in the case of fever earlier, cholera was asserted to be a disease not of the sickly or the very poor, but of 'labourers, shopkeepers and artizans', and a cause of increase, not decrease, in the dependent part of the population and in the population absolutely. The true function of epidemics of all kinds was, however, '*corrective* rather than *destructive*'.[2]

The Second Report on Quarantine was noticeably more circumspect than the first had been. The position taken up with respect to contagion in principle was far less dogmatic, although echoes still appeared of Smith's earlier writings. Medical authority was invoked from time to time (as in the notifications and reports other than the first Quarantine Report), and theoretical issues were more or less avoided in favour of the old pragmatic approach. Authors 'greatly respected' by the Board were found not to agree on some points, but these were largely of a 'purely professional and scientific' nature. There was 'very general unanimity' on the practical question.[3] The authors of the Second Report show an improved dexterity in drawing attention to the undecided state of professional opinion, and then taking advantage of the more limited propositions on which there was some agreement. It must have been clear that the Board had not modified its views on contagion, but these views were less offensive in connection with the little-known exotic disease which was the subject of the Report. Because, unlike cholera,

---

[1] The Cholera Report also included the assertions of the army surgeon Alexander Thom that past epidemics of plague [an inexplicably absent disease], and other mysterious events like sweating sickness, had all been forms of cholera [now, for the nineteenth century, a well-known and obtrusive disease]. This is the same technique as that used before 1830, when those acquainted with it, tended to reduce all the 'doubtful' diseases to plague.

[2] Sutherland, Appendix, p.5, *Report on Cholera*, [p.195].

[3] *Second Report on Quarantine*, p.136.

yellow fever appeared to be confined to and characteristic of certain specific areas of the world, its nature seemed to be closer to that of marsh ague, and it was more acceptably included in the continuous spectrum of intermittent, remittent, and continued fevers which Smith, Maclean, and others had postulated around 1825. There were no repercussions when this Quarantine Report appeared, but it does not seem that the hostile attitude of the profession to the Board was changed by it. This is hardly surprising, since by then the general hostility to the Board was such as to outweigh all other considerations.

3

EPIDEMIOLOGY AS MEDICAL SCIENCE:
WILLIAM FARR

The reports of commissions, and the publications of the General Board of Health, were not the only organs of official opinion on medical matters. Another official source was created with the Registrar-General's Office, established under the Registration Act of 1836. The figures produced by this office, and the use made of them by a wide range of writers over the period in question, are the most obvious manifestations of the 'inclusive' methodology which dominated the century. It was, however, a somewhat broader set of contemporary considerations that led to the enactment of 1836. This had been preceded by other registration bills, most of them abortive; by a Select Committee on parochial registration (1833), as well as by a long-term accumulation of civil disabilities, partial registration, and anomalies in the marriage laws.[1] The legal, actuarial, and medical professions tended to support national civil registration, although in the last case this cannot be demonstrated to have had any direct influence in Parliament.[2] It can be shown that in other areas of government, the need had been felt for a regular flow of information from the provincial centres in particular. Fellows of the Statistical Society of London, and others, not then Fellows, like John Bowring, were actively involved in this tendency, but the official consideration of statistical departments preceded the foundation of the statistical societies, since it can be said to have begun, for the nineteenth century, in 1830.

---

[1] D.V. Glass, *Numbering the People* (Farnborough, 1973); Registrar-General's Dept. [H.M.S.O.], *The Story of the General Register Office and its Origins from 1583 to 1937* (1937); M.J. Cullen, *The Statistical Movement in Early Victorian Britain* (Hassocks and New York, 1975), Ch. 2.

[2] Glass. *Numbering the People*, p.119. For criticism of plans for national registration, see *Lond. Med. Gaz.* 1835-6, ii. 346-50.

A statistical office was set up at the Board of Trade in 1832.[1]

Not surprisingly, the necessity for improved national systems of medical statistics had been recognized well before Bentham's *Constitutional Code* ascribed a 'Health-regarding-evidence-elicitative and recordative' function to its proposed Ministry of Health.[2] Those opposed to it apparently held Chadwick responsible for the 1836 Act, which may have been delayed in order to take advantage of the system of local areas evolved for the administration of the new Poor Law.[3] Chadwick can instead be credited with some part in adding to the Act a requirement for the civil registration not only of all deaths but of the causes of all deaths, this being a desideratum which was consistent with the Benthamite view of the proper basis for inductions. In addition, Chadwick was, at the time the Bill was presented, engaged in questions relating to medical poor relief.[4] With equal consistency, the Provincial Medical and Surgical Association had urged this form of registration in 1833.[5]

This chapter will be chiefly concerned with the ideas and influence of William Farr, who abandoned medical journalism and an unsuccessful medical practice to enter the new office as 'Compiler of Abstracts'. Farr held this position from its inception in 1838 until his resignation in 1880. In his public capacity Farr, although not as close to policy, enjoyed opportunities of dominating official opinion similar to those of Chadwick and Southwood Smith. He was appointed in order that, according to a contemporary, the Registrar-General 'might be enabled to turn to scientific use' the data received

---

[1] L. Brown *The Board of Trade and the Free Trade Movement 1830–1842* (Oxford, 1958), Ch. 5; *Rep. of 3rd Meeting of British Association* (1834), p.483; Cullen, *The Statistical Movement*, Ch. 6 and 7.

[2] Glass, *Numbering the People*, pp.16 ff., 119–20; Bentham, *Works*, ix. 443–7.

[3] Finer, *Life of Chadwick*, pp.124–5; Glass, *Numbering the People*, p.127.

[4] Glass, *Numbering the People*, pp.139–40; *Examiner*, 11 Dec. 1831, p.793. Finer, *Life of Chadwick*, pp. 154–5. For Southwood Smith to Lord Brougham on the need for registration, see Dedication to the 1st edn. of *Philosophy of Health*.

[5] D.V. Glass, 'Some Aspects of the Development of Demography', *J. Soc. Arts*, 104 (1955–6), 854–68: 854. Credit is also given to Francis Bisset Hawkins, author of 'the first English monograph on medical statistics'. See M. Greenwood, *Medical Statistics from Graunt to Farr* (Cambridge, 1948); G. Rosen, 'Problems in the Application of Statistical Analysis to Questions of Health 1700–1800', *Bull. Hist. Med.* 29 (1955), 27–45; Glass, *Numbering the People*, p.140.

and 'especially the facts medically certified to him as to the causes of registered deaths'. Like John Simon Farr himself decided what functions he would perform in his new position.[1] For the first ten years, he published with the abstracts he had made of causes of death, a 'letter' to his superior, the Registrar-General, commenting on the significance of the figures, developing his own ideas and, as Simon did in his reports, dealing in turn with particular problems. In addition, he wrote, often in stirring language, commentaries on the Weekly and Quarterly Returns. In the course of this activity he evolved an 'official' classification and nomenclature of disease.

His influence therefore takes several forms. Contemporaries were impressed by his Life Tables, and welcomed each statistical return as an infallible addition to factual knowledge. Other writers laid more stress on his related contributions to sanitary reform. Characteristic conclusions were drawn by writers and workers like Edmund Parkes, who, on reviewing the public attention lately given to health and State medicine, ascribed this development to the use of statistics, which had made governmental and national indifference impossible.[2] Less obvious is the influence of Farr's own theoretical ideas, which in many ways resembled those of the medical profession rather than those of Chadwick and Southwood Smith. Farr was deeply committed to the sanitary cause; his more exhortative writing seems predictable in content; and on many matters relating to statistics (such as doctrines of population) he echoed and developed convictions also expressed by Chadwick. He supported Chadwick on quarantine, and believed fervently that prevention was better than cure. Many later accounts, in part because of the general tendency to over-simplify sanitary doctrines, discovered no real difference between the ideas of the two men. They were not friends, and biographers have noticed some points of actual dispute; but there were other important differences of method and

---

[1] Simon, *Sanitary Institutions*, p.211. For a statement of intent by Farr, see *Appendix 1839*, pp.63–5; for Farr's own view of the qualifications necessary for his position, see Ch. 4, Appendix 2 of Glass, *Numbering the People*.

[2] E.A. Parkes, *Manual of Practical Hygiene* (1864), p.xviin.

belief.[1] Farr was at pains to be conventionally 'scientific', and made an explicit distinction between theory and practice, while giving content to both. He further maintained that both speculation and analogical reasoning were useful; and that in sanitary practice no single measure (such as sewage removal) was more important than another, and that housing and education were perhaps most important of all.[2] As we shall see, he produced a version of the miasmatic theory which was more or less a criticism of the makeshift ideas given out in other quarters. This theory was dependent not only on the objective discoveries of gas chemistry, but also on a specific view of disease influenced by the work of Justus Liebig. This view was essentially pathological.

Simon described Farr, with some deliberation but not inaccurately, as 'a mind which revelled in generalisation, well-instructed in theoretical medicine according to the earlier lights of the present century ... he had also considerable literary resources and powers'.[3] Of humble birth, Farr was adopted at an early age by the only local man of substance, who also employed his parents.[4] His education was directed largely by himself, until he began receiving practical medical instruction in the nearest town, Shrewsbury. Then, by a seemingly abrupt transition, and on funds left him by his guardian, intellectual and professional resources of the highest quality were made available to him. He spent a period of about two years, from 1829 to 1831, in Paris, attending the lectures of Orfila, Louis, Guillaume Dupuytren, Jacques

[1] Lewis, *Chadwick and Public Health*, pp.32–3; see also the correspondence reproduced in Glass, *Numbering the People*, Ch. 4, Appendix 1; *Br. For. Med. Rev.* 18 (1844), 198.

[2] Finer allows Chadwick to have at first held views of this broader type: *Life of Chadwick*, p.211.

[3] Simon, *Sanitary Institutions*, p.211.

[4] William Farr (1807–1883), L.S.A. 1832, F.R.S. 1855. Supported himself by writing after 1833; adopted by *The Lancet*. Tried unsuccessfully to institute a lecture course on 'hygiology': see Farr, 'Lectures on Hygeine [*sic*]'; see also *Lancet*, 1835–6, i. 10. For biography see *DNB*; F.A.C. Hare, *William Farr* (1883). Selections from his writings were edited, with a memoir, by N.A. Humphreys as *Vital Statistics* (1885). Recent studies are Eyler, 'Farr, An Intellectual Biography'; this is not well represented by idem, 'William Farr on the Cholera: The Sanitarian's Disease Theory and the Statistician's Method', *J. Hist. Med.* 28 (1973), 79–100. See also Cullen, *The Statistical Movement*, especially Ch. 2; V.L. Hilts, 'William Farr (1807–1883) and the "Human Unit"', *Victorian Studies*, 14 (1970), 143–50.

Lisfranc, Georges Cuvier on natural sciences, Geoffroy St. Hilaire and others on comparative anatomy and physiology, Andral on hygiene, and Gay-Lussac and Louis Jacques Thenard on chemistry. At the end of this period, after some unspecified contact with University College, London, Farr returned to Shrewsbury. That he was not appointed to a vacancy in the permanent staff of Shrewsbury Infirmary may have convinced him that he required formal qualifications; he subsequently re-entered University College, attended medical lectures, and in 1832 gained his L.S.A. This remained his only formal qualification; the doctorate by which he was commonly known was an honorary one bestowed by New York University in 1847. During either of his periods of contact with University College, Farr might first have met J.R. McCulloch and possibly Chadwick.[1]

In spite of major recent work, many important points in Farr's early career remain obscure. In the absence of explicit information, it is assumed that his interests in statistics, pathological anatomy, public health, and hygiene all derived from his two years in France. Farr himself dated his interest in medicine, to the fortuitous impression made upon him as a youth of nineteen by the conversation of a well-read and philosophical local practitioner.[2] Previously, partly owing to the limitations of the libraries available to him, his bent had been primarily theological. Farr's involvement in the subject matter of medicine and public health is hardly to be separated from his interests in history, physiology, and anthropology; he was especially interested in the idea of racial degeneration. There is no evidence of his ever having been formally instructed in mathematics; undoubtedly, his fairly limited skills were initially acquired as tools to serve his other concerns. Eyler rightly emphasizes the existence of strong British traditions in the areas of most concern, particularly the

---

[1] Farr continued to attend lectures at University College until 1835: Hare, *William Farr*, p.4.

[2] *Vital Statistics*, p.ix. The practitioner was 'Dr. G. Webster, of the Salop Infirmary'. The influence of Webster warrants further investigation, especially as it immediately preceded Farr's removal to Paris, but Webster himself is surprisingly anonymous. He may have been the George Webster who graduated M.D. at Glasgow in 1798.

statistical, and points to some aspects of Farr's early work which could not have been derived from the less expansive French tradition.[1] Like Chadwick, Farr displayed a good knowledge of the history and literature of British statistics, but more personal points of contact are harder to find. It is possible that the much underestimated James Clark, later Sir James Clark, was one of these.[2] Clark's experience as a naval surgeon, and on the continent, had prompted him to observations on hygiene and to the collection of data which were embodied in *Medical Notes on Climate, Diseases, Hospitals and Medical Schools in France, Italy and Switzerland* (1822), enlarged as *The Influence of Climate in the Prevention and Cure of Chronic Diseases, more particularly of the Chest and Digestive Organs* (1829).[3] Clark took an informed interest in medical education, with particular reference to University College, and in institutions for the promotion of chemistry and other sciences of national importance. The first edition (1843) of Liebig's *Familiar Letters on Chemistry* was dedicated to Clark. He was, in addition, an early advocate of sanitary reform, and the active associate of George and Andrew Combe, John Conolly, and John Forbes.

It seems possible that Clark attended Farr's first wife, who died of tuberculosis, and he apparently employed Farr to revise his work on that disease.[4] Farr's paper of 1838 on cholera was based on a report, lent him by Clark, of cases registered with the Board of Health in Rome.[5] The circumstances leading to Farr's appointment at the Registrar-General's Office, which

---

[1] Hare, *William Farr*, p.5; Eyler, 'Farr, An Intellectual Biography', pp.125 ff., 165-78.

[2] For Clark (1788-1870), F.R.S. 1832, K.C.B., M.A. Aberdeen, M.R.C.S. Edinburgh 1809, M.D. Edinburgh 1817, see *DNB*; *Munk*; *Proc. R. Soc. Lond.* 19 (1871), pp.xiii–xix; P.Huard and M.D. Grmek, 'Les Elèves étrangers de Laennec', *Revue hist. sci. applic.* 26 (1973), 315-37. It is a measure of Clark's habitual anonymity in public affairs that he is not mentioned by Hale Bellot, *University College*.

[3] The 3rd edn. of this influential work (1841) was entitled *The Sanative Influence of Climate*. It may be noted here that the author of *A Medical Guide to Nice* (1841), ascribed by Eyler to the William Farr of this chapter, was instead a William Farr of Nice, M.D. in 1841.

[4] Hare, *William Farr*, p.5. Clark, *Treatise on Pulmonary Consumption*(1835), especially p.167.

[5] Farr, 'On the Law of Recovery in Cholera', *Lancet*, 1838-9, i. 26. For references by Farr to Clark's own work see 'Vital Statistics', pp.588, 600.

might have been thought of as a means to rescue him from a considerable personal and financial crisis, are surprisingly obscure; credit is conventionally given to Chadwick (with Arnott), but Clark's name is also mentioned.[1] Clark was at the time a member of the British Association's 'London committee' on registration.[2] Farr's first substantial published work on statistics, the article for McCulloch's *Account of the British Empire* (1837), did not appear alone, but as one of a sudden rush of contributions on statistical subjects, which Farr might have been encouraged to produce as evidence of his suitability for the new post.[3] Other features of his life and work, which are not capable of explanation in terms of his years in France, are his reverence for Sydenham (very evident in the 1830s), and the overriding influence on his theoretical ideas of the chemistry of Liebig.[4]

It has been claimed elsewhere that a major influence on Farr was Jacob Henle, and that the direction of Farr's research was determined by his awareness of the strengths and weaknesses of Henle's work.[5] Both these claims are based on the circumstance that Farr, in 1840, referred in a footnote to a *British and Foreign Medical Review* judgement of Henle's chapter on contagions and miasms. The journal regarded Henle's case as ingenious, but unproven. It seems fair to suggest that any such display of ingenuity would appeal to Farr, but that he was not otherwise influenced by Henle.[6] There is no evidence, other than his linguistic facility, for Farr's having read Henle's untranslated work. As already indicated, Farr was much more taken with chemical explanations of disease compatible with recent work on the

---

[1] Glass, *Numbering the People*, p.141. Farr was also left £500 (and a library) by his old teacher Webster, but the latter's death did not occur until 1837: *Vital Statistics*, p.xii.

[2] *Rep. of 4th Meeting of British Association* (1835), p.xxxix.

[3] Eyler's bibliography of Farr's works gives three various items for 1835–6; seven for 1837, and four for 1838, most of them obviously statistical: 'Farr, An Intellectual Biography', pp.373–4.

[4] The former point is rightly stressed by Eyler: ibid., pp.174 ff.

[5] G. Rosen, 'Jacob Henle and William Farr', *Bull. Hist. Med.* (1941), 585–9; M. Greenwood, *Epidemiology, Historical and Experimental* (Baltimore and London, 1932), p.13.

[6] *Appendix 1840*, p.18 n.; *Br. For. Med. Rev.* 9 (1840), 398–404.

pathology of the body's fluids. Henle's excursion did not direct his research, for he had decided well before 1840 that smallpox was regulated by definite mathematical laws, and had made what he regarded as similar calculations (including the construction of a 'regular curve') for cholera.[1] His studies of epidemics were preceded by an analogous tabular treatment of the duration, crises, and outcome of disease in individuals, which, when sufficiently elaborate, was taken to provide a sound basis for prediction and prescription by the practitioner.[2] The remark with which Farr turned away from the animalcular hypothesis, that causes might not be known directly but that their nature might be discerned by determining their laws of operation, was no more than conventional with respect to causes.

Eyler, however, is undoubtedly correct in regarding Farr's belief in the regularity of diseased as of healthy functions, as one of the most fundamental of his assumptions. Given Farr's concentration on the application of this belief to the phenomena of the rise and fall of disease in the individual and, later, in the group or population, it seems likely that he owed it as much to Hippocrates, Sydenham, and the English school of topography as to the French statisticians. Farr's belief in the lawfulness of life, although expressed with great richness and variety, was also a belief in the relatedness of medicine and its subject matter to the physical sciences, and as such was a standard tenet among philosophical nineteenth-century practitioners. His 'law of recovery and mortality in cholera' demonstrated that:

Pathological phenomena are as regular in their courses as physical phenomena observed in inorganic matter; and that the instruments of physical investigation are applicable to medicine: for, after due allow-

---

[1] See below. 'On Mr. Farr's Law in Cholera', *Rep. of 8th Meeting of British Association*, Trans. of Sections (1838), pp.126–7, is only a summary of Farr's paper. *The Lancet's* account (apparently not seen by Eyler) is longer and includes a diagrammatic representation of the 'regular curve'. For a similar curve for 'the force of mortality' in smallpox, see 'On Prognosis', *Br. Med. Almanack*, 1838, p.214.

[2] These first tables served the regular professional interests involved in the management of the individual case. Cf. also the work of T.R. Edmonds: e.g. 'Statistics of the London Hospital with Remarks on the Law of Sickness', *Lancet*, 1835–6, i. 778–83. Farr's earliest tables were an investigation of the concept of 'critical periods' and used data derived from Hippocrates and a critic of the concept, Latham: 'Lectures on Hygeine', pp.775–7.

ance . . . it will be found that the facts can be as exactly expressed by formulae, as any facts in the province of natural philosophy . . . If the abstract sciences are every day descending to practical applications, the empirical arts are also rapidly rising into the region of knowledge.[1]

In character, Farr has been described as 'quiet', in the sense of retiring. On the contrary, it seems that although of some simplicity, he was curious, enthusiastic, and occasionally obstinate ('crochety'). In his receptivity to foreign literature he might be compared with Simon, but, in contrast with Simon's rather colder caution, he was suggestible rather than systematic, and inclined to make impulsive and sometimes inflexible commitments. It is perhaps worth noting that, as the debates on fever showed, a reasonable acquaintance with French writers at least was not uncommon in the 1820s; Farr did not begin serious writing until the late 1830s.

Farr stated, when he embarked on his official career, that 'medicine, like the other natural sciences is beginning to abandon vague conjecture, where facts can be accurately determined, and to substitute numerical expressions for uncertain assertions'.[2] Much of his work can be seen as an attempt to bear out this article of the common faith. Wherever possible, he used mathematical formulae, carefully explained. Three characteristic examples may be noted.[3] The latest and best known of these is that relating land elevation and cholera incidence. This elaborate generalization aroused much enthusiasm in the 1850s when it was first put forward, and continued to be of concern to those interested in *Grundwasser* theories; others came to regard it merely as a first approximation to the relation of cholera with water supply. Its main function, however, was as an exemplary or model investigation.[4]

The second example was an explicit attempt to quantify the language of Sydenham, that is to find a mathematical expression for the rate of progress and decline of an epidemic.

[1] Eyler, 'Farr, An Intellectual Biography', e.g. pp.115–17, 137–8, 143–50; Farr, 'On Mr. Farr's Law in Cholera', p.127.

[2] *Appendix 1839*, p.64.

[3] Other examples are described by Eyler, 'Farr, An Intellectual Biography', especially pp.145 ff.

[4] Farr, *Report on Cholera Mortality* (1852), pp.lxi–lxvi. The correlation appears in *Encyclopaedia Britannica*, 8th edn. (1854), vi. 633. For its persistence into the 1870s, see Eyler, 'Farr, An Intellectual Biography', pp.285 ff.

These features were of course well attested, but also among the most difficult to explain. Farr took for discussion a smallpox outbreak of 1837–9, which was not only the most completely documented of recent epidemics, but also the easiest to discuss, since there was no doubt as to the manner in which smallpox was propagated.[1] He took due note of Sydenham's special interest in this disease but, as already suggested, the campaigns for (and against) the eradication by inoculation or vaccination of smallpox, and the relevance of such a prospect to population growth, had already made it the object of systematic study. Smallpox was, in the early nineteenth century, the only contagious disease of well-defined character which also exhibited in some degree the phenomena of extension confined by Southwood Smith to his purely epidemic category. It may have been the suitability of smallpox for quantitative analysis which disposed Farr automatically to regard it as the leading disease in his 'epidemic, endemic, and contagious', and 'zymotic' categories.

Given the fixed character of smallpox, it was possible to speculate more precisely on the nature of the latent cause which, it was assumed, must be responsible for the sudden but periodic extensions of the disease. It did not seem that this cause, which could be either a physical agent or some factor such as an increase in the virulence of the contagious principle, could be discovered directly; therefore it was to be approached by defining its laws of action. These 'may be determined by observation, as well as the circumstances in which epidemics arise, or by which they may be controlled'. Farr concluded after calculation that, although the mortality rates from smallpox varied with population density, incidence of inoculation and vaccination and other factors, it appeared probable that the disease 'increases at an accelerated and then at a retarded rate; that it declines first at a slightly accelerated, then at a rapidly accelerated and lastly at a retarded rate, until the disease attains the minimum intensity and remains stationary'. The calculated rates agreed with those observed,

---

[1] Farr had already produced a study of the earlier type on smallpox: 'On a Method of Determining the Danger of Diseases. Art. I', *Br. Ann. Med.* 1 (1837), 72–9; 'On the Law of Recovery in Smallpox. Art. II', ibid., pp.134–43; 'On Prognosis'.

and the same regularities were shown by figures for other contagious diseases, in so far as these were complete. Farr likened the epidemic's progress to that of a projectile.[1] As with the previous example, these calculations were probably more notable for their inspirational than for their real value.

The third example appeared three years after the second, when work on the census of 1841 had made it possible to estimate the current population of a particular area. Farr first obtained an algebraic expression for 'the mean physiological duration of life in particular circumstances' based on a version of cost of living index, and then showed for certain London districts that their mortality rates increased in the ratio of the sixth root of their densities. This formula or one like it could, he thought, be used to estimate the influence on a population of insanitary conditions by eliminating as a factor the inevitable effect of a high or low density. As early as his first report, Farr had stated his conviction that mortality increased as the density of population increased; he then thought that this was due to the increased concentration of expired gases in the atmosphere. By 1843 he was still convinced of the relation, but explained it rather differently.[2] Farr regarded his density calculations as an 'example of the methods to be employed in estimating the influence of particular agents on mortality' and, more generally, as an illustration of the necessity of the 'scientific approach' in handling the multifactoral problems presented by living matter. A sanitary inquiry, he said, was 'not such an easy matter as some suppose'. Appreciation of this part of Farr's work was expressed many years later by Benjamin Richardson, another sanitary reformer:

Give one of us who has mastered these tables the deathrate of a place and the prevailing causes of death for a sufficient period to prove that the regular deathrate is before us, and we can determine, with fair exactitude, what is the state of the drainage, the water supply, the general condition of the inhabitants and the number of public houses, although we may never have set foot in the place . . .[3]

It will be admitted that nomenclature can create more

---

[1] Farr, *Appendix 1840*, pp.18 ff. That is, a 'regular curve'.
[2] *Appendix 1843*, pp.200 ff.
[3] Richardson in Chadwick, *Health of Nations*, i. p.xlvi.

problems in medicine that in any other science. Nineteenth-century medical writers were well aware of the dangers and difficulties, but this did not prevent the evil.[1] With respect to nomenclature and the associated question of classification, Farr made definite if modest contributions. With one important exception, it does not appear that any of the new terms employed by him passed into common use.[2] His contribution here was the perhaps more useful one of reducing, at least for official purposes, the number of synonyms and fine distinctions, of speculative or extravagant descriptions, and such vague terms as fits, colds, decline, and inflammation (unspecified).[3] In so doing he eliminated much eighteenth-century terminology, as well as the incomprehensible and vulgar (although not the popular, which he respected wherever it was sufficiently precise), and deliberately by-passed important controversies represented in nomenclature, in particular the definition of fevers and epidemic diseases. At all events, a fixed nomenclature was better than one which was not fixed. As Farr pointed out, uniformity in this connection was as important as in weights and measures in other contexts.

Farr's first attempts at classification appeared in 1837, when he presented, in considerably abbreviated form, tables of causes arranged alternatively according to seat, or organs involved, and to the pathological 'nature' of diseases. In the latter case, the majority of the causes of death were divided into fevers and inflammations; consumption was placed under 'serous effusions'. Farr had already repudiated Cullen's nosology, which had been used by John Heysham and consequently by Joshua Milne for the famous Carlisle life tables, and was still in general official use. As Compiler of Abstracts, Farr considered the subject of nosology more deeply, paying particular attention to the efforts of Cullen and of John Mason Good. Like all later nosologies, Farr's differed according to its intended functions. Cullen's classification, he concluded, was unsuitable for statistical purposes (as was any detailed arrangement); it also failed to present

---

[1] See e.g. W. Davies, 'Fever in its Relations to Sanitary Reform', p.70.
[2] As predicted by the *Br. For. Med. Rev.* 18 (1844), 198.
[3] For some years Farr made detailed comments on all unsatisfactory usages found in the registrars' returns. See especially *Appendix 1842*, pp.106–12.

diseases in their 'presumed natural relations'.[1] In drawing up an alternative, Farr was apparently able to please himself. As in the 1850s, there was some consultation of 'eminent members of the profession' and, again as in later years, Farr accepted advice from the Statistical Society of London and from the British Association; which is as much as to say, from friends, since he was himself involved in both organizations. The 1834 meeting of the British Association had set up two committees on civil registration, one in London and one in Edinburgh; from time to time Farr referred to each of these.[2] He claimed, however, to have paid most attention to the old registers, which were not made up according to any 'preconceived idea', and to have considered before anything else the practical sanitary purpose of his nosology.[3] Accordingly, he included in a single 'epidemic, endemic and contagious' category all diseases which 'were of a specific nature, propagated in a peculiar manner and known by experience to become epidemic in unhealthy places and among the sickly classes, at greater or less intervals of time'. These diseases, he said, were the 'index of salubrity'.[4] Other divisions on the same level were similarly 'founded on the mode in which diseases affect the population': after the first group (exemplified by smallpox), came sporadics (cancer was typical of generalized or constitutional affections of this type; pneumonia, of local) and accidents (exemplified by burn). The distinction between 'plagues' and 'sporadics' was of course, as Farr recognized, of some antiquity. The sporadic diseases were divided into the 'natural families' representative of the integrity of organ systems. Though it invited others, this grouping avoided some controversies. Farr further reduced the substance for dispute by acting on the assumption that no general rules could be deduced from small numbers. He

[1] Farr, 'Vital Statistics', pp.594 ff.; *Appendix 1877*, p.227; *Appendix 1839*, p.67.

[2] These committees (subcommittees of the Medical Section) were independent of each other and, as we have already seen, often disagreed. See *Rep. of 4th Meeting of British Association* (1835), pp.xxxviii–xxxix; *Rep. of 5th Meeting of British Association* (1836), pp.251–5.

[3] This intention sufficiently distinguished Farr's nosology from earlier attempts.

[4] Farr, *Appendix 1839*, p.67. Cf. idem, 'Vital Statistics', p.586, where epidemics are specifically excluded from consideration.

left aside diseases rare in England, like the problematic yellow fever and plague; and referred 'all modified forms of fever' (including, in 1842, the 'dothinenteric')[1] to the general heading of typhus.[2]

Other parts of the nosology were drawn up under the combined influence of similar practical considerations, and the findings of the later French pathologico-anatomical school. For instance, Farr made a primary division between diseases referable to particular organs or systems, and diseases of uncertain seat, but this division was also based on the fact that the average practitioner found it much easier to give accurately the site (as demonstrated by symptoms of functional disorder) rather than the nature of the affection. In his own classification, Farr said, he recognized a 'species', 'whenever important pathological states and phenomena were isolated or could be individualised'. Cullen's nosology had been ruled by a primary emphasis on function, both on the general and the local level; Farr referred all local conditions, which included the greater number of diseased states, to a site. He was, nevertheless, as concerned with process ('dynamic disease') as with structure, and warned against the 'violent and improbable hypothesis' of localism, in which all symptoms were referred to a primary and evident anatomical lesion. By way of indicating his views on the 'structure versus function' debate, Farr gave a general discussion on change in the body, making primary reference, in the manner of Liebig, to the blood. As an illustration he explained inflammation, 'one of the most important and most frequent phenomena of disease', in terms of the heat produced by combustion in the blood and tissues. Animal and plant species were distinguished on the basis of structure, but the 'technicalities' of natural history were not to encumber medical science, which had its own principles, and could 'derive more advantages from the methods of chemistry and natural philosophy'.[3]

Farr was obliged more often than his contemporaries to make explicit reference to natural history, and at one point

---

[1] Form of Bretonneau's term for typhoid fever, 'dothiénentérie'.

[2] Farr queried the absolute disappearance of plague, and suggested that sporadic cases did occur and were confounded with typhus: *Appendix 1842*, p.94.

[3] Ibid., pp.112 ff., 114.

he went so far, in a criticism of Cullen, as to deny the reality of species among animals and plants as well as among diseases. The admired Sydenham's conspicuous use of the analogy between diseases and species of organisms was justified, he thought, because zymotics were nearer than other diseases to the definition of species in natural history.[1] Nature produced such diseases in a uniform manner, and they exhibited a regular 'life cycle' in the patient of development and decline. Farr's scattered and seemingly inconsistent remarks on natural history make up a view typical of the partial rejection by English writers of eighteenth-century definitions, combined with a continued dependence, in a different context, on the analogy itself. Farr dissociated himself from 'specific' in the 'strict sense', as he did from the literal connotation of 'fermentation'. He was further typical of his period in rejecting most explicitly for diseases the definitions of specificity depending on reproduction, such as that of Cuvier.[2] This amounted to allowing for diseases their production by means other than a previous case of the same malady.

It is obvious that one basis upon which Farr recognized disease species was that of consensus. Although in advance of the average practitioner in his allegiance to French and German authors, it in no way suited his purpose to present that practitioner with a nosology which the latter found unfamiliar and therefore useless. Hence his deference to English 'habits' and his citation, in annotations to his nosology, of standard English systematic works and English monographs.[3] Farr added that he excluded many foreign works

---

[1] Ibid., pp.112 n.; 121.

[2] Cf. *Appendix 1877*, p.299; *Appendix 1842*, p.114.

[3] Among others Farr recommended Henry Holland on influenza; George Budd on scurvy; his friend R.D. Thomson on dyspepsia; Thomson, Dalton, Liebig, and George Budd on the effects of starvation; Bayle, Laennec, Louis, and James Clark on phthisis; W.P. Alison and R. Carswell (a nosologist and one of Farr's teachers at University College) on scrofula; and in general Hippocrates, Sydenham, K.P.J. Sprengel (1766–1833), J.A.F. Ozanam (1773–1837), Villermé, C.J.B. Williams, and Liebig. On fever he suggested Louis, Christison, and Southwood Smith — the last-named undoubtedly because of his inclusion of statistical material. Statistics published by Smith had been used by Edmonds to reveal regularities in the mortality among patients in the London Fever Hospital: Farr, 'Vital Statistics', p.585; idem, 'On Prognosis', p.201.

only to allow easy reference by the practitioner. The French were well represented still, notably by Andral, Villermé, Louis, and Laennec, some of whom had, of course, been his teachers in Paris, but all of whom would have been at least familiar names to his readers. In these writings, he said, 'will be found the prevailing medical opinions which will for some years guide the medical practitioners of this country in returning the causes of death'.[1] The effect of adopting majority views was further to diminish the number of specific distinctions.

This statistical nosology was first used in 1839.[2] In 1842, Farr reviewed it, answered criticisms, and introduced a complete theoretical justification of the 'epidemic, endemic and contagious' group, based on the work of Liebig. The criticisms received by this stage included the 'friendly' comments of the medical press and of members of the profession, to which Farr responded without going into details. Criticism he was concerned to reject had come chiefly from William Alison and a Committee of the College of Physicians of Edinburgh which had followed the report, given by Alison at the British Association's Dublin meeting in 1835, of the 'Edinburgh Committee' of the Association.[3] Like much of Alison's other public work, these representations were made in view of the possibility of the extension of new English legislation to include Scotland. As in other cases, a distinction was maintained consonant with alleged differences in Scottish conditions. Alison felt obliged to make more allowance for the registration of causes of death by unqualified persons, and wanted only those details recorded which all observers were capable of recognizing in all instances. Thus croup, laryngitis, and quinsy would not be registered as distinct diseases, but under the single heading, 'diseases of the windpipe'. Like Farr's corre-

---

[1] *Appendix 1842*, p.93n.

[2] It was given to registrars in the form of a recommended list of specific diseases, more detailed than the published extracts of returns. When the nosology first appeared it was suggested (by the *Br. For. Med. Rev.* 9 (1840), 352) that copies be sent out to all practitioners. It seems that this was not done. Instead the practitioner was advised to write or call for a copy, which would be provided free of charge: Farr, *Lancet*, 1843, i. 236. The first version of the nosology was publicized in *The Lancet*, 1838-9, ii. 655ff.

[3] Alison, 'Report on the Registration of Deaths', *Rep. of 5th. Meeting of British Association* (1836), pp.251-5.

spondent, the Swiss Jacob-Marc d'Espiné, Alison also wanted the distinction between 'acute' and 'chronic' preserved, whereas English informants were asked instead to make quantitative estimates of the duration of the condition or conditions preceding death. In reply Farr argued forcefully for his own degree of stress on detail, specificity, and economy in the number of columns involved in a registration, and stated uncompromisingly that the Edinburgh method was only the more simple as it was the less scientific. He also urged the desirability of instituting a classificatory practice which could be extended beyond the British Isles to the army abroad, the colonies, and all other dominions. The 'London committee', he implied, had been similarly critical of the Edinburgh proposals. Farr did not think the situation so different in England that he was oversanguine about the number of deaths which would be reported by unqualified informants. Rather, he wanted educated information recorded when it was available, and simple formulae used for the rest.[1]

Farr's 'statistical nosology' is to be seen less in relation to the specialized or learned nosologies produced at the same, later, period, than to the systematic clinical works on which he heavily depended. His classification was in no way enforced, except indirectly, by the rationalization of the returns into official categories, and would not have been used, as were other nosologies, in teaching. However, in many vital areas it dictated the terms of discussion, and here his simplifications and his theoretical excursions were of importance. Farr was concerned to reflect prevailing opinion, but not, as his replies to Alison showed, the lowest common denominator of opinion.

The provisions as to registration in the Act passed in 1836 were defective, but this was apparently partially compensated for by the active interest and co-operation of medical men and professional institutions. Initially, medical men were only bound to give information as to cause of death if applied to within eight days of the decease. In 1845, with the aim of improving the standard and degree of completion of returns, all qualified practitioners were requested to accept an obli-gation to provide a written certificate of the cause of death

---

[1] Farr, *Appendix 1842*, pp.123-9.

in all cases attended by them which ended fatally. Deaths would, thenceforth, be recorded as either 'Certified' or 'Not Certified'.[1] This appeal, accompanied by a veiled threat that all uncertified deaths might be regarded as matters requiring investigation, was apparently rejected by only about fifty of the 10,000 or more qualified practitioners. Although, as with so many similar provisions, medical certification of death did not become compulsory until much later (1874), the percentage of certified deaths was consistently high, and this mode of certification probably led to greater attention being paid to Farr's nosology. In addition, of the 2,193 local registrars appointed by September 1838, 527 were medical men (416 of these being also officers of Poor Law Unions).[2]

After 1842, Farr made no change in principle in his classification for at least twenty years. Review committees were set up only when the question arose of the nosology's being extended to other departments or other countries. It was, as Farr had hoped, found practically useful, although its deliberate generality was found less serviceable by a variety of factions after 1850. There were also some characteristic objections to Farr's work having theoretical content, of that particular or indeed of any kind.[3] Specific changes introduced by Farr included the separation of 'puerperal fever' from 'childbirth' (1847), the inclusion of diphtheria as a condition distinct from scarlet fever (1855), and the division of 'typhus' into 'typhus', 'enteric', and 'simple continued' fevers in 1869. This last innovation was delayed according to Farr's principle that it was better to subsume controversial matter under a broader term, than to invite speculation or challenge the conservatism of many practitioners.[4]

Different conditions combined with different requirements to produce revisions during the movement towards internationalism in public health in the 1850s.[5] Farr himself, in

---

[1] Farr had come to regard this as a necessity by 1842: ibid., p.124.

[2] Glass, *Numbering the People*, pp.140 ff.; *7th Rep. Registrar-General*, PP, 1846, XIX. 249–50, 264–6; *1st Rep. Registrar-General*, PP, 1839, XVI. 3[5].

[3] See e.g. *Lond. Med. Gaz.* 9 (1849), 851–2.

[4] Farr, *Appendix 1877*, pp.229, 230. But cf. his *Report on Nomenclature and Classification* [1856], pp.15–16.

[5] For the later history and difficulties of standardization, see J. Kennedy and C.E. Kossmann, 'Nomenclatures in Medicine', *Bull. Med. Lib. Ass.* 61 (1973), 238–52.

consultation with d'Espiné, revised his nosology at this time with the aim, suggested by the first International Statistical Congress in Brussels in 1853, of producing 'a uniform nomenclature of the Causes of Death, applicable in all countries'. In the new version, Farr maintained the distinction between 'plagues' and sporadic diseases, but introduced more subdivisions: as classes, *Zymotici*, *Cachectici* (constitutional diseases), *Monorganici* (local diseases), *Metamorphici* (developmental), and *Thanatici* (violent deaths). The *Zymotici* were divided into *Miasmatici* (a term Farr derived from the Greek for stain or defilement), *Enthetici*, *Dietici*, and *Parasitici*, of which fever, syphilis, scurvy, and worms respectively could be regarded as the types. The enthetic diseases were those 'properly called contagious', being communicated by direct contact or puncture. In an arrangement highly characteristic of nineteenth-century epidemiology, the miasmatic diseases were defined as diffusible through the air or water, and attended by fevers of various forms; the communicable matter deriving from the human body (as in smallpox) or from the 'earth' (as in ague).[1]

As epidemiological medicine became more self-conscious, its emergent professional bodies (especially the Epidemiological Society, founded in 1850), also began to assume responsibility in areas such as registration and nomenclature. Following an initiative of the Epidemiological Society a top-level Committee on Nomenclature, based at the College of Physicians but involving representatives (including Farr) from all other major official and professional bodies, was set up and began discussions in the late 1850s. A hiatus occurred in the work of this committee between 1858 and 1863, and the College's first *Nomenclature of Diseases* was not published until 1869. The universal application of the College's system was strenuously resisted by the Registrar-General, thus providing, at a late date, an example for this department of the distinction between official and professional belief.[2]

---

[1] Farr, *Report on Nomenclature and Classification*. See also *Sixteenth Annual Report of the Registrar-General* (1856), pp. 71–105.

[2] See A.M. Cooke, *A History of the Royal College of Physicians of London*, iii (Oxford, 1972), 837–40.

The period was, in general, one of regression in the growth of State medicine.

A disease need not be specific to be distinct.[1] As we have already seen, the former term may itself have an analogic rather than a literal meaning, and may be used to refer to the regular course of development characteristic of a disease, rather than to a particular kind of cause or mode of reproduction. It was possible to claim that in all three of Farr's main categories ('epidemic, endemic and contagious'; 'sporadic'; 'accidental') the members were disease states rather than disease entities: 'adjectives rather than noun substantives'. In the normal way the question of essence, or *divinum quid*, arose persistently only in connection with the 'contagious' members of the first group. By forming this group, and citing smallpox as typical of it, Farr was implying that the characteristics of that disease were in some way definitive of all its members. At first, however, he was preoccupied less with pathology than with public health, and said merely that he included in the group, besides contagions and endemics, all diseases which, however much they might differ in other ways, agreed in destroying great numbers in a short time and at uncertain intervals. Farr added that 'epidemic' was not a categorical but a relative term, meaning unaccustomed frequency, which could apply as well to erysipelas in a hospital ward as to cholera in an entire population. Such usage contrasted strongly with Southwood Smith's definitions, but did, apparently, imply a similar stress upon the conditions which caused a disease to prevail excessively in a particular place. Farr, however, proceeded as if referring to an established medical principle, quoting Sydenham as authority for the importance of locality in considering prognosis and treatment. 'The experienced practitioner ... will discover that the characters of disease change, and will not treat a pneumonia in the same way in Whitechapel and in Westmoreland, if it appears, from the causes of death, that the diseases and constitutions of the population present striking discrepancies'.[2]

On the criterion of their undue influence on the public

[1] For a contemporary discussion of the different senses of specificity, see J. Ross, *The Graft Theory of Disease* (1872), Ch. 8.

[2] Farr, *Appendix 1839*, p.63.

health, or rather, of their preventability, Farr included with smallpox such diseases as cholera, dysentery, croup, and erysipelas, all of which were more or less controversial.[1] Alison's Edinburgh College of Physicians Committee thought that if there was to be a group of 'spreading diseases', then the group should be defined by that characteristic alone; and a disease like dysentery should be included only when its behaviour was known to be affected by some incidental 'local and temporary' cause. Dysentery should, therefore, be classified as a sporadic disease, and appear with smallpox only as 'epidemic dysentery'.[2] In reply, Farr referred first to his practical motive of wishing to put together all diseases known to prevail in unhealthy seasons and localities, so that analysis might be made of the operation of such diseases under the greatest variety of circumstances; and second, to the disadvantages of placing a disease sometimes in one group and sometimes in another. He asserted no other motive for including cholera with smallpox.[3] In sum, Farr's use of 'epidemic' comprehended both Southwood Smith's usage, and that of the Edinburgh College of Physicians Committee, which was roughly opposite to that of Smith.

Farr's practical argument must be allowed. On the other hand, he did claim that dysentery was (like smallpox) both specific and contagious, and, at one point, that all the diseases placed in the first class were of a 'specific nature'. Whatever the admixture in his motives in first drawing up this group, the fact remains that he included all its members in the pathological speculations of 1842, when the group name 'endemic, epidemic and contagious' was replaced by the single term, 'zymotic'.

This term, which apparently originated with Farr, was based on the Greek for 'to ferment', and the theory representing the disease process as a form of fermentation or 'zymosis' was an adaptation by Justus Liebig of his own chemical explanation

---

[1] See Greenhow, *Sanitary Papers*, pp.17–18.

[2] According to this procedure, major epidemics of Asiatic cholera would appear as 'epidemic cholera'. All other forms and incidents would be definitively 'sporadic'. The Edinburgh committee categorized as 'epidemic, endemic and contagious diseases' only 'epidemic influenza', smallpox, measles, scarlatina, whooping cough, 'epidemic continued fever', syphilis, and hydrophobia.

[3] Farr, *Appendix 1842*, p.126.

of putrefaction, fermentation, and decay.[1] Liebig's work will be discussed in detail in the next chapter, but it must be dealt with here for its relevance to Farr. The other ground for the latter's speculations was the argument by analogy from the effects of poisons. This approach will also be dealt with later. Farr's statement of principle with respect to his zymotic group was that 'the blood is probably in the greater number of them, the primary seat of disease; and they may be considered, by hypothesis, the results of specific poisons, of organic origin, either derived from without, or generated within, the body'.[2] A poison like arsenic, he stated, caused death only by bringing about a state of the body called arsenic poisoning, or, as he proposed, 'Arsenicia'. Various of the features of Arsenicia might also occur as the effects of other poisons, but, *in toto*, a characteristic picture was presented which pointed to a particular agent. Correspondingly, the state called smallpox or variola was owing to a specific matter or transformation of matter called varioline, and cholera, to cholerine. Farr's procedure was to suppose the existence of an 'exciter' for every disease still described as distinct, even if (as in the cases of puerperal fever and erysipelas, and of yellow fever and marsh fever) several diseases were thought to be caused by one poison.[3] Arsenic produced different effects according to the dose, the individual and many accidental circumstances; in this complexity the poison itself was the one essential factor. Similarly, the 'exciter' typhine produced different forms, typhus and Louis's *fièvre typhoïde*. Again, although the primary phenomena were constitutional, poisons and exciters affected particular organs more extensively and frequently than others, and thus gave rise to 'specific pathological formations or secretions'.[4]

The analogy with poisons was familiar enough to Farr's

---

[1] See *OED*. In a note Farr stated that the verb and its derived noun were to be found in Hippocrates but were used there in a different sense: *Appendix 1842*, p.120.

[2] *Appendix 1842*, p.93.

[3] At this time it was possible on epidemiological and pathological grounds to ascribe a case of puerperal fever not only to other cases of the same kind but also to erysipelas or any previous 'animal poison' case, including typhus: *Appendix 1843*, pp.187 ff.

[4] Farr, *Appendix 1842*, p.20. 'Exciter' was Liebig's term.

readers, and served more to justify his proceedings than to inspire them. His point of departure was the diseases propagated 'either by inoculation and contact (contagion) or by inhalation (infection)', in which there was a perpetuation of the morbid principle. This was proved by inoculation as in hydrophobia or smallpox. The diseases of this class, said Farr, 'have been frequently spoken of as fermentations; and Liebig has now opened the way to the explanation of their nature by a reference to the phenomena attending the transformations of organic compounds, excited by the action of other compounds simultaneously undergoing analogous transformations'. Farr justified this excursion, which involved supposing the existence not only of the agent, but also that of a corresponding matter in the blood, by finding a 'very similar' theory in the classic English writers, Sydenham, Richard Morton (1637–98), and Thomas Willis (1621–75). All these, he said, had taken the zymotic hypothesis for the basis of their pathology, anticipating Liebig's views to an extent unappreciated by that writer; and yet they were not 'mere chemiatric theorists', but had 'studied diseased action as assiduously, and with as much sagacity, as modern chemists have studied fermentation'. All had extensive clinical experience. Sydenham, according to Farr, based his famous methods of treatment on 'experimental' investigation, and tested them by their results; and yet in his exposition of therapeutic principles he kept his theory of commotion (fermentation) constantly in view. Here Farr was clearly seeking to convince the medical profession firstly, that he was not speculating irresponsibly, secondly, that good practice was related to theory, and thirdly, that medical men had nothing to fear from the chemists, or others who might contribute to the ideal of 'experimental medicine'. Farr completed the case for his own defence with the following:

A single word, such as *Zymotics*, is required to replace in composition the long periphrasis 'epidemic, endemic and contagious diseases'; with a new name and a definition of the kind of pathological process, which the name is intended to indicate, persons who have not made themselves acquainted with the researches of modern chemistry can scarcely fall into the gross error of considering this peculiar kind of diseased action, and vinous fermentation, absolutely identical; or of considering that others entertain that opinion. Liebig draws a distinction between fermentation and putrefaction; the reasons are more urgent for distinguishing the pathological transformations from fermentation and putrefaction, while it is admitted that they are of a chemical nature, and analogous to fermentation; by which they are moreover to a certain extent explained . . .[1]

Liebig's counter-explanations of fermentation were first published in 1839; his views on fermentation and disease in 1840. That Farr had at least noticed the former is perhaps indicated by a passing metaphorical reference to 'acid fermentations' in his first 'letter' or Appendix. During the next year he noted, through the *British and Foreign Medical Review*, Theodor Schwann's and Henle's biological explanations of fermentation.[2] The attraction of Liebig's speculations must have lain partly in his emphasis on general laws and on the applicability of these laws as much to organic and living as to inorganic matter. Farr's receptivity in this regard is indicated in his preparatory statement that 'the human body consists of atoms of various kinds in certain degrees of proximity — in a polarity — and in relative positions — which probably determine the properties of the organism, considered in reference to its various parts and to the external world; from which it is constantly receiving, and to which it is incessantly rendering, its elements'.[3] The apparent vindication offered at the same time by what he saw as Liebig's reformulations of the doctrines of Hippocrates and Sydenham, would also have appealed to Farr, being parallel to his own successes in detecting fixed laws behind Sydenham's observations. Although aware, like Chadwick and Southwood Smith, of the tendency of the medical profession to be soothed by the names of its forefathers, Farr's interest in Sydenham was far more than expedient.

Given Liebig's particular attention to opinion in England, nothing beyond this need be supposed in order to account for Farr's immediate acquaintance with his ideas. None the less, it is, perhaps, worth stressing Farr's interest in normal metabolic physiology as an aspect of the individual and his connections with his family, race, and environment;[4] and,

---

[1] Ibid., pp.120, 122.

[2] *Appendix 1839*, p.65. Farr's notice of Schwann and immediate adoption of Liebig follow very closely the reactions of the *Review*.

[3] *Appendix 1842*, p.112. Farr's state of receptivity probably owed a good deal to Daltonian atomic theory.

[4] Farr's early 'Lectures on Hygeine' were dominated by the theme of racial degeneration. *Appendix 1842* gives space to Liebig's theories of respiration, digestion, etc.

further, Farr's long-standing friendship with Robert Dundas Thomson, nephew of Thomas Thomson, who first studied chemistry under his uncle in Glasgow, and who was working under Liebig at Giessen in 1840. R.D. Thomson conducted research into the food of animals, in particular the chemical aspects of the relationship between selective intake and different animal systems, and established some reputation first in humoral analysis and then in the analysis of airs and waters for sanitary purposes. During the late 1830s he was physician to a London dispensary, lecturer in chemistry at the Blenheim Street medical school (which he had helped to found), and co-editor with Farr of the *British Annals of Medicine*. He also published some work on poisons.[1]

The aetiological (or essential) mode of defining the epidemic, endemic, and contagious diseases removed for Farr as classifier the awkwardness of the fact that such a disease usually showed both constitutional and local effects, that is, was at once of indefinite and definite seat. It also brought a new unity to the group. Each was 'excited by organic matter in a state of pathological transformation'. However, Farr could not allow specificity in the strict or literal sense even for the diseases due to agents reproduced in the body, since he felt obliged to admit the possibility of spontaneous generation.[2] 'Epidemic', 'endemic', and 'contagious' were in part superseded by 'zymotic', and in part given a new meaning related to the hypothetical disease process and to inferred properties of the various exciters. Diseases which were neither contagious nor infectious, like marsh ague and yellow fever, were those in which the exciter was destroyed as soon as it was made. This might have seemed an unnecessary assumption, since such diseases could be simply explained in toxical terms; but Farr, like many of the profession, and unlike Southwood Smith, believed that diseases might be sometimes contagious and sometimes not, and he could use the zymotic hypothesis to explain this by supposing that,

---

[1] For Thomson (1810–64), M.D. Glasgow 1831, F.R.S. 1854, M.R.C.P. 1859, F.R.C.P. 1864, first Medical Officer of Health for St. Marylebone, see *DNB*; J.B. Morrell, 'The Chemist Breeders: The Research Schools of Liebig and Thomas Thomson', *Ambix*, 19 (1972), 1–46: 25 and *passim*.

[2] Farr, *Appendix 1842*, p.120. As *The Lancet* in 1825; and John Snow.

under certain conditions, the fresh exciter was not destroyed or, alternatively, not produced. He therefore explicitly rejected the purely toxical hypothesis.[1]

These pathological explanations, although suggestive, partly avoided and partly begged the questions of the contagiousness of any disease and of its ability suddenly to extend itself. This was in many ways desirable, since it was preferable by this time that discussion should centre on the body rather than on the environment; and the question of epidemic extension was in fact unanswerable. This is, however, to use hindsight. Farr was conscious of the difficult questions left unanswered in abandoning one set of causes for another. He also knew that some diseases did not fit well into his categories. He reserved the important questions of contagion and mode of propagation for inquiry 'when the laws of those epidemic diseases which the registers enable us to investigate, are under discussion', and concluded that 'upon the present occasion it will be sufficient to state that no diseases have been placed in the class which have not been propagated by inoculation, proved to be infectious, or described by good authorities as endemics or epidemics'.[2]

Farr gave some further attention to the problems of propagation with his study of the effects of population density. At the outset, he made a strong defensive statement of his position: 'It is a property of zymotic diseases to prevail more at one time than another; to become epidemic, endemic or contagious in certain circumstances; but as this does not alter their essential nature, they have been invariably classified under the same head.' In 1839, Farr referred without reserve to poisonous atmospheres formed of the gases of exhalation and organic decomposition. By 1843, he had a different view of the influence of insanitary conditions or, more precisely, of the causes of the higher mortality rates of towns. This change was attributable largely to his adoption of the zymotic hypothesis, but Farr first attempted to disprove his earlier view. Thomas Graham's work on the diffusion of gases meant, he said, that a gas like carbonic acid gas would not accumulate

---

[1] *Appendix 1842*, p.121.
[2] Ibid., p.122. The implied discussions never really took place. See also Eyler, 'Farr, An Intellectual Biography', p.148.

in the atmosphere even though produced in great quantities by animal respiration.[1] On the contrary, it dispersed automatically even without the help of air currents, and was eventually fixed by plants. All other gases, including the sulphuretted hydrogen frequently suspected by sanitarians, dispersed in a similar manner and, because produced in lesser quantities, at an even greater rate. This application of Graham's conclusions was justified by the lack of direct evidence of excessive concentrations of the 'sanitary gases'.[2]

Farr therefore concluded that the high mortality of towns was caused not by gases, but by matters suspended in the atmosphere: zymotic matters, since the effects of other sorts of particles were mechanical (for example, abrasive) or localized. Zymotic particles floated in the air, 'forming a morbid atmosphere, the density of which will be in proportion to the proximity of the bodies by which it is given off, and to the greater or less facility for escape'. This was the basis of the long-established importance of ventilation and other practical measures. Such particles did not disperse of themselves, and in a confined space adhered to all exposed surfaces. With regard to their physical and chemical properties, these had, Farr observed, been little investigated by the English; until they were, he was prepared to accept the 'well supported hypothesis' of Professor Graham. This was to the effect that contagious or infectious matters were not likely to be simple volatile substances, but rather, 'highly organised particles of fixed matter' analogous to the pollen of flowers. To the zymotic particles in the air of towns were added the putrid particles given off by the skin and lungs. The proof of this long-standing assumption had been provided by Liebig, who obtained ammonia, a product of the putrefaction of animal matter, in experiments on atmospheric air. Farr's summing up of this position is an excellent example of his own blend

---

[1] *Appendix 1843*, p.179. For Graham (1805–69), of Glasgow and University College London, F.R.S. 1836, Master of the Mint, see *DNB*; *DSB*; Hale Bellot, *University College*, pp.127–30. First paper on gas diffusion, 1829.

[2] These conclusions could have been arrived at earlier; that they were not might argue that Farr in the 1830s gave less attention to sanitary and miasmatic theory, and to this part of chemistry.

of feeling and sanitary science.[1] It would seem that, although like all his contemporaries uncertain of the relationship between putridity and disease, Farr took decomposing organic matter to be either a predisposing cause only or a link in a chain of causation dominated by a zymotic exciter.

Farr went on from this point to establish the density relation already described. This he qualified as being no direct representation of the role of the zymotic atmosphere, since density of population was not a strict measure of the density of this atmosphere, which varied according to a great variety of local conditions for any one situation. Furthermore, the density relation could not, given that the matter of which zymotic atmospheres was formed was a kind of poison, express the relative doses inhaled in a stated time, nor was it in accordance with analogy that mortality should increase in the simple ratio of the dose. The effect of increasing dosage was not fully investigated even for ordinary poisons, but it seemed that there was a range of smaller doses which could be taken with equal impunity, until a level was reached fatal to certain individuals or characteristic of that particular poison. Farr ended, predictably, with an appeal to the chemists for more research.

These early speculations determined the character of Farr's writings for at least fifteen years. Later chapters will show the extent to which Liebigian notions of ferment were current among the profession and elsewhere. Part of the credit for this must be Farr's, for his formulations came early, and in an influential form, however speculative they may have appeared. As we shall see in the next chapter, his special terminology was sometimes resented as an imposition; but criticism also resulted from the increasingly imprecise usage which followed its adoption for practical purposes.

Farr's first report on cholera was not published until 1852, three years after the second epidemic. This presented for the first time in such a case a record of every death, rather than

---

[1] Farr, *Appendix 1843*, pp.206-7. Farr was quoting from Graham's *Elements of Chemistry* (1842), p.282. Note that Farr's own language, being picturesque, can also be misleading. See e.g. *Appendix 1840*, p.16.

simply of those occurring in the worst affected areas.[1] From these data Farr constructed shaded maps of cholera fields, and showed among other things that the disease had followed the same track as in 1832, though with differences in intensity, and that three times as many deaths occurred on the coast as in the interior. The most sophisticated of these generalizations was, of course, that relating to elevation. This Farr placed in the context of some speculation about other diseases, and the moral and physical superiority of races occupying high ground. Over all, his intention was 'to show, independently of the theories, that the conditions in which cholera is or is not fatal may be determined, and yield important practical deductions'. The most significant of the latter was that 'although elevation of habitation, with purity of air and purity of water, does not shut out the cause of cholera, it reduces its effects to insignificance'. The measures recommended by Farr included not only those traditionally designed for avoiding constitutional weakness and miasmata of all kinds, but also the full set of precautions urged by John Snow.[2] Farr relegated Snow to his section on 'Theories and Analogies', but drew out in his discussion of the effects of elevation the obvious relation between that factor and water courses.

The section just referred to included accounts of half a dozen prominent theories of cholera because, Farr said, the conflict of theories often produced useful results; and 'the theorist, however speculative he is, may by tracing . . . analogies, often open the way to a happy generalization, which admits of practical applications, and is the explanation of the facts'.[3] Farr's appreciation of Snow did not alter his adherence to the zymotic hypothesis. Instead of discussing his earlier commitment as if in the light of new data or a new discovery, he merely referred the reader to appropriate portions of the 1842 Appendix. There was, none the less, a broadening of the concept of zymosis more specifically to include environ-

---

[1] From the returns of deaths Farr selected all choleraic and diarrhoeic diseases. All those put down to 'cholera' or 'choleraic diarrhoea' were referred to cholera; those ascribed to any complications of choleraic or diarrhoeic disease struck out; all the rest were counted as diarrhoea, which was taken as a constituent of the epidemic.

[2] Farr, *Report on Cholera Mortality*, p.ci.

[3] Ibid., p.lxxv.

mental factors. The cause of cholera was some 'specific chemical modification of matter', a variety of which was produced in India under certain unfavourable circumstances; this had the property of propagating and multiplying itself in air, water, and food. That cholerine was an organic matter, Farr said, could not be doubted, but 'great questions' remained, for example was cholerine produced in the human organism alone and propagated by external matter? Was it produced and propagated in dead animal or vegetable matter, or mixed effusions of excreta and other matter out of the body? Was it propagated by water, air, contact, or through all these channels? Too little work, he concluded, had been done on these points, although this was, of course, partly owing to the impossibility of experimenting on the human subjects of the disease.

Farr's notion of specificity was again defined by his allowing the idea of 'spontaneous development' of cholera: there were some facts which importation could not explain. However, he was more inclined to resort to some predisposing cause which had operated on the population since 1836, producing the progressive increase of diarrhoeal affections observed since that date. Any 'cholerine' added to this promising state of affairs could be expected to produce cholera on an epidemic scale.

Farr's later work, especially his report on the cholera epidemic of 1866 (published in 1868), and his activities in connection with the cattle plague, also of 1865-6, is of great interest, especially for its adaptation of his earlier ideas according to changes in theoretical context; but this phase of his life has received much stress elsewhere, and does not fall within the period of interest of this book.[1] Further attention will, however, be given to Farr in the chapter on John Snow.

It is Farr's consciously and conformably scientific approach, and his interest in pathology and process, which separate his work from that of Chadwick and Southwood Smith in the later period. A third and related characteristic is his sensitivity to the feelings and prejudices of the profession. When Farr

---

[1] See especially J. Brownlee, 'Historical Note on Farr's Theory of the Epidemic', *Br. Med. J.* 1915, ii. 250–2, and Eyler, 'Farr, An Intellectual Biography'. The latter perhaps overstates the interest of some later developments.

and Chadwick or Smith wrote upon the same points, Farr was markedly more conciliatory.[1] In other respects, Farr is identifiable with the profession, or at least with its van — in his contingent contagionism, his respect for the specificity of disease, and his combination of chemico-medical theory and sanitary practice.

In view of the structure of his career, and in spite of his own opinion of the qualifications required for his position, it cannot be said that Farr was ever part of the medical profession, but he regularly showed signs of wishing that he were so. It was not the closed world of the London physician that attracted him, but the liberal-minded, structured merit-ocracy aimed at by most of the reformers of the 1830s.[2] He was friendly with Wakley and Forbes, both of whom edited journals (*The Lancet* and the *British and Foreign Medical Review* respectively) which campaigned for reform, and was involved in the short-lived 'British Medical Association' of the same period. He felt a proprietary concern for medical ethics or morality, and took, as shown by his knowledge of Sydenham's period, a more than antiquarian interest in the history of the profession. Like Chadwick, he rejected Malthusian doctrines, but he placed more stress than Chadwick on the effectiveness of medicine in prolonging the mean dur-ation of life. Medical men were, past, present, and future, the guardians of public as of private health. 'Sanative' rules and habits (by which Farr meant the mode in which the individual managed his own and his family's health) were, where they existed at all, those inculcated by a previous generation of medical men, and had as yet been little mitigated by the praiseworthy efforts of the present generation, Southwood Smith, Andrew Combe, and others, to acquaint the population with the laws governing their own bodies. Governments could do little by direct enactments for the diminution of sick-ness, but public health could be promoted by changes in the national education, in medical education and the manner of remunerating medical men, and by 'placing the medical institutions of the country on a liberal scientific basis'. That

---

[1] See e.g. Farr on the need for medical statistics, *Appendix 1839*, pp.63–4.
[2] Farr, 'Medical Reform', *Lancet*, 1839–40, i. 110.

Farr identified with the often purely professional interests of medical practitioners is best illustrated by his taking that side with respect to their employment under the new Poor Law.[1]

In its theoretical aspect, Farr's approach may usefully be compared with that of Edmund Parkes. His views were concerned with, and originated in, a consideration of disease in the individual as well as in the group; and, in the meantime, his sanitarianism was of the classical kind, which saw environmental factors as combining in no particular order to undermine the constitution. His position and opportunities were unique, but his dependence on the universality of natural law, and on statistical evidence as the most reliable basis for the elucidation of such laws, was typical of his generation of laymen and medical men alike.

[1] Farr, *Appendix 1843*, p.186; idem, 'Vital Statistics', p.601; idem, 'Medical Reform', pp.105–6.

4

MORBID POISONS AND PROCESS:
JUSTUS LIEBIG

I

In the previous chapter, two analogies were introduced: the one relating disease to the action of poisons, and the other, to fermentation. Each has a long history, and a special currency in the period under discussion. Each seems to imply the designation of a specific and material agent occupying a position among the conditions regarded as causing disease, strictly parallel to that of organisms in the modern theory. This chapter will indicate how far these ideas should be thought of as preparatory in this way. The main contention will be that the fermentation analogy which became dominant in the 1840s was adopted because it offered not a chance of identifying, but a notion of the process brought about by, the agent or agents of disease.[1] As already indicated in relation to Farr, we come in discussing these analogies closer to the interests of the profession as distinct from the doctrines of the sanitarians.

It is difficult to imagine a time at which comparisons were not drawn between poisons and the (hypothetical) agents of disease, and the content of this analogy therefore varies according to context.[2] Since it was always an obvious analogy on empirical grounds alone, its terms could be used familiarly, without implying very much. In the nineteenth century 'morbid poison' was used like an algebraic expression in some arguments, just as 'epidemic influence', or 'epidemic atmosphere',

---

[1] Cf. e.g. R.H. Shryock, *The Development of Modern Medicine* (Philadelphia, 1936), p.267.

[2] L.G. Stevenson, *The Meaning of Poison*, Logan Clendening Lectures, 7th series (Lawrence, Kansas, 1959), depends heavily on A.R. McIntyre, *Curare* (Chicago, 1947). For toxicology in its philosophical aspect, with stress on its 'most intimate connexion' with both 'the science and art' of medicine, see W.B. Carpenter, 'Taylor and Copland on Poisons', *Br. For. Med. Chir. Rev.* 2 (1848), 172–201. See also A.W. Blyth, *Poisons* (1884); Earles, 'Early Theories of Action of Poisons'.

was in others. Even with a new equivocal disease like cholera it was possible to apply the analogy in a commonsense kind of way. As Thomas Michael Greenhow of Newcastle wrote in 1849: 'if by the term poison is intended to be expressed matter, whether solid liquid or aerial, which being received into the human system produces morbid actions or suspends vital functions, then the physical cause of cholera must be poison'.[1] Shades of usage have already been found in Southwood Smith.

As the reaction to the General Board of Health's Quarantine Report showed, the inclination of the profession in England was, by 1845, towards some sort of specificity in disease. This was owing partly to pragmatism and an ingrained respect for clinical observation, and partly (among the more than practical practitioners) to their own work in pathological anatomy. It was, of course, possible to explain specific diseases physiologically, without supposing the entrance into the body of some deleterious material.[2] But once an epidemic disease was allowed to be specific, it was natural to relate it more closely to those diseases which had always been so regarded. Of this group smallpox was the definitive member; and as already indicated, this disease appeared, almost regardless of theoretical context, to be the result of the reception into the body of a *materies morbi* and the subsequent resolution and elimination of a material capable of producing identical effects. Parkes assumed that 'cholera, like other epidemic and contagious diseases, must result from the action of a specific agent, rather than any temporary combination of atmospheric influences'. He then set out to determine the source of the 'poison', arguing of necessity from what were taken to be its effects: that is, the behaviour of cholera in the field as well as its pathology. Persons attempting this approach were encouraged by the analogy of smallpox because the nature of the disease had been inferred in the same way, without direct demonstration of the agent.[3] However, the

---

[1] Quoted in *Braithwaite*, 20 (1849), 412. In cholera, in particular, the analogy was directly suggested by the gastrointestinal character of the disease and by the sudden onset and rapid progress of the symptoms.

[2] As e.g. cholera was explained by R.D. Thomson: *Lancet*, 1850, i. 154–5.

[3] Parkes, 'Inquiry', p.251 n.

range of environmental and personal factors determining the behaviour of a disease like cholera seemed so wide that the tasks bore little relation to each other in practice. A less straightforward approach, and one more likely to reveal something of the pathology of such diseases, was to turn from mere terminology to the bases of the poison analogy; that is, to argue analogically from what was known of the nature and effects of true poisons.

The notion of specific poisons in disease was, in the nineteenth century, often ascribed to Giovanni Maria Lancisi (1654–1720), but Lancisi's agent was envisaged only for endemic fevers or agues, and was of exclusively vegetable origin (whence 'paludal poison'). The term 'morbid poison' was applied primarily to the 'increasing' agents of contagious diseases.[1] Its usage in the nineteenth century was probably promoted by the definition of John Hunter, whose views in this connection were amplified, developed, and publicized after his death by his pupil Joseph Adams.[2]

Hunter's interest in defining morbid poisons was probably in part a reflection of his resistance to the then common notion that the blood was a passive material, constantly tending to putrefaction.[3] He distinguished morbid from the known vegetable and mineral poisons, and also, though not so completely, from the 'natural' poisons produced by animals, such as venoms.[4] Hunter imagined that the blood became tainted, that any products of the blood could transmit the poison, and with it, the power of poisoning others. His emphasis was on pathology, rather than epidemiology; he divided 'the manner of receiving and the manner of being affected by' morbid poisons, into 'simple', and 'compound', terms which his disciple Adams replaced by 'contagious' and 'infectious'.[5]

---

[1] Simon, Lecture XII, *Lancet*, 1850, ii. 227. But cf. Carpenter, 'Taylor and Copland on Poisons', pp.196–7.

[2] For Adams (1756–1818), M.D. by diploma, Aberdeen 1796; Extra-L.R.C.P. 1796, physician to Smallpox Hospital, 1805, L.R.C.P. 1809, see *Munk*; *DNB*.

[3] J. Adams, *Memoirs of Hunter* (1817), pp.83–4; idem, *Observations on Morbid Poisons* (1807), p.6. For Hunter on morbid poisons, see Ch. 23 of his lectures on the principles of surgery as given in the *Works* (1837), i, especially pp.611–17. See also Ch. 9, ibid., pp.299–316.

[4] See Adams, *Observations on Morbid Poisons*, p.8.

[5] Hunter, *Works*, i. 313, 616; Adams, *Observations on Morbid Poisons*, p.6.

Hunter's notion of morbid poison derived less from the effects of poisons like arsenic and more from the fact that some animals manufactured poisons of their own. Other authors, however, later in the century, based their assumptions on the work of toxicologists such as Robert Christison of Edinburgh. The great interest in toxicology evident in the early nineteenth century, of which Christison's treatise of 1829 may be regarded as the most successful product, was a popular as well as scientific phenomenon, with forensic toxicology forming the ground in common.

Christison's approach was justifiably pragmatic, and he purposely avoided giving any definition of poison. Similarly, he found no system of classification satisfactory, but settled for a modified version of Orfila's categorization according to human symptoms.[1] He was much impressed by the new theories of absorption, but since he wished to preserve the doctrine of the 'sympathetic operation' of certain quick-acting poisons, he still maintained that these agents could bring about local impressions through a purely nervous mode of communication. The debate over the means of transmission of poisonous influence continued, as one reflection of major developments in physiology. By the middle of the century, consistently with the 'new humoralism', the circulatory system was thought to act almost to the exclusion of the nervous.[2] On morbid poisons, Christison remarked that these were usually excluded from works on toxicology; but he dealt briefly with the poisons (nature unknown) formed by putrefaction in food and in the body after death, which did not produce specific effects like the poison of smallpox, but which seemed capable of producing a general febrile state.[3] This, he thought, clearly had some bearing on the apparent

---

[1] Christison, *Life of Christison* (1885–6), ii. 168. For a self-evident discussion of the difficulties of definition, see Hunter, *Works*, i. 611 ff. Christison regarded Mathieu Orfila (1787–1853) as the founder of systematic toxicology. Orfila's major work was *Toxicologie générale* (1813–15; 5th edn., 1852); his chief contribution was to locate poisons in organs other than the stomach. See Blyth, *Poisons*, p.16. Classification was still difficult in the 1880s: ibid., p.24.

[2] Christison, *Treatise on Poisons* (1829), p.5; *Rep. of 4th Meeting of British Association* (1835), pp.xxxviii–xxxix; Carpenter, 'Taylor and Copland on Poisons', p.176.

[3] In this connection the reference was as usual to the experiments of Gaspard and Magendie.

tendency of putrid effluvia to engender epidemic fevers in man.

Christison's work was extensively quoted in the most detailed and systematic treatment of the analogy between poisons, and the agents of epidemic disease to appear at this time. Robert Williams's intention in *Morbid Poisons* (1836–41) was avowedly practical and non-speculative; his procedure was to show that the varied details of the behaviour of epidemic disease could be made to fall under the established laws governing the behaviour of poisons generally.[1] The most important of these common laws was that all poisons had certain 'definite and specific' actions. Secondly, all poisons lay latent in the system for a period of time, the length of which was characteristic of each, before those actions were set up; thirdly, the phenomena resulting from the poison when roused into action varied according to the dose and the predisposition of the patient. Two more minor laws were, that the specification of the poison depended on the affinity existing between the liquids and the solids of certain parts of the organism and the poison ingested; and that this specific action ceased on the elimination of the poison from the system.

On the face of it, this would seem to have been a procedure of some promise, but Williams was able to justify all his laws without going beyond what was gained by accepting the implications of the phenomena of smallpox. He was, indeed, ascribing the whole spectrum of diseases from smallpox to ague, to a single class of agents, but this was achieved simply by arguing that all diseases were like smallpox in showing constant clinical appearances. Moreover, in attributing both ague and smallpox to a morbid poison, Williams was merely creating a class of substances which incorporated, respectively, both a substance which was a product of vegetable decomposition, and a substance which was apparently produced only by the human body. Whether or not this was justifiable become a real question rather later, when it was given some

---

[1] For Williams (d. 1845), M.D. Cantab. 1816, F.R.C.P. 1817, President of the Royal Medical and Chirurgical Society in 1841 and 1842, see *Munk*; *DNB*; his friend W.F. Chambers in *Lancet*, 1846, i. 291; 'B.G.', ibid. 1842–3, i. 759–60. Cf. Baas, *Outlines of Medical History*, ii. 911, on the introduction of potassium iodide.

basis by developments in organic chemistry. It arose particularly in relation to the belief in contingent contagionism, although it did not occur to every holder of that belief. There was no reference to the known properties of poisons in Williams's treatment of the question. The book ended in defining not disease agents, but regularities of behaviour and of morbid appearances; hence its usefulness to the discerning reader.

The laws of poisons, Williams stated, were more important than their *modus operandi*. He did, however, give their mode of action some consideration in view of recent research, and here the analogy was operative. He assumed that the experiments of Magendie and others showing the absorption of poisons by the blood and the relative contributions of the circulatory and nervous systems in the transmission of the poisonous influence, applied directly to the morbid poisons also; and the detection of substances like alcohol and iodine in the blood and secretions added conviction to other experiments in which a diseased state was produced in one animal using blood and other matters from another specifically diseased, and in which no specific matter was ever demonstrated. Although the most obvious implication of an analogy drawn between the effects of poisons and morbid poisons was that the latter also consisted of chemical substances in principle detectable, Williams placed no emphasis on this.

Finally, it should be said that while poisons as then known appeared to have few or no properties over and above those also possessed by morbid poisons, the latter, as Williams recognized, had certain characteristics 'wholly unknown' to medicinal and poisonous substances. The first of these was that in diseases like smallpox the effects produced did not appear to be related to the dosage, since the most diluted smallpox matter was as likely to produce a severe case as a mild one. A second peculiar law of morbid poisons, Williams said, was 'the faculty which the human body possesses of generating to an enormous extent a poison of the same nature as that by which the disease was originally produced'.[1] Thirdly, and even more remarkably, many morbid poisons 'possess the

---

[1] Williams, *Morbid Poisons* (1836–41), i. 13.

extraordinary property of exhausting all future susceptibility, in the constitution of the party affected, to any similar action of the same poison'. Lastly, the intensity and specific action of some of them could be modified by climatic conditions.

With respect to reactions to Williams's work, it may be remarked of it as of theories of disease causation in general, that to many medical men of the period any such systematic exercise was dubious, and to few of them would *Morbid Poisons* have appeared as other than armchair reading.[1] This meant, not so much that Williams's work was seldom read, but that its relation to daily professional life and practice was thought of as limited. That Budd was aware of the tendency of his contemporaries to segregate the theoretical and the practical, is shown by his insistence on the practical implications of his own speculative views. As it happened, the greater part of Williams's book was as little speculative as he had claimed; so that John Simon, who greatly admired it, could recommend it to his pupils as 'occupying the highest rank in the practical literature of this country'.[2] For present purposes it is relevant as having set out in full and deliberately, the resources that Williams's contemporaries used piecemeal and often without regard for their logical implications. It is also a demonstration of the lesser emphasis placed at the time on those aspects of causation given first priority by modern readers.

The impression should not be given that the poison analogy was a resource the usefulness of which was exhausted by the middle of the century. Part of Williams's difficulty was that he was writing in the middle, rather than towards the end, of a period of enthusiastic investigation into the action of poisons, and before that investigation could be assisted by the period of most rapid advance in organic and inorganic chemistry. W.B. Carpenter, who was also interested in the poison analogy, could consequently maintain at the end of the decade, in 1848, that Williams's treatise was 'a work of

---

[1] For a dubious reaction, see *Br. For. Med. Rev.* 13 (1842), 89.

[2] Simon, Lecture XII, *Lancet*, 1850, ii. 227. Williams's work was also appreciated by Watson (*Principles and Practice of Physic*, ii, 713); William Baly (in his Gulstonian lectures on dysentery, 1847); W.A. Guy (*Public Health*, 1870–4, Pt.I, p.107); etc.

sterling merit', in advance of its time, which had 'to a very remarkable degree anticipated the pathological views now prevalent'. Work on poisons was never easy. One of the problems given much space by Carpenter, was the lack of relation which modern research had revealed between the ordinary physical and chemical properties of substances, and their action on the body.[1]

The application of the poison analogy suggested rather little about the nature or mode of action of the so-called morbid poisons, but it did isolate those facts likely to prove most difficult to explain in chemical terms, and which nevertheless had to be accounted for if such an explanation was to prove acceptable. This feat was accomplished in the early 1840s by Liebig, who explained the disease process in terms of fermentation, and fermentation, putrefaction, and decay in terms of a mode of change characteristic of organic molecules. Liebig's aim was to establish both for these organic processes and for other actions called catalytic an explanation in terms of the basic properties of matter. By doing this he hoped to demolish first, those explanations which referred to the alleged peculiar properties of living matter, which Liebig considered to be no explanations at all; and second, that view of catalysis, developed by Berzelius, which posited as its agent a specific catalytic force.[2]

These explanations were an important part of the conspicuous contribution made by Liebig to the advent and development of organic chemistry at this period. His view of catalysis was consistent with his over-all approach, which asserted the continuity, in real chemical terms, of organic matter. This basic premiss was most acceptably demonstrated to his contemporaries by his explanation of how the food of animals was elaborated from elementary constituents by plants. The processes of excretion and decomposition could be added to complete the cycle.

There were, Liebig claimed, compounds so unstable that changes in temperature and electrical condition, or friction, or contact with bodies of apparently totally different natures,

---

[1] Carpenter, 'Taylor and Copland on Poisons', pp.197, 181 ff.

[2] Graham, *Elements of Chemistry*, pp.195, 723; J.R. Partington, *A History of Chemistry*, 4 vols. (1961–70), iv. 261 ff.

caused such a disturbance in the attraction between their constituents that the latter entered into new forms, without combining with the acting body or catalyst. Organic molecules were unstable because they were large, and therefore prone to such forms of decomposition, three of which were fermentation, putrefaction, and decay. Putrefaction occurred spontaneously in nitrogenous substances in the presence of water, by the impingement of oxygen molecules. After an initial exposure, air was no longer necessary. Liebig gave this definition: 'All those processes of decomposition which begin in a part of an organic substance from the application of an external cause, and which spread through the whole mass, with or without the co-operation of that cause, have been called processes of putrefaction.' The constituents of a putrefying animal or vegetable product arranged themselves in compounds according to their natural affinities, in place of the uneasy alliance imposed upon them in the organism by Liebig's vital principle. Since organic molecules could be disrupted by motion being imparted to their particles, it followed that before this event, and in the absence of the vital principle, the stability of such molecules was due to inertia.

If mechanical motion was enough to cause change, one body in motion could effect change on another; as according to what Liebig called the law of Claude Louis Berthollet and Pierre Simon de La Place, only recently applied to chemistry: 'A molecule set in motion by any power can impart its own motion to another molecule with which it may be in contact'.[1] It was a very remarkable fact, said Liebig, that very small quantities of organic matter in a state of putrefaction possessed the power of causing unlimited quantities of similar matters to pass into the same state: for example, a spot of fermenting grape juice, when added to inert grape juice, fermented the whole mass, and the same thing happened when putrefying blood was added to fresh blood. The type of all fermentations was that effected by yeast, which Liebig asserted was not a self-multiplying vegetable organism as

---

[1] Liebig, *Organic Chemistry* (1842), p.365; Partington, *History of Chemistry*, iv. 302.

Cagniard La Tour, Schwann, and Kützing had claimed, but a nitrogenous substance, derived from the vegetable product gluten, which underwent decomposition or putrefaction on its own account following an initial exposure to air. When added to a solution of sugar, a non-putrescible substance, the molecules of yeast imparted 'intestine motion' to those of the sugar, causing it to decompose according to the natural affinities of its particles into alcohol and carbonic acid gas. This reaction ended in the disappearance of both substances, unless one was in excess. Liebig stated:

Yeast produces fermentation in consequence of the progressive decomposition it suffers from the action of air and water ... during the fermentation of sugar by yeast, both of these substances suffer decomposition at the same time and disappear in consequence. But if yeast be a body which excites fermentation by being itself in a state of decomposition, all other matters in the same condition should have a similar reaction on sugar, and this is in reality the case ... Yeast and putrefying animal and vegetable matters act as peroxide of hydrogen does on oxide of silver, when they induce bodies with which they are in contact to enter into the same state of decomposition ...[1]

But if a substance related to yeast were added, such as gluten, new yeast was formed from it by the action of the particles of the old yeast upon its similar constituents; and the new yeast continued in its turn to bring about the decomposition of the sugar. However, there was mutual action, since after the old yeast had declined, the continued production of yeast was dependent upon the decomposition of the sugar; for in cases where the sugar had completely disappeared, any gluten which remained did not suffer change from contact with the new yeast, but retained all the characters of gluten. The new yeast did not become active until nudged by oxygen. After this explanation, Liebig concluded, the idea that yeast reproduced itself as seeds reproduced seeds, could not for a moment be entertained.[2]

He then went on to relate these explanations to effects on the body. There were, he said, many compounds from inorganic nature and from animals and vegetables that produced peculiar changes or diseases in living beings. He outlined a

---

[1] *Organic Chemistry* (1840), quoted in *Harvard Case Studies in Experimental Science*, ed. J. Conant, 2 vols. (Camb., Mass., 1957), ii. 461.
[2] *Organic Chemistry*, p.366.

scale of activity, in which poisons came last after nutrients and medicines. These categories referred to processes rather than to substances, since most substances could be included in more than one category according to the effects of quantity or to the intensity of their actions. The action of inorganic substances was easily explained; they either 'destroyed the continuity' of particular organs, as did sulphuric acid, or they operated chemically by forming more or less stable combinations with constituents of the body. There was, however, 'a class of substances generated during certain processes of decomposition, which acted on the animal economy as deadly poisons, not on account of their power of entering into combinations with it, or by reason of their containing a poisonous material, but solely by virtue of their peculiar condition'. Clearly, the poison of ill-cooked Würtemberg sausages, the effluvia from decaying organic matter, pus, and similar substances could all be assumed to be in a state of putrefaction, and therefore capable, even in very small amounts, of inducing change in the constituents of the blood and body. This corresponded to the reaction of sugar solution and yeast in the absence of gluten. The specific contagious diseases, in which there was an increase of morbid material, were comparable to the same process when gluten was present. Liebig gave the theory of this process as follows:

. . . a body in the act of decomposition (it may be named the *exciter*), added to a mixed fluid in which its constituents are contained, can reproduce itself in that fluid, exactly in the same manner as new yeast is produced when yeast is added to liquids containing gluten. This must be more certainly effected when the liquid acted on contains the body by the metamorphosis of which the *exciter* has been originally formed. It is also obvious, that if the *exciter* be able to impart its own state of transformation to one only of the component parts of the mixed liquid acted upon, its own reproduction may be the consequence of the decomposition of this one body.[1]

Among Liebig's major ambitions was the formation into a completed cycle of the scattered observations and theories concerning the material exchanges which took place between the organism and its environment.[2] One condition of this

[1] Ibid., pp.364, 366–7.
[2] See F.L. Holmes, 'Elementary Analysis and the Origins of Physiological Chemistry', *Isis*, 54 (1963), 50–81.

attempt was his view of the blood as a highly complex matter uniquely susceptible to change; so that (for example) each organ might attract from the blood the elements necessary for its function and maintenance. From this it followed that the molecules of the blood would be particularly vulnerable to the motions of the molecules of decomposing matters (including contagions) whose constituents had once been part of the blood, or which had actually been formed in the blood.

An obvious and important implication of Liebig's explanation of contagious diseases was that there were at least two peculiar constituents of the blood corresponding to the sugar and the gluten, one of which was exhausted to produce immunity. Since little was known about the waste matters in the blood, Liebig was able to make inferences which no one was then in a position to disprove; for example, susceptibility to some contagious diseases was highest in childhood, and Liebig supposed this to be due to the presence in the blood of wastes from the growth processes unique to that period of life.[1] In any case, Liebig did not think it necessary to postulate matters greatly different from the known constituents of the blood, since the properties of an organic compound could differ a great deal simply according to the arrangement of its atoms.

Ancillary evidence for Liebig's view of disease came from the knowledge that putrefaction, fermentation, and 'morbid' matters were affected by disinfectants or oxidizers, although the effects of these inside the body were less predictable. Some infective matters also appeared to decompose and lose virulence in the presence of moisture and air; and the incidence of the non-contagious diseases appeared to depend upon conditions of temperature and humidity. It will be remembered that for Liebig morbid viruses were by definition in the act of decomposition; this process went on to completion in the presence of water and oxygen. Lastly, Claude Bernard was reported as having produced a supposed state of fermentation in the blood experimentally. There were, however, as many negative as positive results of this kind.[2]

---

[1] *Organic Chemistry*, p.385.

[2] *Br. For. Med. Chir. Rev.* 4 (1849), 153. Bernard thought of fermentation as a process of organic destruction, and as extracellular: J.M.D. Olmsted, *Claude Bernard Physiologist* (1939), Ch. 17.

Two of the phenomena of contagious diseases that distinguished their hypothetical agents from the ordinary poisons, were the increase in the agent and the immunity which folowed an attack. We have seen that in Liebig's theory one was dependent on the other. Liebig had no difficulty in explaining the continual replacement of the so-called exciter in the disease process, but he was forced to attribute its over-all increase to a slower rate of decomposition compared with that taking place in the other constituents of the blood.[1] The over-all increase was, therefore, a subsidiary rather than a primary phenomenon, although it was in principle possible in all forms of fermentation.

Liebig was not interested in deciding questions of the specificity or contagiousness of various diseases. He took for granted the general categories of 'poison, contagion and miasm', and might not have dealt with these concepts at all, if others had not sought to explain fermentation and putrefaction 'vitalistically', and subsequently to exploit the long-standing analogy between these processes and disease, in order to explain epidemic diseases in the same way.[2] To imagine that life itself constituted a sufficient explanation of these phenomena was to Liebig as stultifying as to think that bodily processes could not be explained in chemical terms because they took place in a living organism. A second motive was his desire to demonstrate the scope or universality of his principle of 'contagious molecular action' (a demonstration which for Liebig would go far towards establishing the validity of that principle), and to show that his vital force belonged to the same, accessible class as the chemical forces. Both motives served the ideal of 'Newtonianism', which for Liebig meant that effects were not to be referred merely to like causes, but rather to laws comprehending a wide range of phenomena.[3]

II

Liebig took up chemistry on his own initiative, although he eventually received financial assistance from his father and

---

[1] Liebig, *Organic Chemistry*, p.384.
[2] Liebig, *Animal Chemistry* (1846), p.212.
[3] Ibid., p.189. For Liebig on method, see ibid., pp.157 ff.

from the Grand Duke of Hesse.[1] In Paris he was discovered by von Humboldt, became the only pupil of Gay-Lussac, and joined forces with Wöhler and Dumas. On his return to Germany he was installed by the Grand Duke, against some local opposition, as extraordinary (or 'assistant' — *ausserordentlicher*) professor of chemistry at the small University of Giessen. By 1825, he had set up a teaching laboratory which was to serve as a model for Britain and the rest of Europe.[2] His first years were spent in teaching and in the evolution of the first simple and rapid techniques of organic analysis. Many of his research results were published in his own *Annalen der Pharmacie*, founded in 1832. By 1837, his international reputation was such that he was invited by Thomas Thomson and the British Association for the Advancement of Science to deliver at the Liverpool meeting of the Association a report on the state of organic chemistry. In 1840, the first part of this report was published (in English and German) as *Organic Chemistry in its Applications to Agriculture and Physiology*. At about this time Liebig abruptly switched part of his interest to biochemistry and physiology, and as a result produced, as the second part of his report, *Animal Chemistry, or Chemistry in its Applications to Physiology and Pathology* (1842).[3]

From the first Liebig had felt a mission towards the practical applications and benefits of chemistry, and his energies became increasingly involved in the reform of agriculture and

---

[1] Justus von Liebig (1803–73), Ph.D. Erlangen, M.D. Giessen (hon.), Corresp. F.R.S., was b. Darmstadt. For biography see *DSB*; J. Volhard, *Justus von Liebig*, 2 vols. (Leipzig, 1909); W.A. Shenstone, *Liebig, His Life and Work* (1895). For a bibliography, see C. Paoloni, *Justus von Liebig. Eine Bibliographie sämtlicher Veröffentlichungen* (Heidelberg, 1968). For contemporary reactions see A.W. Hofmann, *Life-Work of Liebig* (1876); J.L.W. Thudichum, 'On the Discoveries and Philosophy of Liebig', *J. Soc. Arts*, 24 (1875–6); M. von Pettenkofer, 'Liebig's Scientific Achievements', *Contemporary Review*, 29 (1877), 865–87. For recent assessments of his contribution to physiology, see *Animal Chemistry*, ed. F.L. Holmes (1964); G.J. Goodfield, *The Growth of Scientific Physiology* (1960). On Liebig and agriculture, see F.R. Moulton (ed.), *Liebig and After Liebig* (Philadelphia, 1942).

[2] Morrell, 'The Chemist Breeders', pp.32–3. On practical instruction in chemistry, see also W.A. Smeaton, 'The Early History of Laboratory Instruction in Chemistry at the École Polytechnique, Paris, and Elsewhere', *Ann. Sci.* 10 (1954), 224–33; Pettenkofer, 'Liebig's Scientific Achievements', p.873.

[3] Cf. Holmes, 'Elementary Analysis and Physiological Chemistry', pp.73–4.

dietetics and the advancement of German industry.[1] Agriculture (British as well as German) received the greatest part of his attention. He took a related interest in scientific education, and his success as a popularizer and teacher was prodigious. His best-known popular work, *Familiar Letters on Chemistry*, reached thirteen editions in eight languages between 1843 and 1850.[2]

In 1845 he was created a hereditary baron, and in 1852 moved to Munich at the request (conveyed to him by Max von Pettenkofer) of the King of Bavaria. There he lectured, but took no more laboratory pupils. He became the associate of Pettenkofer, Karl Thiersch, and others, and figured as a member of the group sometimes referred to by English physicians as the 'Munich chemists'. While at Munich, however, Liebig took rather more interest in medicine and animal physiology.[3]

His character was a determining factor in the reception of his work. He was exceedingly energetic; dedicated, but impulsive; warm, yet forbidding; generous, yet resentful. A similar dichotomy, between varieties of speculation and analysis, may be seen in his methods of working. He was also his own best publicist, but in defending his views he often alienated even his supporters.

Liebig's ties with Britain were many.[4] His influence there may be seen as part or a reflection of the general impression which German thought and institutions were then making on the British, but the relationship as well as being a reciprocal was also a personal one. Liebig visited Britain three times after 1837 (1842, 1844, 1845); he was the friend as well as the admirer of Michael Faraday (with whom he was compared by English writers); and the majority of his foreign

---

[1] This did not mean for Liebig an interest in applied rather than pure science. See his 'Lord Bacon as Natural Philosopher', *Macmillan's Magazine*, 8 (1863), 261 ff.

[2] Liebig took great care over the *Familiar Letters*: see H.E. Roscoe, 'Justus Liebig', *Nature*, 8 (1873), 28.

[3] L.F. Haber, *The Chemical Industry During the Nineteenth Century* (Oxford, 1969), p.67.

[4] For Liebig himself on his feeling for England, see his 'Was Lord Bacon an Impostor?', *Fraser's Magazine*, 75 (1867), 484 ff.

students were British.[1] Most of these students became ardently loyal to Liebig and his ideas, and formed, on their return to Britain, a most efficient propaganda machine. They translated his works, which from 1840 appeared in England almost as soon as they did in Germany, and wrote works of their own in his support. Liebig himself edited and contributed largely to several editions of *Turner's Elements of Chemistry*. His most indefatigable disciple and editor in Britain was William Gregory, professor of chemistry and medicine at Aberdeen; his best representative was August Wilhelm von Hofmann, his relation by marriage as well as his pupil, and a man of winning personality. During his twenty years in England (1845–65), Hofmann taught not only British but German students.[2] Liebig's closest contacts were probably with members of the British Association, but he was also (for example) a corresponding fellow of the Royal Society, and an honorary member of the Manchester Literary and Philosophical Society. Although Liebig's adjutants in Britain were often men of scientific training (for example, Lyon Playfair), his efforts at conversion were directed as much, if not more, at manufacturers and landowners, and the wider relevance of his work was appreciated by economists and prominent laymen with interests in socio-economic questions. Some idea of his celebrity in Britain may be obtained from an account in *The Lancet* of a great dinner in his honour in Glasgow at which he was given the freedom of the city. One of the tributes to the guest of honour came from the clergy, who praised him for providing ways of increasing the means of subsistence to meet the increase in population. A more personal reaction is that of William Budd, who met him in 1842, and later wrote an account of it to his brother:

... Don't you envy me? He is a charming fellow. Quite a young man

---

[1] Liebig's last visit coincided with the failure, on religious grounds, of his candidature for the professorship of chemistry at King's College, London: T. Holmes, *Sir Benjamin Collins Brodie* (1898), pp.79, 232–4. For his British pupils, see Roscoe, 'Justus Liebig', p.27; Morrell, 'The Chemist Breeders'; and cf. Haber, *The Chemical Industry*, p.75.

[2] Hofmann (1818–92) was encouraged to come to England by the Prince Consort and James Clark, who were instrumental in founding the (Royal) College of Chemistry. In addition to *DSB*, see J. Bentley, 'Hofmann's Return to Germany from the Royal College of Chemistry', *Ambix*, 19 (1972), 197–203.

— not over 37 — like myself, a very lean creature . . . Thoroughly impregnated with tobacco as all other Germans. — I had him to myself for nearly four hours. In that time we went through the whole range of his own topics. You may fancy how intensely interesting and improving the conversation was for me — I left him having a higher opinion than ever of his profound talent . . .

The popular appeal of Liebig's explanations was manifested in the sale of little 'aquaria', called 'Liebig's World in a Glass Case'. These illustrated the 'simple rotation of matter in animated nature'.[1]

Later in life Liebig offended English opinion by mounting a full-scale attack on Francis Bacon, criticizing both the place given to him in history and the methods adopted in his name by Liebig's contemporaries. This took place after Liebig had become exasperated by his disputes with English agriculturists. Some time earlier he had stated to Faraday that Germans were only theoretical, the English only practical.[2] Liebig's wish was to redress the balance in each case, since he believed as strongly in the (Baconian) notion that science should improve the quality of man's lot, as in the necessity for pure science.

To the medical profession Liebig was at first known only as a chemist. Few of his British pupils, whatever their early training, became other than professional chemists. The *British and Foreign Medical Review* seemed almost to introduce him to its readers before reviewing *Organic Chemistry*, which it found a very striking piece of work. With *Animal Chemistry*, however, Liebig achieved an instant notoriety. Medical men were both appalled and exhilarated by the simplicity and breadth of his interpretations of physiological phenomena. Members of the Royal Medical and Chirurgical Society discussed at length a paper on his views, before arguing over the propriety of presenting a paper about 'peculiar doctrines which were not, in fact, before the society'. *The Lancet* adopted him, hailing him as 'a man of a century'. This journal had already given some indication of its attitude: in a

---

[1] *Lancet*, 1844, ii. 170; Budd Papers, William to Richard [5 Sept. 1842]; Pettenkofer, 'Liebig's Scientific Achievements', p.877.

[2] Shenstone, *Liebig, His Life and Work*, p.201. As usual, the 'English geniuses' were excepted from this. The philosopher to whom Liebig explicitly avowed allegiance was John Stuart Mill: *Animal Chemistry*, Author's Preface; 'Was Lord Bacon an Impostor?', p.484.

review of two earlier works by Liebig it had stated that 'there is far more chemistry in medicine, — there is far more of exact science in medicine, than physicians are inclined to believe'. This may be seen as part of the journal's general stand on medical reform and the deficiencies of existing forms of medical education.[1] *The Lancet* published in 1842 and 1843 a series of lectures by Henry Ancell, explaining Liebig's views, and in the following year, a series adapted from his own course of instruction by Liebig himself, whose enlistment as lecturer *The Lancet* described as 'our efforts to establish a new era in medicine'. Ancell, a dispensary surgeon, lecturer in jurisprudence and *materia medica*, and medical reformer, had already (1839–40) published lectures on the blood in *The Lancet*.[2] He had intended expanding these into a treatise, but delayed doing so in order to benefit from the judgement of the profession on the cell theory and on *Animal Chemistry*. Finding the latter widely misunderstood, Ancell undertook on his own initiative to explain Liebig's views. His lectures were later translated into German and approved by Liebig. Ancell's own work was governed by the conviction that the blood was of 'primary importance' in disease.[3]

At this juncture, what his contemporaries meant by 'Liebig's theory of disease' was not primarily his view of contagions and miasms, but rather the physiological speculations contained in a chapter of *Animal Chemistry* bearing that title. There Liebig compared the body to a self-regulating steam engine and stated:

Every substance or matter, every chemical or mechanical agency, which changes or disturbs the restoration of the equilibrium between the manifestations of the causes of waste and supply, in such a way as to add its action to the causes of waste, is called a *cause of disease*. *Disease* occurs when the sum of vital force, which tends to neutralise all causes of disturbance (in other words, when the resistance offered by the vital force), is weaker than the acting cause of disturbance . . .

---

[1] *Br. For. Med. Rev.* 11 (1841), 436; *Lancet*, 1842–3, ii. 129–30; ibid. 1841–2, ii. 485, 519–20; ibid. 1838–9, ii. 264. For this journal's claim to a special relationship with Liebig, see an obituary, ibid. 1873, i. 613.

[2] Ibid. 1843–4, i. 486. For Ancell (1802–63), L.S.A. 1828, M.R.C.S. Edinburgh 1831, see obituary, ibid. 1863, ii. 637; Baas, *Outlines of Medical History*, ii. 911, 912; McMenemey, *Charles Hastings*.

[3] Ancell, 'Liebig, his Chemistry and Reviewers', *Lancet*, 1842–3, i; idem, *Treatise on Tuberculosis* (1852), Preface.

To the observer, the action of a cause of disease exhibits itself in the disturbance of the proportion of waste and supply which is proper to each period of life.[1]

These views are not relevant here except insofar as they drew attention and determined reactions to Liebig's writings in general, and as they developed and made apparent attitudes which were implicit in his earlier speculations.[2]

The cardinal virtue of Liebig's work was not its originality (which was in many respects only apparent), but its combined comprehensiveness and simplicity.[3] Not only did Liebig reveal the continuity of phenomena in terms of the elements involved; he also provided mechanisms based on the accredited properties of matter. Explanation in 'Newtonian' terms was not unwelcome to physicians and medical philosophers, who had since the seventeenth century hoped that medicine would some day find a firm foundation in the properties of matter and the methods used to arrive at these. Such a foundation would justify their faith in the uniform operations of nature, which they grasped as their due in the particularly complex maze of phenomena presented to them. 'Newtonianism' also constituted their ideal of rational knowledge. Moreover, progress in organic chemistry, and increased study of the body fluids, had induced a notion of 'dynamic disease' to which Liebig's speculations were well suited. On this occasion, however, their feelings were mixed, and this was not owing simply to the fact that Liebig's argument as well as his evidence could be faulted in many respects.[4] Firstly, the physicians had no desire to return to the crudities of mechanism or iatrophysics. Secondly, few would allow (while welcoming the giving over of increased areas to 'objective' definition) that what occurred *in vitro* adequately corresponded to proceedings

---

[1] Liebig, *Animal Chemistry* (1842), p.254.

[2] Some indication of their operation in a medical context may be gathered from H. Bence Jones's work, *On Gravel, Calculus and Gout: Chiefly an Application of Professor Liebig's Physiology to the Prevention and Cure of These Diseases* (1842), and from reactions to it: see *Br. For. Med. Rev.* 15 (1843), 500; *Lancet*, 1842–3, i. 442.

[3] *Animal Chemistry*, ed. Holmes, Introduction, pp.viii–ix; Holmes, 'Elementary Analysis and Physiological Chemistry'.

[4] *Animal Chemistry*, ed. Holmes, pp.xxxi ff. That Liebig never carried out a physiological experiment was both a strength and a weakness: Pettenkofer, 'Liebig's Scientific Achievements', p.883.

in vivo, and they were not placated by Liebig's version of the vital principle. The true relation of chemistry to medicine, said the *British and Foreign Medical Review*, was that the former had nothing to say of the vital functions of the organized tissues. Vital laws were the province of the physiologist, whom the organic chemist could best serve by investigating such areas as nutrition. At this time the issue of the relationship of chemistry to medicine was raised as if it were a new question. Long reviews in the medical journals traced the progress of chemistry from its former alleged position of dependency on medicine, to its current claims to being a science in its own right; and discussed, usually with caution and sometimes with misgiving, its entry into areas of medicine other than the pharmaceutical. The *British and Foreign Medico-Chirurgical Review* remarked temporizingly in 1849: 'the chemist has been enabled to give an interpretation of many of the phenomena of disease, and he has been bold enough to construct hypotheses, which, with a little modification, may, perhaps, bear the test of further investigation'. At the same time Golding Bird, one of the best-known chemical physicians, stated of Gerardus Johannes Mulder's correlation of fever with the production of oxyprotein that 'like all chemical theories of health or disease [it] should be admitted with caution as a more melancholy error can scarcely be committed, than that of explaining the phenomena of the animal organism too exclusively on chemical principles.'[1] The reader will recall the care taken by Farr in introducing his chemical theories to the notice of physicians. These attitudes belonged to a situation which Liebig had, of course, helped to produce.

Underlying the physician's attitude to the chemist was some concern for professional prerogatives.[2] Practitioners were, for instance, indignant at the fact that many of Liebig's 'laws' seemed to ride roughshod over the conclusions which they themselves had arrived at by dint of experience. They

---

[1] *Br. For. Med. Rev.* 14 (1842), 494. This review was by W.B. Carpenter: *Nature and Man* (1970), Appendix. *Dublin Review*, 25 (1848), 189; *Br. For. Med. Chir. Rev.* 4 (1849), 152; *Lond. Med. Gaz.* 1843–4, i. 619.

[2] As Holmes shows, the reception of *Animal Chemistry* was dependent upon a wide range of factors: *Animal Chemistry*, ed. Holmes, pp.lxv ff.

resented any attempt to derive principles of treatment from these laws. Ironically, but understandably, they found the reduction of disease to one or a few expressions reminiscent of quackery, and clung to a multifactoral view of health and disease. Thus one finds that reviewers dwelt on any section of *Animal Chemistry* rather than the 'Theory of Disease' chapter. Even *The Lancet*, and Ancell, confined themselves to quoting large portions of it or directing the reader to make up his own mind.[1]

In neither the case of *Animal Chemistry*, nor that of *Organic Chemistry* (in which Liebig had taken fewer risks), should it be assumed that the hostility of readers was equivalent to indifference. As the *British and Foreign Medical Review* confessed, who could resist exploring the guesses of a Liebig? Even at his most suspect, he was suggestive, and his two major works between them provided a programme for research. This was a matter of methods and standards as well as of ideas. As Holmes points out, the most important group in Liebig's audience was formed of those who took up one part and criticized another.[2] As will become clear, the principle of 'contagious molecular action' as deployed by Liebig achieved a particularly wide currency, and plainly answered a need.[3] The *Dublin Review*, in a largely chiding account of Liebig's works, gave its most unqualified approval to Liebig on nutrition, and to his explanation of fermentation, putrefaction, and decay: 'the doctrine of metamorphosis has, we believe, been generally considered creditable to its author'.[4] *Animal Chemistry* was notorious but not popular, and physiology proved less tractable than Liebig had anticipated; *Organic Chemistry*, on the other hand, went through seventeen editions in eight languages before 1848. It was the 'theory of the contagiousness of chemical action' which J.S. Mill used as an 'admirable example' of the spirit of the Deductive Method: 'The recent speculations of Liebig in organic

---

[1] See e.g. Carpenter, *Br. For. Med. Rev.* 14 (1842), 492 ff. *Lancet*, 1841-2, ii. 519; Ancell, 'Liebig, his Chemistry and Reviewers', p.732.

[2] *Animal Chemistry*, ed. Holmes, p.xc.

[3] Partington traces this idea back to Francis Bacon, Willis, and Stahl (*History of Chemistry*, iv. 302); A.K. Balls to Stahl in particular (Moulton, *Liebig and after Liebig*, p.31).

[4] *Dublin Review*, 25 (1848), 196. See also *Lond. Med. Gaz.* 1840-1, i. 876-8.

chemistry show some of the most remarkable examples since Newton of the explanation of laws of causation subsisting among complex phenomena, by resolving them into simpler and more general laws.' Mill stressed the way in which Liebig had resolved the special laws of fermentation (caused not by yeast itself, but by 'yeast in a state of decomposition') into several more general laws, and yet subsumed these under a single law, that of the contagiousness of chemical action.[1]

It might, perhaps, be wondered whether the deployment of Liebig's ideas by the medical profession was affected by the different view of fermentation offered by Cagniard La Tour, Theodor Schwann, and Jacob Henle. It is safe enough to say that most British *medical* writers, in the early 1840s at least, were scarcely aware of the disagreement except in so far as Liebig himself brought it before them; and he, while expending a good deal of energy in opposition, gave no very precise idea as to the names and ideas of his opponents.[2] It is doubtful whether the medical reader knew of Schwann's earlier papers at all, unless he had been interested enough to follow up the references given by the *British and Foreign Medical Review*, whose articles were then probably as much the sole means of access to Schwann as they were to Henle. The *Review* attributed to Schwann an English reputation gained by his work with Müller on digestion (1836). It added as complement a description of the yeast fungus taken from *Comptes rendus* and 'tested' by the reviewer. The account given was uncritical. On the question of fermentations which did not involve any addition of yeast, the view was taken that

---

[1] Mill, *A System of Logic* (1843), i. 562; and, in general, Chs. 9 and 13, unchanged in the 3rd edn. (1851).

[2] See Partington, *History of Chemistry*, iv. 304 ff. It can be assumed that the French sources were better known than the German. Schwann's major work, *Mikroskopische Untersuchungen* (1839), which briefly sets out his argument for yeast's being organized, and the agent of fermentation in consequence of that organization, was not translated until 1847, although previously well known among physiologists: Schwann, *Microscopical Researches*, trans. H. Smith (1847); the second edn. of William Baly's translation of Müller's *Handbuch der Physiologie des Menschen* (*Elements of Physiology*, 1840); the 2nd edn. of W.B. Carpenter's *Principles of Physiology* (1841), especially p.74. Idem, 'Report on the Microscope in Anatomy and Physiology. Pt. II: On Cells', *Br. For. Med. Rev.* 15 (1843), 259-81, discussed Schwann's, Schleiden's, and other cell theories. On cell theory in general, see A. Hughes, *A History of Cytology* (1959).

higher organisms might, under peculiar circumstances, develop from their own tissues forms like those of lower organisms. This account of fermentation seems to have been almost literally superseded by the review in the following year of *Organic Chemistry*, in which Liebig's statement of the gratuitousness of the Schwann–La Tour hypothesis was simply paraphrased. The review of Henle described his deployment of the yeast fungus hypothesis.[1]

That Liebig did not always deny that yeast was a living organism was scarcely to be detected in the rush of his attack on the second proposition, that the yeast fungus caused fermentation by its multiplication and growth. It was sufficient for Liebig that belief in the former proposition seemed to be a characteristic of those physiologists who doubted his principle of the sufficiency of chemical explanation in other areas. He continued to use two lines of argument: first, that what was known of living organisms conflicted with the phenomena of which they were said to be the cause; and second, that to attribute the phenomena to the presence of organisms was to leave them as mysterious as before. Although Liebig took the various phases of yeast fermentation as typical, his aim was to arrive at laws covering all fermentations, including those not brought about in the presence of living organisms. Thomas Mayo proved an apt pupil:

How unlike, in the important particular of referring phenomena to general laws, is Schwann's cell theory of fermentation to Liebig's reference of that process to the contagious influence of chemical action – a law so widely instanced in the decomposition of substances held together by weak chemical forces. By this law, truly a chemical one, we are enabled to accept the primary influence of the cells, as being in a state of chemical action . . .[2]

There is no reason to suppose that Liebig's influence would have been less had Schwann and others been, for some reason, well known. Liebig offered a view of the organic world; Schwann offered, or so it appeared, a curiosity. Schwann himself was clearly aware that there were disadvantages in

---

[1] *Br. For. Med. Rev.* 9 (1840), 495 ff., 479, 398 ff.; ibid. 11 (1841), 446.

[2] Liebig, *Familiar Letters on Chemistry* (1844), pp.202 ff.; Mayo, *Sequel to Outlines of Medical Proof* (1849), p.29. For Mayo (1790–1871), M.A., M.D. Oxon., F.R.C.P. 1819, F.R.S. 1835, President of the Royal College of Physicians 1857–62, see *DNB*.

using his view of fermentation to support his general theory of forms.[1] It is a mistake, too, to look for the strident incompatibilities of the Pasteur years in the earlier period, in spite of Liebig's own attempts to polarize the discussion. As cell theories became established, many adopted what might be called a 'bio-chemical' view of fermentation, that is, a view combining the two different interpretations.

The concept and appearances of putrefaction have always been part of medicine.[2] In the early modern period, Boerhaave (1668–1738) stated that putrefaction could occur in the body as a result of the action of alkaline humours produced by faulty digestion. John Huxham (1694–1768), a pupil of Boerhaave, applied the latter's principles to the explanation of fever. As well as the states caused in the body by laxity and rigidity of the fibres, Huxham invoked a third, the tendency towards putrefaction. He divided fevers into three kinds: inflammatory, low nervous, and putrid. The latter two characters were often found blended. John Pringle adopted contemporary pathology, but paid unusual attention to environmental factors, including 'noxious air'. The best example of his approach is his work on scurvy, which he thought of as a 'beginning corruption of the whole habit' brought about by purtrid food, foul air, and other such causes. He carried out many experiments to determine the 'septic and antiseptic' properties of substances. For Pringle, as well as for similar writers, the appearance of *petechiae* or spots indicated an attempt by the body to eliminate humours now become putrid, and an alteration in the nature of the fever to 'pestilential' (contagious and malignant). The 'antiseptic' method of the famous Christoph Ludwig Hoffmann (1721–1807) was based on an assumption of the putridity of those normal products of the body which became the excretions. If retained, these septic or acid substances acted as irritants on the solid parts.[3]

---

[1] Schwann, *Microscopical Researches*, p.197 n.

[2] For some discussion see O. Temkin, 'An Historical Analysis of the Concept of Infection', *Studies in Intellectual History* (Baltimore, 1953), pp.123–47.

[3] See J. Pringle, 'Improvements in Preserving the Health of Mariners' (1775), in *Six Discourses* (1783), pp.143–200. For Pringle's experimental work on antiseptics see Appendix to his *Observations on Diseases of the Army* (1765). Baas, *Outlines of Medical History*, ii. 623.

Gilbert Blane (1749–1834) regarded putrefaction as by definition incompatible with life, and consequently posited as one of his 'energies peculiar to life' an 'antiseptic power' or Conservative Principle.[1] In this he was following John Hunter, who had given his 'Living Principle' the function of constantly opposing the 'natural' septic tendencies of matter. A similar concept of resistance was an integral part of the 'eliminative' views of the earlier writers. Liebig's vital force may now be seen as a version of it. Blane's problem of the incompatibility of putrefaction with life was solved by the special vulnerability which Liebig attributed to the blood.

The long theoretical and empirical history of the concept of putrefaction as a chief mode of change or degradation in matter was reflected in nineteenth-century terminology. The term 'putrid' could be used to describe *sequelae*, complications, or severe forms; to classify fevers; to indicate that group of diseases or conditions which might include anthrax ('malignant pustule'), fever, pyaemia, and erysipelas; or it could be used more widely of all diseases thought to be dependent upon insanitary conditions. Well before the second quarter of the nineteenth century physicians had been accustomed to think of the phenomena of putrefaction as establishing some kind of continuity between the body and its environment. Putrefaction was readily imagined as a process depending on contiguity more or less irrespective of the substance involved. It could be regarded as a state, preceding or coming after other states; or as a substrate upon which were imposed more specific conditions. The putrefactive condition was useful experimentally, since it could, apparently, be readily induced in the lower animals by the introduction of purulent matters (which were, of course, easily obtained and recognized).

The sanitarians made no very precise use of this essentially pathological, but also experimental tradition.[2] Liebig, however, depended upon it, rationalized it, and thus made possible

---

[1] G. Blane, *Elements of Medical Logick* (1819), pp.25 ff.

[2] As we have seen, Southwood Smith made some attempt. The *Essai d'hygiène générale* (1841) of L.C.A. Motard was evidently a more sustained (although eclectic) effort: see *Br. For. Med. Rev.* 14 (1842), 449.

some parts of a sanitary pathology, or, more accurately, a pathology of those diseases regarded (by the profession) as contingently contagious — a term which indicated, it will be remembered, multifactoral causation and relatedness to the environment.[1] Illustrations may be found in papers by C.W. Bell (1849)[2] and W.B. Carpenter (1853).[3] Carpenter accepted both Liebig's explanation of fermentation and the viability of the analogy with disease process, and he wrote with the intention of giving the latter valuable support.[4] His general proposition was that 'all the recognised predisposing causes of zymotic disease tend to produce in the blood an undue accumulation of azotised [nitrogenous] matter, already in a state of *retrograde metamorphosis*, and therefore precisely in the condition in which it is most readily acted on by ferments'. This 'doctrine' was suggested to Carpenter by the liability of the parturient female to become the subject of zymotic disease. Forms of puerperal fever could be induced not only by transfer from other cases of the fever, but by other kinds of *materies morbi*. It occurred to Carpenter that this susceptibility could be caused by waste matters which were present as a result of uterine activity and breakdown. He went on to examine the traditional and recently stressed causes of predisposition: famine, the ingestion of putrid food and water, and overcrowding. 'The *modus operandi* of the generally recognised predisposing causes of zymotic disease', he concluded, was such that these were all 'reducible to one of three categories':

---

[1] See a survey of the external evidence for Liebig's theories, *Br. For. Med. Chir. Rev.* 4 (1849), 152 ff.

[2] Bell, 'Address in Medicine'. Bell (?1811–62), M.D. Edinburgh 1833, nephew of Sir Charles Bell, physician to Persian royal household, etc., moved to Manchester, 1845: see W. Brockbank, *The Honorary Medical Staff of the Manchester Royal Infirmary 1830–1948* (Manchester, 1965), pp.25–7; *Surgeon–General's Catalogue.*

[3] W.B. Carpenter, [signed] review of M. Marchal on epidemics, *Br. For. Med. Chir. Rev.* 11 (1853), 159–77, of which the substance may be found in *Organic Chemistry*, pp.386–7, where Liebig deals briefly with 'accidental' conditions for contagion.

[4] For William Benjamin Carpenter (1813–85), L.S.A, M.R.C.S, M.D. Edinburgh 1839, F.R.S. 1844, son (and pupil) of Dr. Lant Carpenter, editor of *British and Foreign Medico-Chirurgical Review* 1847–52, Registrar of University of London from 1856, see *DNB*. Prolific and influential popular and philosophical writer. For a memoir, bibliography, and selected essays, see Carpenter, *Nature and Man.*

1. Those, namely, which tend to introduce into the system decomposing matter that has been generated in some external source [the eighteenth-century *ingesta*].
2. Those which occasion an increased production of decomposing matter in the system itself; — and
3. Those which obstruct the elimination of the decomposing matter normally or excessively generated within the system, or abnormally introduced into it from without [the eighteenth-century *retenta*].[1]
All the unsanitary influences could be subsumed under these headings, and all, it could be seen, had the same effects.

Charles William Bell's address was faithful to Liebig, but (as could be expected) still propounded an individual view of epidemic disease. Bell was particularly concerned to account for the 'doubtful' diseases: that is, he said, those caused by poisons which were formed outside the body and yet were capable of reproducing themselves in the blood and of communicating the disease to others. He was, as already noticed, anxious to refute the dogmatic anticontagionism of the General Board of Health. Bell's claim was that if all the facts then known about the so-called epidemic diseases were reviewed 'with the aid of that knowledge of the chemical actions which influence the decomposition of organic bodies, inculcated by Liebig', it would be found that these diseases were the product of one or a combination of three causes: specific poison, putrefaction, and epidemic influence. With the last of these Liebig might have (perhaps) little to do; but in the case of the two former, the processes involved were rendered by Bell in terms culled directly from Liebig's work. Bell's solution to the caprices of a disease like cholera was to suppose that when epidemic, but not contagious, it was the effect of specific epidemic influence alone; but that when epidemic and contagious it was the effect of epidemic influence combined with non-specific but contagious putrid fever. This, and Bell's account of seasonal variations in disease types, were deliberately reminiscent of Sydenham. Bell is, therefore, a good example of the combination of current interests referred to elsewhere. Putrefaction, according to Bell, acted on the whole blood rather than on a special material associated

---

[1] Carpenter, *Br. For. Med. Chir. Rev.* 11 (1853), 175.

with that fluid; and its action, though communicable, did not necessarily originate in the living blood.[1]

Bell's account of unsanitary predisposing causes varied from Carpenter's in placing more emphasis on 'dynamics', although this was a matter of degree: Carpenter also stressed process rather than substance, stating that the influence of the ferment was to be regarded as 'not material but dynamical'.[2] 'The low putrid fever, endemic in our towns' Bell regarded simply as 'the struggle of the vital powers against the tendency to decomposition'. The action of the particles of (for example) tainted air, was constantly resisted by 'the antiseptic chemistry of life'; predisposing causes like starvation, cold, and debauchery depressed the vital powers, and this made it possible for the decomposing agent to become active in the blood. If the compounds thereby produced were not eliminated, death resulted.

It is, perhaps, a measure of how far Liebig's speculations on miasms and contagions were prompted by what he saw as the vices of the biological or parasitic theories of disease, that he made no use of the statistical generalizations of the English sanitarians.[3] At some points he appears to have come close to doing so; for example, when he stated that 'it is a universal observation that the origin of epidemic diseases is often to be traced to the putrefaction of large quantities of animal and vegetable matters'; but this was an (acknowledged) quotation from Henle, having as much reference to the traditional view of marsh ague as to the doubtful diseases, and occurring in a passage in which Henle's aim was to demonstrate that the agent of miasmatico-contagious diseases must be a form of the organisms which caused decomposition. Liebig's response was to argue that

... according to all the rules of scientific investigation, the conclusion is fully justified, that in all cases where a process of putrefaction precedes the occurrence of a disease, or where the disease can be propagated by

---

[1] Bell, 'Address in Medicine', pp.6–7.

[2] Ibid., pp.18–20; Carpenter, *Br. For. Med. Chir. Rev.* 11 (1853), 163.

[3] Liebig was certainly interested in such matters as the proper disposition of sewage etc., but his concern was for agriculture rather than public health. Not surprisingly he or his work was consulted by Chadwick on various occasions, though without much agreement: see e.g. Chadwick's evidence in *Report of Committee on Sewage Manure*, p.106 [648]; Lewis, *Chadwick and Public Health*, p.353.

solid or aeriform products of disease, and where no nearer causes of the disease can be discovered, the substances in a state of decomposition or transformation must be regarded as being, in consequence of that state, the proximate causes of disease.

Nevertheless, he did, as is not surprising, contribute to what might be called sanitary chemistry. The *British and Foreign Medical Review* stated that what it deduced from *Organic Chemistry* was 'totally opposed' to the idea that inorganic gaseous substances were capable of producing diseases with regular phases. Liebig conducted experiments in faecal chemistry; described experiments for examining organic matters found in the atmosphere, and indicated that a test for ammonia (a nitrogenous substance, easily detected and an 'invariable product' of the decomposition of animal matter) was a means of establishing the presence of decomposing organic substances.[1] He also suggested that ammonia might be the 'means through which the contagious matter received a gaseous form': that is, the gas molecules served as a vehicle for the passive particles of organic matter.[2]

As already indicated, Farr's thorough adoption of Liebig's argument by analogy was one of the first and most important positive reactions to take place in the medical world. Farr modified his source very little. He did not, however, refer at that time to the alternative parasitic (or biological) hypothesis,[3] and he did, if only by his nomination of the different exciters, place more emphasis than had Liebig on the specificity of disease. Similarly, Farr's account gave greater encouragement to the reader to think of the agents of epidemic disease as forming a class in some way unique. In so far as his formulations were suggestive, they emphasized substance as much as process, and the simple smallpox model of poison and subject rather than the multifactoral structure of the doubtful

---

[1] Liebig, *Animal Chemistry*, pp.204–5; Henle, *Miasms and Contagions*, pp.958 ff. *Br. For. Med. Rev.* 11 (1841), 445. Carpenter, *Br. For. Med. Chir. Rev.* 11 (1853), 172; Liebig, *Organic Chemistry*, p.392. For the further significance of the presence of ammonia, see Liebig as quoted by *Br. For. Med. Chir. Rev.* 4 (1849), 154.

[2] This suggestion was taken up by Sir William Burnett (PP, 1847–8, LI. 408), and by Budd (*Typhoid Fever*, 1873, p.96); cf. J. Haygarth (*Letter to Percival*, 1801, pp.48 ff.).

[3] See only *Appendix 1842*, p.121.

diseases. Liebig emphasized on the other hand that the exciters were ultimately derived from the blood, and that they exerted their actions 'solely by virtue of their existing condition'. He was, consequently, able to cite the failure to find peculiar matters in either bad sausage or smallpox virus as evidence for his own view.[1]

An additional feature of Farr's account was his reference to the classic English authorities, Sydenham, Morton, and Willis, and his stress on the resemblance between their pathological views and those of Liebig. However slight the real resemblance, this was a happy reminder, since two other current interests, humoral pathology and the interaction of epidemics, were, as we have seen, already bringing Sydenham to mind as an authoritative source. English writers proved very willing to see Liebig as Sydenham (or Hippocrates) either modernized or vindicated. In some cases this may be put down to the desire of an author to recommend a valuable idea which, owing to its source, his readers might otherwise disregard. In others, the writer was simply concerned to appropriate the idea in the national interest, which indicates some degree of approval.[2]

Reflections of Liebig's theories are to be found in a variety of quarters apart from those already mentioned. (Sir) Thomas Watson (1840-2), Thomas Graham (1842), Bransby Cooper (1847), General Board of Health (1849), J. Hughes Bennett (1852), and John Snow (1853) are familiar names which can be given as examples from within the period 1840 to 1855.[3] Many little-known names could also be given.[4] No uniformity will be found among these authors, and this is by no means a function of the different dates of writing. Some differences

---

[1] Leibig, *Organic Chemistry*, pp.369, 371.

[2] See e.g. Golding Bird, quoted in *Br. For. Med. Chir. Rev.* 4 (1849), 154.

[3] Watson, as first published in *Lond. Med. Gaz.* 1841-2, ii. 662-4. Cf. the edn. following the publication of *Animal Chemistry: Principles and Practice of Physic*, ii. 665-8, especially p.668. Graham, *Elements of Chemistry*, pp.723 ff.; Cooper, Lecture 5 of a course in surgery at Guy's Hospital: *Lond. Med. Gaz.* 5 (1847), 49 ff.; *Report on Quarantine*; Bennett on the 'present theory' of eruptive fevers, quoted in *Braithwaite*, 26 (1852), 6; Snow, *On Continuous Molecular Changes* (1853).

[4] e.g. J.W. Tripe, quoted in *Braithwaite*, 20 (1849), 1. John William Tripe (1821-92) was first Medical Officer of Health for Hackney District, with a special interest in medical meteorology. See *Surgeon-General's Catalogue*.

are particularly relevant here, and may be illustrated by the appearance in different contexts of Farr's word 'zymotic'. There was little research which can be construed as following along the lines suggested by Farr's list of 'exciters', unless it were Benjamin Richardson's experiments of a rather later date.[1] The more philosophical physicians, like Bennett and Carpenter, used 'zymosis' in the pathological sense given by Farr; but in general, Farr succeeded better in his second object, which was to bring the term to signify the whole range of preventable diseases.[2] It was used in this sense by the General Board of Health, and 'zymotic poison' came to mean on some occasions the indeterminate product or products of decomposition, which, with epidemic influence, were thought to cause all epidemic disease. Thus one finds in *The Lancet* references to the 'dim zymotic visions' of Southwood Smith, and in the *Morning Chronicle*, the demand that the Board substantiate its 'zymotic theory' by chemical analysis of the atmosphere. Elsewhere the Board appeared to adopt something of the actual mechanism defined by Liebig, not in relation to the body as much as to the environment:

It may be observed that the diseases here termed zymotic are synonymous with the class of epidemic, endemic, and contagious diseases, and they are called zymotic or *fermenting*, from the notion that one disease of this nature acts as leaven thrown into a mass prepared for, that is having the conditions for taking on, the fermentive action. The existence of diseases of this class indicates the presence of certain impure conditions of the atmosphere, just as the barometer indicates the presence of certain natural conditions of it.

In another place the Board was more precise, but also more metaphorical:

a single infected person, and much more a large body of infected persons, localising themselves in the midst of a population already

---

[1] See e.g. B.W. Richardson, 'On the Theory of Zymosis' *Trans. Epidem. Soc.* 1 (1859–60), 20–30. Richardson (1828–96), M.D. and M.A. St. Andrews, M.R.C.P. 1856, F.R.C.P. 1865, F.R.S. 1867, was well known as an imaginative and fluent writer, sanitarian, humanitarian, and activist for the temperance movement. See *DNB*; Richardson, *Vita Medica* (1897). A 'life' by his daughter prefaces his *Disciples of Aesculapius*. A.S. McNalty, *A Biography of Sir Benjamin Ward Richardson* (1950) includes a bibliography, but gives no useful account of Richardson's experimental and speculative work.

[2] 'Zymotic disease' remained in use well after 1870 as a synonym for 'filth disease' or 'preventable disease'. *OED* gives 'generally, of typhus', and an instance from *Household Words*.

predisposed to disease and actually under an epidemic influence, may act on that population zymotically, that is, as the leaven which sets in action the fermenting mass.[1]

By this time, the popularity of Liebig's formulations was such that they were, according to the *British and Foreign Medico-Chirurgical Review*, 'freely admitted and confidently discussed in most of our modern works in practical medicine', and it is not surprising that one of the Board's staff, John Sutherland, showed unmistakable signs of having been influenced by them.[2] It is not clear from Sutherland's brief remarks whether he imagined the process by which the poisonous essence impressed itself on other organic matter to take place in the body, outside it, or both. It will be remembered that Farr in his report on cholera was equally undecided. What is certain is that sanitarians in general found Liebig's notion of 'contagious molecular action' extremely useful as a hypothesis of the connection between remote and environmental causes. In 1855, the Committee for Scientific Enquiries set up by the President of the then Board of Health to investigate the cholera epidemic of 1854–5, reported as follows:

The doctrine of epidemic cholera which has gained almost universal acceptance, does not affect to explain what may be . . . the exciting cause of epidemic manifestation . . . But with this mystery still unsolved, there has grown more and more into shape a doctrine which is both intelligible and practical; — that the undiscovered power in its wanderings acts after the manner of a ferment, that it therefore takes effect only amid congenial circumstances, and that the stuff out of which it brews poison must be air and water abounding in organic impurity.[3]

The practicality of this doctrine lay in its entailment of standard sanitary practices; but any credit for intelligibility must be Liebig's. It remains true that Liebig's influence was felt over-all less upon sanitary than on experimental science; relevant areas of investigation being the body fluids, the excretions, and the artificial production of disease. None the

---

[1] *Lancet*, 1849, ii. 97; *Morning Chronicle*, 24 Aug. 1849. *Report on Quarantine*, pp.89–90, 54–5. For rather more explicit comments on the current trend, see Southwood Smith, *Results of Sanitary Improvement*, p.14; idem, *Epidemics Considered*, p.23.

[2] *Br. For. Med. Chir. Rev.* 4 (1849), 154; Sutherland, Appendix to *Report on Cholera*, p.198.

[3] Report of Scientific Enquiries Committee, p.48, PP, 1854–5, XXI.

less, his work reduced for most physicians the dichotomy between sanitary generalization and medical science; it served a number of current interests, especially humoral pathology; and his theory of continuous molecular action, in its precarious position between inorganic chemistry, natural philosophy, and biology, did establish a common and flexible notion of process for all epidemic, endemic, and contagious diseases.

5

THE CHOLERA-FUNGUS CONTROVERSY OF 1849

In the last chapter some indication was given of the nature of relevant changes in medical science over the period between the first cholera epidemic (1831–2) and the second (1848–9). These changes were related, directly or indirectly, to the development of chemistry, and helped to form the desired 'scientific link between epidemiology and pathology'.[1] The present chapter deals in part with a second influence, that of microscopy, and in particular with the 'cholera-fungus' controversy of 1849. Besides this I would like to give a broader picture of the nature of professional activity at and around the time of the second cholera epidemic. Analysis of the various stages of the controversy will show something of the interaction of professional institutions, and in particular the way in which these were proliferating and competing with one another.

The approach of cholera was first noticed in the journals early in 1847.[2] Except to enthusiasts for a particular theory or remedy, it did not seem that the profession was better equipped to meet the problem than it had been in 1831, although there was a vague but real feeling that it could now be tackled 'more scientifically'.[3] There were standard clinical descriptions of the disease, and some agreement had been reached as to the effect of such factors as age, sex, and class. However, the matter which dominated all preliminary discussion was treatment, and on this there was no agreement at all.[4] Many physicians believed, with the General Board of Health, that cholera could be prevented or cured in the first

---

[1] Clark, *College of Physicians*, ii. 675.

[2] The first undoubted case in the British Isles occurred in London on 28 Sept. 1848: Parkes, 'Inquiry', p.258.

[3] See e.g. the 'research programme' outlined by the *Mon. J. Med. Sci.* 8 (1847–8), 595.

[4] See e.g. *Lond. Med. Gaz.* 5 (1847), 677. For a selection of opinions, see *Braithwaite*, 18 (1848), 385 ff. See in general Howard-Jones, 'Cholera Therapy'.

stage (premonitory diarrhoea), but this did not solve their real problem, which was that of the individual patient with a fully developed case of the disease. They felt, and said, that the sanitary generalizations established since 1832 represented a major advance, but this was not seen as affecting their role, except perhaps to expand it.[1] In general, it was hoped that treatment would be more rational, that is, dependent on a well-founded pathology or aetiology, rather than empirical, that is, pragmatic. In an emergency, however, no resource is neglected, so that the modern reader will detect little difference in treatment between one epidemic and the next.

The contagion question has already been discussed in some detail. The sanitarians give, as they intended, the impression that opinions had radically changed. However, it is by now clear that even if (as is proper) the discussion is confined to a particular disease, it is wrong to make out any such change without considering the dichotomy between medical theory and sanitary practice. Even the Royal College of Physicians, which Chadwick quoted in his own support, expressed itself to this effect. It did not so much reverse a previous opinion on cholera as agree on a 'practical conclusion' (that cholera 'appears to have been very rarely communicated by personal intercourse'), 'without expressing any positive opinion with respect to its contagious or non-contagious nature'.[2]

As cholera became established, the flow of ideas on the subject increased. Such diversity was not encouraging: after examining a batch of seventeen pamphlets, books, and reports (among them William Budd's first published work on cholera), the *London Medical Gazette* concluded that, whatever their individual merits, these works 'presented collectively but little novelty and threw little if any additional light either on the pathology or the therapeutics of cholera'. *The Lancet* stated to its correspondents that it would refuse to publish further essays on cholera unless they were 'supported by facts that have been demonstrated, or admit of being demonstrated'.[3]

---

[1] See e.g. the deliberations of the Bristol profession: *Bristol Gazette*, 21 June 1849.

[2] Recommendations published by the Royal College of Physicians, *The Times*, 3 Nov. 1848. See College Cholera MSS., Minute Book, 28 Oct. 1848.

[3] *Lond. Med. Gaz.* 9 (1849), 719–28; *Lancet*, 1849, ii. 494.

The cholera-fungus theory will provide examples of the difficulty of meeting this seemingly straightforward demand. If a work won praise in the journals, it was for being unpretentious, 'ingenious', or useful to the novice. Some works were given space so that they could be suitably dismissed. 'Theories of cholera' does not cover the total output, since many writers were concerned only with treatment, and some few others confined themselves to symptomology or pathology, or simply to nominating one of the traditional predisposing causes. To deal with 'theories' of causation (especially if proximate causes, or physiology and pathology, are excluded) is inevitably to deal with the fringe areas of medicine, in terms both of the resources used, the time spared to such speculations by the average practitioner under normal conditions, and the precarious respectability of such theories.

A convenient summary of 'theories of cholera' listed the following: the telluric, electric, and ozonic theories; the animalcular and fungoid; the zymotic or humoral; and the theories naming ingesta, or putrid effluvia, or a specific poison as in smallpox.[1] Budd appears as an exponent of the fungoid theory, Snow, being then among those called 'modest', does not appear in this context at all.[2] To the list may be added some other products of the current influence of chemistry: the 'deficiency' theories of Tunstall and Blacklock. James Tunstall based his theory on the observation of John Davy that the air expired by cholera patients contained an abnormally low proportion of carbon. He thought of the excretion of carbon as having an antiseptic action in the body, and deduced that available carbon was deficient (rather than unexcreted) from reports of the therapeutic value of petroleum.[3] 'Carbon theories' were not uncommon, and may usually be traced to

---

[1] 'History of the Origin, Progress and Mortality of the Cholera Morbus', *Lond. Med. Gaz.* 1849, ii. 507–11, 556–9, 600–2; reprinted from *The Times*. The journals of other countries could have drawn up almost identical lists: see e.g. C.E. Rosenberg, 'The Cause of Cholera: Aspects of Aetiological Thought in Nineteenth Century America', *Bull. Hist. Med.* 34 (1960), 331–54. Most of the items were of course traditional, e.g. the telluric theory (meaning, 'of the earth'). The volcanic theory was a variant of the telluric, as the ozonic was to an extent a variant of the electric.

[2] See *Lond. Med. Gaz.* 9 (1849), 466.

[3] J. Tunstall, 'Petroleum in Asiatic Cholera', *Prov. Med. Surg. J.* 12 (1848), 390–1; 471–2. Tunstall was then attached to Bath General Hospital.

Liebig's *Animal Chemistry*. Blacklock, writing in India, attributed cholera to the 'continued use of a diet deficient in sulphur'. Sulphur was necessary to maintain the body in its normal electrical condition, and its absence gave rise to 'morbid ganglionic excitability'.[1]

The animalcular and fungoid theory is the main concern of this chapter, but the electric and the ozonic deserve some attention. Many people found it difficult to believe in a material cause which could not be detected by known chemical means. Electricity was a little-known force, which varied in the earth's atmosphere, and yet seemed in some way to be among the basic properties not only of matter itself but also of living beings, since it appeared to be analogous if not identical to nervous energy, or even the vital principle itself. Most importantly, it could be experimented with and measured. Consequently it was a popular component of cholera theories, either as a sufficient cause or, more frequently, as a cause in combination with other causes. The pundit on electricity and cholera seems to have been Sir James Murray, whose work, *Electricity as a cause of cholera & other epidemics, & the relation of galvanism to the action of remedies* was reviewed in the *London Medical Gazette* and elsewhere.[2] Blacklock combined electrical with chemical factors; others envisaged swarms of organisms being attracted or even generated by electrical force. Electrical explanations of the potato blight of the 1840s had been just as popular, as a naturalistic explanation of a similar phenomenon (famine), which could also be regarded as a judgement, enforced indirectly through natural laws.[3]

The ozonic theory was sponsored in England by Robert

[1] A. Blacklock, professor of surgery at Madras Medical College in 1854. Quoted in *Braithwaite*, 20 (1849), 422 ff. 'Sulphur' was also a feature of some seventeenth- and eighteenth-century physiological theories but for the nineteenth see Holmes, 'Elementary Analysis and Physiological Chemistry'.

[2] See Carpenter, *Nature and Man*, pp.48 ff., for some contemporary speculations; as a reflection of them, see Cowdell, below. Medical galvanism was a widespread interest of the last quarter of the eighteenth century. In the nineteenth century, *Naturphilosophie* made a particular use of the phenomenon. Murray's work was published in Dublin; n.d. *See Lond. Med. Gaz.* 9 (1849), 725.

[3] Many regarded the two plagues as a single judgement, or even assumed the potato blight to be a form of cholera: R.N. Salaman, *The History and Social Influence of the Potato* (Cambridge, 1970), p.290.

Hunt, who was active in the British Association, and who was for many years chief scientific writer for the *Athenaeum*.[1] Schönbein, the discoverer of ozone, had remarked that its incidence in the atmosphere seemed to vary in exact ratio with the electrical intensity, and that it was formed during all combustion processes.[2] Hunt drew attention to its great powers of oxidation and disinfection, and also to observations by Quetelet which indicated that over the cholera period the electrical intensity of the atmosphere had been abnormally low.[3] Hunt concluded that under normal circumstances ozone was designed by nature to prevent poisons forming during decomposition, and that cholera epidemics were the result of a deficiency of ozone caused by the low level of electrical activity. As support for his theory he gave the example of Birmingham, whose puzzling exemption from cholera could, he said, be explained by supposing that the great industrial fires of the city had maintained the level of ozone in the atmosphere. He added that T. Moffatt, another member of the British Association, had on the basis of similar correlations suggested that influenza epidemics might be caused by an excess of ozone. As may be imagined, these theories were easily criticized, but remained attractive if only for the reason that they suggested feasible kinds of research and verification.[4]

---

[1] Hunt, 'The Probable Causes of Pestilential Cholera', *Lond. Med. Gaz.* 9 (1849), 473-5. Reprinted from the *Athenaeum*. For Hunt (1807-87), F.R.S. 1854, an expert on mining and photography, see *DNB*.

[2] Christian Friedrich Schönbein (1799-1868), professor of chemistry at Basle from 1828. Identified ozone as the source of 'electrical smell', 1840: Partington, *History of Chemistry*, iv. 190-6.

[3] It was provisionally assumed that ozone was a 'peculiar volatile compound of oxygen and hydrogen'. Hunt therefore adduced evidence of the oxidizing properties of hydrogen peroxide. Ozone continued to be regarded as the active element in the best disinfectants: see Condy, *Disinfection and Prevention of Disease*, p.12.

[4] For criticism, see *Lond. Med. Gaz.* 9 (1849), 462; for an experimental test, see a letter by J. Williams of Nottingham, *Morning Chronicle*, 10 Oct. 1849. See also correspondence between 'Antizymosis', 'Antiozonozymos', 'Medicus', and others in the *Chronicle* for September and October 1849. By 1852, ozone was thought to be a kind of electrified oxygen. For a discussion of the subject in its medical aspect by Schönbein, see 'On some Secondary Physiological Effects produced by Atmospheric Electricity', *Med. Chir. Trans.* 34 (1851), 205-20, communicated by Faraday: *Letters of Faraday and Schönbein* (1899), pp.193, 199. For a later survey of the whole subject, see C.B. Fox, *Ozone and Antozone* (1873).

The ozonic and fungoid theories offered different kinds of explanation, but were comparable in other respects. Each named a discoverable entity as the agent, and the fungoid theory reflected the influence of the new microscopy as the ozonic did that of chemistry. To some extent rival interests were involved. Contemporary views of the limits and peculiar virtues of microscopy were often made out in comparison with the capabilities of chemical analysis.[1] The organic chemists had shown animal and vegetable substances to be composed of the same limited range of elements, and this to a microscopist was an argument for making form the basis of classification. Knowledge of the chemical constitution or properties of the lower forms of life was minimal. Some of the earliest workers to investigate adulteration and pollution regarded the microscope as the finer tool, partly because smaller quantities were required for analysis.[2] The proponents of the cholera-fungus theory at first depended almost entirely on microscopical evidence; later in the debate they were criticized for this, and some points were decided on chemical grounds. Chemists and microscopists met in defining the conditions in which the 'cholera-bodies' were found. Some writers, arguing from analogy, claimed that certain of these conditions provided a sufficient explanation of the presence of the bodies.

The belief that progress is a definitive characteristic of science is most persistent in the biological and medical sciences, where basic entities are (apparently) directly observable, and where cure and control seem to provide obvious proof of advance. In these sciences 'thresholds' are defined with the greatest simplicity by the capabilities of instruments or techniques. The period under present consideration, however, lies between two thresholds.[3] By 1850, the best English microscopes were capable of achieving a resolution which was not significantly improved upon until, over a decade later, a better understanding of the principle of high numerical

---

[1] See e.g. J.S. Wilkinson, *Lancet*, 1849, ii. 448.

[2] See John Quekett, in *Trans. Microsc. Soc.* 2 (1849), 151; *Q. Jl.Microsc. Sci.* 5 (1857), 229.

[3] Hughes, *History of Cytology*, pp.7, 10, warns against relating the development of microscopy too directly to technical improvements.

aperture had been reached, and immersion lenses introduced. On the other hand, the period made remarkable by globulism and other errors had ended in 1830, when Joseph Jackson Lister produced designs for the correction of spherical and chromatic aberration in compound microscopes.[1] After ten years of application the full potential of this improvement had been realized.[2] None the less, because of the erratic past of the instrument, devotees and detractors alike were very wary of inferences which were at all speculative. In addition, it must be stressed that other than optical criteria governed the successful use of the microscope. Except for a very few methods, techniques of fixing and colouring material for examination were severely limited, in terms of their diffusion if not of their discovery, until after 1860. The innovations in practice, which began in the 1850s and 1860s, took place almost exclusively on the continent.[3]

English microscopes of this period were excellent, but English microscopy at first could not rival what the Germans achieved with inferior instruments. Schleiden, assuming (*c*. 1840) that a country which had produced Robert Brown could scarcely lack good observers, thought that the English lagged behind because their instruments were inferior.[4] W.B. Carpenter called the English tradition 'desultory', and criticized the 'mere collectors' spirit' which pervaded it.[5] These strictures were perhaps too severe. The English were not so much negligent in the pursuit of microscopy as interested in a particular class of objects, often the comparatively gross independent organisms, or plants. Such studies could, through a fortuitous choice of subject, yield far-reaching conclusions, but these achievements were necessarily occasional, and could not compare with the steady rate of progress of German

---

[1] For a short contemporary history of the microscope, *see Edinb. Med. Surg. J.* 73 (1850), 161 ff.; for a less parochial view, see Hughes, *History of Cytology*, Ch.1.

[1] For a graphical representation, see G.L'E. Turner and S. Bradbury (eds.), *Historical Aspects of Microscopy* (1967), p.189.

[3] See J.R. Baker, 'The Discovery of the Uses of Colouring Agents in Biological Micro-technique', *J. Quekett Microsc. Club*, 4th series, 1 (1938–43), 256–75; Hughes, *History of Cytology*, pp.13 ff.

[4] Quoted by E. Lankester, *Trans. Microsc. Soc.* 7 (1859), 67.

[5] Carpenter, ibid. 3 (1855), 54, 44.

microscopists in the more difficult areas of cytology and embryology.

In English science, the unit of organization was the society. The membership, concerns, and attitudes of English microscopical societies bore far more resemblance to those of the broadly based 'philosophical' and 'philosophical and literary' organizations, than to those of specialist societies. The busy medical practitioner (or clergyman) was encouraged in his use of the microscope by the belief that his observations, sporadic though they might be, would help to form the broad inductive base essential to valid generalization.[1] Either that, or he might one day discover a new species, and be able to put his name to it. Thus much microscopical observation in England was done by persons with no deep, or shared, scientific commitment. Even where effort was sustained it was directed towards an exhaustive study of a single class of objects. This situation is another reflection of the absence in England of the professionalism of German science. No Englishman without independent means could afford to take up microscopy as his main pursuit.[2] The economic aspect of course reflects the differences in institutional and vocational organization. Collaboration was limited to committees on special subjects, which seldom came to fruition.[3] It was mainly as a member of a society that a man had access to the better instruments, which could cost £50 or more. The amateur character of English science is to be seen first, in that the microscope was sponsored chiefly by a society; and second, in that contemporaries regarded this society as unscientific, because it consisted of a combination of men at work with an instrument.[4]

The Microscopical Society of London (chartered 1866) originated in the activities of a 'band of brothers' led by James Scott Bowerbank. Credit may also be given to Edwin Quekett; he died in 1847 and his brother John's long service

---

[1] See the editors' reasons for including a section for memoranda, *Q. Jl. Microsc. Sci.* 1 (1853), Preface.

[2] Carpenter, *Trans. Microsc. Soc.* 4 (1856), 20.

[3] See e.g. ibid. 2 (1854), 87.

[4] Asserted of his contemporaries by Lankester, ibid. 7 (1859), 64; for evidence, see e.g. *Br. For. Med. Rev.* 28 (1842), 489.

to the society is better known.[1] Monthly meetings began in 1840 under the presidency of Richard Owen, who had gained his reputation by being the first to apply the microscope to teeth, and who was later to risk it in connection with the fungus alleged to cause the potato blight. Membership of the Society reached 177 in 1841, 180 in 1852, and 276 in 1859.[2]

Within the membership of microscopical societies the microscope was applied not to medicine, but to geology and natural history.[3] Many medical men (or persons with medical qualifications) belonged to these societies, but it is plain that most did not associate the instrument particularly with medical research, or engage in such research themselves.[4] In its early years the Microscopical Society of London had few relations with medical societies, with the possible exception of the Pathological Society, which was not founded until 1846. It appears that those interested in medical microscopy spent the period of isolation in writing full-scale treatises or in translating those which seemed to them most important.[5] At the end of the decade 1840–50, the membership of this small group of experts was almost unchanged, but microscopy itself had become much more broadly based. This development inevitably caused tensions, which were added to

<hr>

[1] For Edwin John Quekett (1808–47), F. Linnaean Soc. 1836, of University College London, and a surgeon in Whitechapel, see *DNB*. John Thomas Quekett (1815–61), L.S.A. and M.R.C.S. 1840, F.R.S. 1860, F. Linnaean Soc. 1857, followed Edwin to London and University College. Asst. conservator of Hunterian Museum at the Royal College of Surgeons, 1843; made *ad hominem* professor of histology, 1852. Secretary of Microscopical Society 1841–59; President, 1860. Because of his interests and position Quekett was regularly consulted by members of the profession. See *DNB*; E.P. Herlihy, *J. Quekett Microsc. Club*, 4th series, 4 (1957), 331–8 (includes a bibliography); M.V. Salmon, 'The Quekett Sale Catalogue', ibid. 29 (1962), 9–11.

[2] On the foundation see J.B. Reade, *Mon. Microsc. J.* 3 (1870), 113. For a history with biographies, see A.D. Michael, *Jl. R. Microsc. Soc.* 2nd series, 15 (1895), 1–20.

[3] See an analysis of 130 papers published in the (select) *Transactions of the Microscopical Society of London* between 1840 and 1857: Lankester, *Trans. Microsc. Soc.* 7 (1859), 68.

[4] The inconsistency did not go unnoticed: see e.g. G. Jackson, ibid. 2 (1854), 88; G. Shadbolt, ibid. 5 (1857), 140.

[5] A review of English treatises on the construction and use of the microscope mentioned only three as appearing before Quekett's *Practical Treatise* of 1848: *Edinb. Med. Surg. J.* 73 (1850), 179.

those ensuing from the microscope's being the property of popularizers as well as of philosophers.[1]

The General Medical Council did not recommend until 1869 that the student himself be taught microscopy, but lectures and demonstrations were given to some students and qualified men from 1840 onwards. At St. Thomas's Hospital, Richard Grainger applied in 1843 for an instrument, and began demonstrations (with George Rainey) in 1847. In the same year (1847) John Simon was appointed as the hospital's first lecturer in pathology, and he introduced, not without opposition, the entry into record books of both chemical and microscopical analyses. John Quekett began giving annual courses in microscopy to members of the Royal College of Surgeons before 1849. Earlier in the decade, Henry Acland and others, at the urging not of their medical teachers but of Richard Owen, had gone to Quekett (then Owen's assistant) as private pupils. In spite of the presence in Edinburgh of such eminent early advocates as J.H. Bennett, Acland's personal possession of a microscope distinguished him, on his arrival there in 1844, among teachers and pupils alike.[2] However, teaching, and some teachers, undoubtedly lagged behind the tendency of some students to acquire instruments of their own.[3]

The microscope was much more readily introduced into medical research than into the professional life of the practitioner. On Owen's offering to have a cheap microscope made for him, Acland's first response was that he 'did not think to use a microscope now. I intended and desired to be a practical physician, and if I began to amuse myself with microscopical researches I should fail in them, and be no

---

[1] See e.g. *Lancet*, 1849, ii. 456. The popular aspects of microscopy included the religious, the commercial, and the didactic: see e.g. the Religious Tract Society's *Curiosities of Animal Life* [1848].

[2] See Newman, *Evolution of Medical Education*, p.104; J.D. Comrie, *History of Scottish Medicine*, 2 vols. (1932), ii. 607–8. W.D. Foster and J.L. Pinniger, 'The History of Pathology at St. Thomas's Hospital', *Med. Hist.* 7 (1963), 330–47: 332. J.B. Atlay, *Sir Henry Wentworth Acland . . . A Memoir* (1903), pp.86, 98 ff., 110, 123–4.

[3] e.g. Carpenter; William Budd (Budd Letters, January 1841–3); Joseph Lister, who was provided with an instrument by his father, J.J. Lister: Joseph Lister, *The Third Huxley Lecture* (1907), p.6.

physician either.'[1] Many medical men had yet to be convinced of the relationship of research to practice.[2] Any suggestion that persons whose primary interest lay elsewhere (be it chemistry or microscopy) could effectively define and solve medical problems was bound to be unwelcome. This mistrust was not simply a profession's concern for its own interests, but was also the reflection of a definition of medical problems which precluded 'simple' solutions or specifics. Finally, even with achromatic microscopes, skill came only with time and perseverance. To John Brown, writing in 1849, the microscope had contributed to a situation in which chemistry and physiology had become 'to all men above forty, impossible sciences'.[3]

Prominence has so far been given to the Microscopical Society of London, and in what follows its members play an important part. Our point of origin, however, is not London but Bristol.[4] Carpenter was lecturing on microscopy to the Literary and Philosophical Institution there in 1842; a Microscopical Society was founded a year later. Among its members were the main exponents of the cholera-fungus theory, as well as Carpenter and the eminent G.H.K. Thwaites.[5] It would appear that this society enjoyed a continuous existence from 1843 to 1905.[6] The thirteen founding members

---

[1] Letter from Acland to his father, quoted in Atlay, *Acland, A Memoir*, p.99.

[2] For an attempt to carry conviction, see a review of James Paget's *Lectures on Surgical Pathology* (1853): *Q. Jl. Microsc. Sci.* 2 (1854), 197. Paget had earlier produced the much praised *Report on the Chief Results Obtained by the Use of the Microscope in the Study of Human Anatomy and Physiology* (London, 1842). Like Carpenter's companion piece of 1843, this was necessarily a survey chiefly of continental developments.

[3] Brown, 'Locke and Sydenham', p.81.

[4] On Bristol's history and environment in general, see C.M. McInnes and W.F. Whitland (eds.), *Bristol and its Adjoining Counties* (Bristol, 1955).

[5] George Henry Kendrick Thwaites (1811–82), L.S.A. 1844, M.R.C.S. 1846, Ph.D, F.R.S. 1865, was b. and educated in Bristol. Lecturer on botany at Bristol School of Pharmacy, 1846; then at Bristol Medical School. March 1849, appointed to botanical post in Ceylon: *DNB*. Contributed largely to botany of cryptogams: J.R. Green, *A History of Botany in the United Kingdom* (1914), p.447.

[6] A second society of the same name was formed very shortly afterwards and persisted until 1958. The first society's library of 250 books passed to the Bristol Naturalists' Society (founded 1862); 3 vols. of Transactions (1844–52) and manuscript vols. of abstracts (1850–77) appear lost. Some arrangement was made with the *Quarterly Journal of Microscopical Science* for the publication of transactions; accounts of proceedings appear in the *Monthly Microscopical Journal* from 1869.

included Budd, A. Prichard, J.G. Swayne, and J.B. Estlin. The society came to an early maturity which Estlin, speaking as president, attributed to the 'knowledge, method and energy' of Thwaites, the first treasurer and secretary. There is no evidence that the primary role in the foundation was played by Budd.[1] By the end of the first year the numbers had increased to an extent that made it necessary for the monthly meetings to be held in the Bristol Institution. In 1849, the society was described as being 'as large as any in the provinces', which, given its context, indicates not only the high incidence of such societies, but also that, in spite of its apparently early date of foundation, the Bristol society was not the first of these.[2] It seems doubtful that the metropolitan society had any part in its beginnings.[3]

The Bristolians may have been inspired by the great geological and palaeontological wealth of their area, but it is also possible to talk in terms of contact between individuals. Carpenter belonged as much to London as to Bristol; George Busk, President of London's Microscopical Society in 1849, was acquainted with William Budd through Budd's brother George; and there were such instances as the exhibition at the Bristol society of specimens lent to a member by Richard Owen.[4]

The discovery of the 'cholera-fungus' was made as a result of the liveliness of another Bristol institution, the Bristol Medico-Chirurgical Society, which was said to comprise 'a

---

See H.M. Hatherly, 'A Short History of the Bristol Microscopical Society', *The Microscope*, 11 (1958), 251–3. Scattered published and manuscript records are held by Bristol Central Library, including a prospectus, *Bristol Microscopical Society*, for 1878, and some items in the Estlin collection, e.g. *Rules of the Bristol Microscopical Society, established 1843* (Bristol [1844]) (printed sheet). See Appendix: Bristol Societies, of the thesis on which this book is based.

[1] Bristol Central Library, Estlin Collection, Gen. Box 1, 'Bristol Microscopical Society' (newspaper slip, giving account of annual meeting of 1844). Cf. C.E. Dolman, art. 'William Budd' in *DSB*. The ultimate source for this claim is Augustin Prichard, *Bristol Roy. Inf. Reps.* 1 (1878–9), 361.

[2] J.G. Swayne, *Lond. Med. Gaz.* 9 (1849), 862.

[3] In 1868 the then President of the Royal Microscopical Society urged that it was 'a matter of regret that we have no relation or connection with the many good microscopical societies which are in existence in nearly all our large towns': *Trans. Microsc. Soc.*, 16 (1868), 83.

[4] Bristol Central Library, Estlin Collection, 'Bristol Microscopical Society'.

vast majority of the faculty of the city and neighbourhood'.[1] The growth of Bristol's medical institutions was rapid, but not atypical.[2] Its largest hospital, the Infirmary, was founded in 1734; its medical school was consolidated in 1832, and was, by 1835, the largest in the provinces after Birmingham and Manchester.[3] Bristol students had the reputation of doing well in the London examinations, but the school and the infirmary naturally had the same difficulty as those of other towns in extracting recognition from the Royal Colleges. In 1840, the foundation of a 'medical university' in Bristol was regarded as a feasible proposition.[4] Bristolians were active in the formation of the Provincial Medical and Surgical Association (1832, at Worcester), and formed their own branch in 1840.

Dr. John Beddoe, arriving in the 1850s, found the city very much an intellectual centre, and in this the older generation of medical men, which included J.C. Swayne, J.C. Prichard,

---

[1] 'A Surgeon', *Bristol Mirror*, 20 Oct. 1849. This society is not mentioned by A. Batty Shaw, 'The Oldest Medical Societies in Great Britain', *Med. Hist.* 12 (1968), 232–44. The present body of the same name dates from 1874: G. Parker, 'The Foundation of the Bristol Medico-Chirurgical Society and the History of Military Medicine in England', *Bristol Med.-Chir. J.* 33 (1915), 129–49. The earlier society may have been continuous with a third such society founded in 1812 and apparently in existence in 1825: G. Munro Smith, 'Notes on some Bristol Medical Societies', ibid. 32 (1914), 268–86: 272. However, Augustin Prichard spoke of Budd as a founder of a 'Pathological Society', by which he evidently meant the Bristol Medico-Chirurgical Society active in 1849: *Bristol Roy. Inf. Reps.* 1 (1878–9), 361. In this case, the society of 1849 could not have begun before 1841. Letters by Budd of 1841 and 1842 mention 'the Bristol [or 'our'] Medical Society', and these may refer to the society of 1849: Budd Letters, William to Richard, December 1841; idem to idem [n.d.]; idem to idem [Tagged, '1842']; but perhaps instead to the 'Bristol Medical Library Society', founded first as a subscription library in 1832: see A.E.S. Roberts, 'On the History and Growth of the Bristol Medical School Library', *Bristol Med.-Chir. J.* 85 (1970), 93–100.

[2] On Bristol's medical and other societies, see Appendix in my thesis, cited above, p.vii. On provincial medical institutions, see E.M. Brockbank, *The Foundation of Provincial Medical Education and of the Manchester School in Particular* (Manchester, 1936), pp.118 ff.; W.J. Bishop, 'Medical Book Societies in England in the Eighteenth and Nineteenth Centuries', *Bull. Med. Libr. Ass.* 45 (1957), 337–50.

[3] 1734 is early, but not remarkably so. For a comparative table, see J.D. Harris, *The Royal Devon and Exeter Hospital* (Exeter, 1922), pp.1–2. On the Bristol school, see G. Parker, *Schola Medicinae Bristol* (Bristol, 1933). For a prospectus for 1832, see A. Prichard, 'The Bristol Medical School', *Bristol Med.-Chir. J.* 10 (1892), 264–6.

[4] By a local man, admittedly. See J.C. Prichard, *Farley's Bristol Journal*, 20 June 1840.

and J.A. Symonds, had played a considerable part. Their coherence and activity as a group were owing not merely to the shared professional interests of its members, but also to their being, in many cases, of dissenting persuasions. This allied them to men of the stature of Dr. Lant Carpenter, and led them to undertakings such as the founding of the Bristol College (1831).[1] This shortlived but notable proprietary school educated a whole generation of prominent Bristolians, including F. Brittan, A. Prichard, and J.G. Swayne. Family continuity in terms of place as well as of occupation is common in the medical profession, but it is so marked in Bristol among obviously talented families as to be indicative of the quality of the city's non-medical as well as medical institutions.

Irrespective of these and other advantages, Bristol was an unhealthy town, and suffered from cholera in 1849 as it had in 1832.[2] By 10 June 1849, undoubted cases had occurred there, and a few days later the Medico-Chirurgical Society called all the local medical men together to agree on a statement to be issued to the public.[3] Afterwards the Society held weekly and then fortnightly meetings to consult on the emergency, and at one of these, on 7 July, there were appointed subcommittees to investigate specifically pathological aspects of the disorder. The Microscopical Subcommittee consisted of Dr. James Fogo Bernard, chairman;[4] Dr. John Cash Neild,

[1] J. Beddoe, *Memories of Eighty Years* (Bristol, 1910), p.248. J.G. Swayne *et al.*, 'In Memoriam Augustin Prichard', *Bristol Med.-Chir. J.* 16 (1898), 1. The College was non-denominational and taught science as well as classical subjects: Bristol Central Library, Estlin Collection, manuscript draft of memorial for an appeal [1841].

[2] Appendix, *Second Report of Health of Towns Commission*, PP, 1845, XVIII. 73 [209]; J.A. Symonds, 'Remarks on the Progress and Causes of Cholera in Bristol', *Trans. Prov. Med. Surg. Ass.* 3 (1835), 170–93. For conditions in Bristol in general, see A. Carrick and J.A. Symonds, 'Medical Topography of Bristol', ibid. 2 (1834), 148–80.

[3] For this and further statements, see *Bristol Gazette*, 21 June 1849. For the comparable proceedings at this stage of an epidemic in other large towns, see Longmate, *King Cholera*.

[4] Bernard (1806–78), b. Bristol, father also a physician there, brother (Ralph Montague) a surgeon at the Infirmary. Educated Paris, Edinburgh, London, Dublin. M.D. Cantab. 1836; F.R.C.P. 1838. Physician to Bristol Infirmary 1843–56 and to Bristol Dispensary for Diseases of the Skin. A founder of the Bristol Medical School; lecturer in *materia medica* 1835–43. See *Venn*; G. Munro Smith, *A History of the Bristol Royal Infirmary* (Bristol, 1917), p.304; *Munk*.

secretary;[1] Dr. William Budd; Dr. Joseph Griffiths Swayne[2] and his father John Champeny Swayne;[3] Dr. Augustin Prichard;[4] (Dr.) Frederick Brittan (then practising as a surgeon);[5] and an extraordinary member, Dr. John Addington Symonds,[6] who may have been co-opted at a later date.[7] Probably several subcommittees were formed, as well as a general committee; of these it is likely that one was to have concerned itself with chemical investigation, but although such work was under-

[1] Neild (b. 1814), M.R.C.S. 1839, L.S.A. 1840, Med. and Chir. Doct. Berlin 1839: *De pseudarthrosi quae ossium fracturas sequitur*. Surgeon to Bristol General Hospital. It is possible that Neild spent the latter part of his career in Australia.

[2] J.G. Swayne (1819–1902), b. Bristol, of a large medical family. Educated Bristol, London, Paris. M.R.C.S., L.S.A, 1841; M.D. London 1845. F. Obstet. Soc. of Lond. Later professor of midwifery at Bristol University Medical School. Author of *Obstetric Aphorisms for the Use of Students*, 1856; 10th edn. 1893; Japanese edn. 1880. Swayne's appointment as physician-accoucheur to Bristol General Hospital in 1853 was alleged to be the first of its kind outside London. For obituary and bibliography, see *Bristol Med.–Chir. J.* 21 (1903), 193–202. Swayne began, but never completed, a *Manual of Anatomy* illustrated with his own etchings of his own dissections; see below, p.162 n. 1.

[3] J.C. Swayne (d. 1852), M.R.C.S. 1808, lecturer in midwifery at Bristol Medical School, Hon. Member of Physical Society of Guy's Hospital, London. Surgeon accoucheur. Active in the foundation of Bristol College. See Prichard, 'Bristol Medical School', pp.269–70.

[4] A. Prichard (1818–98), L.S.A., M.R.C.S. 1840; M.D. Berlin; F.R.C.S. 1849. Son of James Cowles Prichard (1786–1848), M.D. Edinburgh 1808, F.R.S. 1831, physician to the Bristol Infirmary 1816–43, pioneer anthropologist and author of *Researches into the Physical History of Man* (1813; facsimile edn., ed. G.W. Stocking, 1973); a Commissioner in Lunacy, 1845. On the elder Prichard, see Stocking's introduction and bibliography, ibid. Augustin Prichard was educated Bristol, London, Berlin, Vienna, and Paris. Surgeon to Bristol Infirmary, 1850–70; also surgeon to Bristol Eye Dispensary. See A. Prichard, *A Few Reminiscences* (1896); Swayne *et al.*, 'Augustin Prichard'.

[5] Brittan (1823–91), M.B. and B.A. Dublin 1842, M.R.C.S. 1844, M.D. Dublin 1845. B. Bristol, educated Bristol, Dublin, Paris. 1848–68, lecturer at Bristol Medical School; 1856–73, physician to Bristol Infirmary. 'Began work' by translating the *Manuel de médecine opératoire* (1834) of J.F. Malgaigne. For an obituary see *Bristol Med.–Chir. J.* 9 (1891), 67–70.

[6] Symonds (1807–71), M.D. Edinburgh 1828, M.R.C.P. 1853, F.R.C.P. 1857. B. Oxford, of long-established medical family; himself father of critic and art historian of the same name. President of British Medical Association, 1863. Physician to Bristol General Hospital, etc. Prolific occasional writer. Shared J.C. Prichard's belief in the doctrine of moral insanity. See D.H. Tuke, *Prichard and Symonds in Especial Relation to Mental Science* (1891); *Munk*; J.F. Nicholls and J. Taylor, *Bristol Past and Present* (Bristol, 1881).

[7] *Lancet*, 1849, ii. 368.

taken by several Bristolians, no record of committee activity exists.[1]

The eight members of the Microscopical Subcommittee could not be called typical of the approximately 140 qualified medical men who then practised in and around Bristol. Rather, in their varied backgrounds, training, and abilities they epitomized what the Bristol profession had to boast of at this time. Only two had not had a period of study at a foreign university.[2] All were, in degrees appropriate to their ages, entrenched in the medical school and in the three main hospitals: St. Peter's, the Infirmary (nicknamed the Lower and Upper Houses respectively, because of the established route from one to the other), and the General Hospital. Bernard, the elder Swayne, and Symonds (in spite of his comparative youth) represented the older type of practitioner, whose merit was said to lie in his clinical acumen, and the skills with which he established his authority over the patient; Prichard and Budd the new type, the 'scientific' practitioner.[3] Of the group, only Budd was primarily interested in the explanation of epidemic disease. Bernard's interest was in skin diseases;[4] Prichard's in ophthalmology. Joseph Swayne

[1] Ibid.; 'A Surgeon', *Bristol Mirror*, 20 Oct. 1849. Chemical analyses were undertaken by the well-known toxicologist William Herapath and his sons William Bird and Thornton J. Herapath, but also by Budd and other members of the Microscopical Subcommittee.

[2] An analysis of the *Medical Directory* for 1849 shows that two-thirds of Bristol qualified practitioners were either M.R.C.S. and L.S.A, or only M.R.C.S, or only L.S.A. Of approximately thirty-five medical degrees, ten were from Edinburgh, ten from other Scottish universities, five from Oxford or Cambridge, one from Dublin, and from London, three M.B.s and two M.D.s. Four more were qualified at foreign universities. Of the thirty-five, at least four (all from the Microscopical Subcommittee) had studied in Paris; there may have been others as the *Directory* did not give such information. For other analyses, see above, p.5 n.1.; W.D. Foster, 'Dr. William Henry Cook: the Finances of a Victorian General Practitioner', *Proc. R. Soc. Med.* 66 (1973), 46–50 (for Tunbridge Wells). The population of Bristol was estimated in 1851 as 137,328: *Population (Great Britain) England and Wales: Pt. I*, PP, 1852–3, LXXXV, p.cxxvi.

[3] A. Prichard, 'Bristol Medical School', pp. 270–1; Smith, *Bristol Royal Infirmary*, pp.344, 342. 'Scientific' is in this case a contemporary description.

[4] This may explain why Bernard was able to instruct Budd in the lower forms of plant life, although Budd himself also had some interest in skin diseases: Budd, *Malignant Cholera* (1849), p.11, note; Budd Letters, William to Richard, 30 Nov. 1843 [Tagged, 'Skin Diseases, 1843'].

devoted himself to obstetrics.[1] Symonds, besides having an immense practice, reserved his special attention for mental diseases. Brittan was interested in a great many things, one of which was epidemic disease.[2] Of the group only two (Symonds and Bernard) are known to have had experience of cholera during the first epidemic.[3] Bernard was a member of the local Board of Health in 1832. He took official part again in 1849, acting as Sutherland's guide in the latter's inspection of the city. Symonds had arrived in Bristol just before the first outbreak in July, 1832. He was made a 'Commissioner of Health' and then honorary secretary to the Board of Health. In his account of the Bristol epidemic, Symonds embraced a form of contingent contagionism, stating that 'concentration of human effluvia had unquestionably been the most influential agent in propagating the disease, once established'. His conclusions were, he said, limited because very few post-mortems had been performed.[4]

Given the absence in the other members of any commitment like Budd's, their forming the subcommittee becomes indicative of a value placed on pathological research and on microscopical research in particular. The existence of a Microscopical Society (of which all but Symonds were members) makes their activity less surprising, but as we have seen the microscope, though highly recommended, was still at this time the interest of experts and addicts rather than the tool of the general practitioner. Moreover, though even the Bristol investigations are better described in terms of individuals rather than institutions, concerted research activity of any kind is unusual at this period. Bodies such as the Provincial

---

[1] Swayne early accepted the findings of Semmelweis and others and therefore as an obstetrician felt obliged to give up all post-mortem investigation although it had been his 'favourite pursuit': Swayne, *Medical Diagnosis* (1880), p.6.

[2] There are references after 1849 to further microscopical analyses by Brittan: see below, p.221 n. 1. An address of 1874 showed him as an adherent of the then germ theory: *Blood Diseases and Blood Germs* (1874). His lecturing appointments at the Bristol Medical School appear to show great versatility: *Bristol Med.-Chir. J.* 9 (1891), 68.

[3] Of the others, only Budd and the elder Swayne were old enough. Budd was studying in Paris before and after the first epidemic; it is not definitely known what he was doing in the years between.

[4] [G. Parker], 'Dr. Symonds and the Cholera in Bristol', *Bristol Med.-Chir. J.* 50-1 (1933-4), 57-8; Symonds, 'Remarks on Cholera in Bristol', p.170.

Medical and Surgical Association and the Royal College of Physicians thought first of enquiries, often of a statistical type, which aimed at a consensus of opinion on clinical points or on treatment. In 1833, the Association's founder had urged members to 'set up committees, after the excellent example of the British Association'. Subjects suggested were the state and progress of anatomy, the chemistry of animal fluids as illustrative of pathology, and vaccination.[1] Topics of enquiries actually carried out included the treatment of burns and scalds, influenza (1837), and the uses of cod-liver oil in phthisis. In 1849, a 'consensus-enquiry' was carried out into cholera, but some difficulty was experienced in attracting contributions.[2] As we shall see, the College's experience was similar.

Too much stress should not be placed on the medical aspect of the Bristol subcommittee's inspiration. It is worth noting that Budd had lectured in 1845 in the Bristol Literary and Philosophical Institution on the equally topical, but less immediate, subject of the potato disease, and that he had based this lecture on an extensive display of drawings and microscopical preparations.[3]

On 9 July the Microscopical Subcommittee convened at the house of William Budd. The latter had obtained from two of his patients at the temporary cholera hospital samples of the characteristic 'rice-water' evacuations, and Brittan and the younger Swayne were asked to examine these microscopically. Budd himself reserved some of the fluid for chemical investigation. Brittan and Swayne made their examinations separately, and when on the following day each reported his results they were found to 'coincide perfectly': 'Both our drawings and specimens showed certain bodies in considerable abundance, and so singular in appearance, that we expressed our opinion that they were characteristic of the evacuations of cholera, if not the very agents causing the disease. In this

---

[1] McMenemey, *Charles Hastings*, p.100.

[2] For the questions see *Lancet*, 1849, ii. 622; for the report, *Prov. Med. Surg. J.* 14 (1850), 505. For a similar exercise on the part of the King's College Medical Society, see *Lancet*, 1849, ii. 484.

[3] Budd Letters, William to Richard, 16 Nov. 1845 [Tagged, '1845. His gt. losses'].

opinion the other members coincided.' Other versions exist of the response of the other members to the exhibits.[1] The coincidence was no doubt striking, and certainly held a peculiar appeal for Budd, but it is probable that, as the *Morning Chronicle* hoped, Swayne was 'putting forward for the other members more than they would assert for themselves'. Brittan agreed with the *Chronicle* that Swayne had gone 'rather too far'.[2] Nevertheless it was deemed worth while to present the findings to the parent society, which was done on 14 July. When the Microscopical Subcommittee produced its own report (which it did not do until much later), it described the general impression on this occasion as being that 'the bodies in question were *sui generis*, and had never before been observed in any part, or in any secretion, of the human body'.[3]

The Bristol Medico-Chirurgical Society was usually given credit for initiating these investigations, and its members later expressed gratification at the publicity their society had received.[4] In the closing stages of the controversy its meetings were again used as an arena for this particular series of events, but for the most part the business was carried on by individuals, not only independently of the Society but, to a large extent, independently of each other. This was grounds for complaint in at least one quarter, and Swayne was later to admit that it would have been better to have published their results under the aegis of the Society. As we shall see, the medium chosen was often that of the daily press.

After the meeting on 14 July, the investigations were continued by Brittan alone. Between 9 July and 30 July he examined thirty-three samples of evacuation from twenty patients in the Bristol hospitals, 'date of evacuation after seizure' (i.e. onset) being anything from two hours to seven days. In each of six cases he made comparative observations of evacuations produced at different times during the illness.

---

[1] 'Report of the Microscopical Subcommittee', *Prov. Med. Surg. J.* 13 (1849), 601; J.G. Swayne, 'An Account of Certain Organic Cells', *Lancet*, 1849, ii. 369; idem, *Morning Chronicle*, 25 Sept. 1849.

[2] *Morning Chronicle*, 25 Sept. 1849.

[3] 'Report of the Microscopical Subcommittee', p.600.

[4] *Farley's Bristol Journal*, 15 Dec. 1849.

As well as noting the incidence of the 'annular' or 'cholera' bodies, he recorded, qualitatively, the character of the evacuation, the incidence of 'granules' and 'granular cells', of 'muscular and vegetable tissue', and of 'crystals, blood and epithelium'. He also noted the presence of 'animalculae'.[1] Encouraged by the almost invariable appearance of the annular bodies in what appeared to be different stages of development, he went on to examine healthy stools and the stools of 'typhus and other diseases'. He obtained negative results except in the ambiguous case of 'severe choleraic diarrhoea'. On the basis of these positive and negative instances he was 'led to the necessary inference that these bodies were peculiar to the evacuations of cholera patients, and must have some essential relation to the disease'.[2]

Well before the end of this series of examinations, Brittan had begun other experiments with, as he admitted, the aim of determining whether the 'essential relation' was one of cause and effect. He had already made two decisions in favour of this conclusion: first, that the objects were unlike any known bodily products; and second, that they could be found in different stages of development. Since those in the vomit appeared to be at an early stage, it could be inferred that they were introduced from without. All these propositions were open to objection,[3] but the argument seemed of little moment beside the direct evidence which Brittan obtained, of the existence of the bodies in 'cholera atmospheres'. On 19 July, using an apparatus designed by Bernard, he condensed a small quantity of fluid from the atmosphere of a house from which five cholera patients had been removed the day before.[4] In this and similar samples he found annular bodies like those he had already observed.

As he had apparently established that the cholera bodies were not only peculiar to choleraic matters, but always to be

---

[1] e.g. 'vibriones', and *sarcina ventriculi.*

[2] Brittan, 'Report of a Series of Microscopical Investigations', *Lond. Med. Gaz.* 9 (1849), 531.

[3] On the problems of elucidating the life-cycles of fungi see J. von Sachs, *History of Botany 1530–1860* (Oxford, 1890), pp.204 ff.

[4] For a description of an apparatus said to be similar to Brittan's see T. Herapath, *Lond. Med. Gaz.* 9 (1849), 845. Herapath repeated Brittan's experiments with negative results.

found in them, Brittan's 'second discovery' seemed highly significant. According to Swayne it was on the strength of this 'subsequent discovery of cells in the atmosphere' that he and Budd conceded priority of publication to Brittan. Budd, who had also confirmed Brittan's first results, assisted him in a successful repetition of the experiments on air, and as a consequence felt encouraged to examine samples of water from affected areas. Budd's results were also positive; he detected, he said, 'the same organisms in almost every specimen of drinking water' which he was able to obtain from cholcra districts. He further examined a 'great number of specimens of water from healthy quarters' without finding the cholera-bodies.[1]

Brittan published nothing until 21 September, nearly two months after the date of his last recorded examination. Waiting allowed him to add to his own results a second series, obtained by Swayne from an examination of twenty-seven samples from twenty-one patients.[2] Brittan also went to London, to submit his findings to his professional superiors. This was not merely a matter of displaying drawings and preparations. Brittan substantiated his findings with 'examples furnished by these gentlemen themselves'. From these latter, he received decisive encouragement. An announcement by the *London Medical Gazette* of the imminent publication of Brittan's paper read in part:

The results of Mr. Brittan's observations have been submitted to the judgment of the most eminent microscopic pathologists of the metropolis, as well as those gentlemen who have acquired great repute for their researches on cholera, and they, considering them of a novel and most interesting character, have urged Mr. Brittan to give them immediate publicity.[3]

It will become clear that in order to give this kind of encouragement the experts had no need to agree on the exact terms in which the significance or even the nature of these bodies should be described, and there was, in fact, no such agreement. Most of the experts remained unidentified throughout, exceptions being John Quekett and William Baly. Quekett's

---

[1] Swayne, *Lancet*, 1849, ii. 410; Budd, *Malignant Cholera*, p.4.

[2] Tabled in Brittan, 'Report of a Series of Microscopical Investigations', pp.537–40.

[3] Ibid., p.530; *Lond. Med. Gaz.* 9 (1849), 499.

contribution was important because it was his word as published by Brittan, rather than any statement of Brittan's, which established that the cholera-bodies were 'fungoid'.[1] With this support, Brittan gave in his paper for publication. This was the more desirable in that the epidemic could be expected to subside completely within a month or six weeks.

The main forum of discussion was the London press. Most medical societies were in recess from April or May to October, or even later; a very few (for example the Westminster Medical, the South London Medical) held emergency meetings at this time, but usually to discuss treatment or the progress of the disease. It would have been quixotic for Brittan to have published elsewhere, if only because the only 'local' medical journal of national importance, the *Provincial Medical and Surgical Journal*, was put out fortnightly. There were as yet no daily newspapers in the Bristol area. The Bristol weekly papers, although assuming in various degrees responsibility for reporting the progress of the local outbreak, were almost entirely dependent upon reprints from London papers for their account of the cholera-fungus controversy. This did not, of course, prevent their taking a proprietary attitude. Of London journals, Brittan chose the *London Medical Gazette*; it was therefore inevitable that Swayne's rival claims should appear in *The Lancet*. More interesting, perhaps, is the part played by the lay press.[2] *The Times* published Budd's first communication and some others, but did not itself take part in the controversy, except to print a lengthy, anonymous review of the cholera-fungus theory. In general, this newspaper concentrated on sanitary matters and grievances, constituting itself the most freely available source for official information on disease incidence and for proceedings of official bodies responsible for the public health. Its editorials, then as later, were confined to the assumption that disease was preventable by appropriate official action based on

---

[1] Brittan, 'Report of a Series of Microscopical Investigations', p.542.

[1] For a substantial treatment of the activity of the lay press with respect to 'scientific' questions, see A. Ellegård, *Darwin and the General Reader* (Göteborg, 1958).

obvious sanitary principles.[1] Its series on 'The History of the Origin, Progress and Mortality of the Cholera Morbus' is an illustration of its informative policy.[2] By contrast, the *Morning Chronicle*, like *The Lancet*, took an active part. This newspaper pursued a more radical (and sensational) policy, and its pages at this time were remarkable for a series, by Henry Mayhew, describing 'sanitary walks' in the worst parts of London.[3] The existence of the cholera-bodies was personally demonstrated to the *Chronicle* staff, and the paper printed an announcement simultaneously with the *London Medical Gazette*. Thereafter, the *Chronicle* became possessive of Brittan, and did much to raise the temperature and pulse of debate.[4] In the first weeks it made perhaps the boldest claim for Brittan's discovery being one predicted by and complementary to earlier theoretical formulations. This forward behaviour was naturally criticized by the medical journals.[5]

In public-health matters the profession saw itself as prepared to enlist the aid of the press, both in provoking government to action and in educating the public, for example, as to the significance of premonitory diarrhoea. However, such licence extended only to matters in which the public could be expected to help themselves, and this affords further evidence of the distinction made by the profession between public health and medical practice. The deepest corporate concern of the profession was (and is) that it should not be seen to contradict itself. This concern is apt to appear interested as well as hypocritical, but there can be behind it an awareness of the part that may be played by skill and experience in a case where there is no prescribed course of action, and also of the part played in recovery by the patient's

---

[1] 'The Fungoid Theory of Cholera', *The Times*, 5 Oct. 1849; note conclusions. On *The Times* and public-health questions see Lambert, *John Simon*, and Gibson, 'The Public Health Agitation, A Newspaper and Parliamentary History'.

[2] Reprinted in *Lond. Med. Gaz.* 9 (1849), 507–11, 556–9, 600–2.

[3] A selection from the series published in the *Chronicle* by Mayhew between 1849 and 1850 has been edited by E.P. Thompson and E. Yeo, *The Unknown Mayhew* (1973). For the *Chronicle* and issues relevant here see Thompson's introduction.

[4] See e.g. *Morning Chronicle*, 25 Sept. 1849.

[5] Ibid. 21 Sept. 1849. See *Lond. Med. Gaz.* 9 (1849), 759, for the most unbridled criticism.

confidence in his attendant. Who shall decide if doctors disagree? Therefore, as one physician put it, 'results and not processes are for the public eye'. Occasionally the laity can be seen to take the role of censor on to itself.[1]

None the less, the emergency created by the epidemic seemed to justify different behaviour. Others besides Brittan saw the daily press as a proper medium for publication (and adjudication) at this time.[2] Thus, when because of its real lack of knowledge it was the more necessary for the profession not to appear inconsistent, its members were prompted by the same state of ignorance to give maximum publicity to individual insights. Doubtless the crises created by nineteenth-century epidemics accelerated the process by which, as medical practice became less a matter of skill than of science, medicine seemed to cease to be 'the mystery of a caste'. The *Morning Chronicle* approvingly noted, as a remarkable feature of the recent epidemic, 'the sudden flood of information as to medical treatment which . . . poured in upon us in good, homely, honest English instead of the technical phrases and latinised obscurities in which the science of physic was heretofore shrouded'.[3] However, this in many respects temporary fragmentation of the professional interest was also owing to the movement for medical reform and the rising strength of institutions outside London.

The first reactions to Brittan's findings were nearly all claims to a share in the discovery, or to the discovery itself. One of those to claim a share was Swayne. Charles Cowdell of Dorchester, author of a *Disquisition on Pestilential Cholera*, wrote to point out that Brittan's work seemed likely to provide a demonstration of his own long-held views, and also that, although these views had not been based on any microscopical evidence, he had since discovered 'protophytic' bodies in the sweat of cholera patients. These investigations were incomplete, he added, but he was publishing them in order to avoid charges of plagiarism later.[4] Others from

---

[1] *Lond. Med. Gaz.* 9 (1849), 636; 'The Cholera in Bristol', *Bristol Gazette*, 21 June 1849.

[2] See e.g. H. Lamplough, *Morning Chronicle*, 18 Sept. 1849.

[3] Simon, *Sanitary Institutions*, p.x; *Morning Chronicle*, 28 Sept. 1849.

[4] Cowdell, *Lond. Med. Gaz.* 9 (1849), 555.

among the minority of medical men who had made similar observations in a variety of situations in the past without thinking much of it, were tempted to publish rather hasty contributions. It was difficult to charge any of them with irrelevancy, since Brittan had deliberately refrained from hedging his observations about with theory. What these observers, and possibly those experts who urged Brittan to publicize his 'novel' discovery do seem to have displayed, is the 'collector's spirit' which Carpenter deplored in English microscopy.

William Budd also hastened into print during the first week, having apparently agreed to delay publishing his fully-developed theory of cholera only until Brittan had made his announcement. Budd's letter to *The Times* is evidently a contraction of his pamphlet, which he dated 27 September, but which he could not have expected to appear until after 28 September, Brittan's publication date.[1] Budd did not contest Brittan or Swayne's right to the discovery of the cholera-bodies; rather, he laid claim to a set of conclusions constituting a theory of cholera. He was careless about dates and other details of the discovery itself, but went to the extent of placing the evidence for his theory with the president of the Royal College of Physicians until it could be published. The investigations of his colleagues, Budd said, did much to show the existence of a relation between the cholera-bodies and cholera, but they 'were not enforced by any arguments to that effect'.[2] Budd, on the other hand, was prepared to state definitely that: the cause of malignant cholera was a 'living organism of distinct species', which seemed to be of the fungus tribe;[3] these organisms were taken in by swallowing; their presence and infinite multiplication in the intestinal canal caused the peculiar flux of cholera, and thereby all the

---

[1] Budd, *The Times*, 26 Sept. 1849; idem, *Malignant Cholera*, p.27. Goodall saw in 1936 a (printed) variant of this pamphlet dated 25 Sept., which I have been unable to trace. It made several confident assertions which the version of 27 Sept. omitted or modified: Goodall, *William Budd*, p.145. Budd's letter to *The Times* may have been a last-minute substitute for the earlier version of the pamphlet.

[2] Budd, *The Times*, 26 Sept. 1849; idem, *Malignant Cholera*, p.4.

[3] Budd had at first thought that the organisms were algae: ibid., p. 11 n. However it was, he added, 'well known to naturalists that these two families run into one another by insensible gradations'.

essential features of the disease; and, though preserved for a time in air, they rapidly decayed or were consumed in water, which was the 'chief vehicle' of their diffusion. This last point Budd considered had been proved by the researches of Snow, to whom he further granted all the merit of its discovery.[1]

The remainder (and greater part) of Budd's letter set out procedures for the control of cholera by the use of fungicides. The pamphlet shows a similar depth of feeling for the practical consequences of his theory.

The pamphlet added to the letter in *The Times* details of the argument but little evidence. Budd's description of the cholera-bodies, while agreeing in essentials with that of Brittan, was cursory, and there was no table of observations. Stress was placed not so much on the presence of the bodies, but on their being present 'in infinite numbers'; the different appearances they presented were important in allowing the assumption that they were a species of living organism. The fact and assumption combined allowed Budd to describe cholera as a form of the known, if not familiar, phenomenon of elective parasitism. The fungus multiplied in the human gut, which was its peculiar habitat.[2] This was sufficient to explain both the damage done to the body and the puzzling phenomena of propagation outside it. Budd stressed his ability to explain the rapid subsidence of epidemics, which had been 'a stumbling block in the way of all previous theories'. Indeed, Budd could state that 'the facts already brought to light are not only sufficient to enable us to account for all the chief phenomena which mark the course and spread of the disease, but actually to show that these phenomena must necessarily happen as a direct consequence of such conditions'. In this connection he emphasized the role of air as well as water carriage.[3]

After the letter appeared in *The Times*, Brittan wrote correcting his colleague 'on some inaccuracies as to dates', but

---

[1] Budd, *The Times*, 26 Sept. 1849; idem, *Malignant Cholera*, p.19 n. Snow's own pamphlet was dated 19 Aug. and was reviewed by the *London Medical Gazette* on 14 Sept.

[2] This point is enlarged upon in a letter (Budd, *Lancet*, 1849, ii. 399) written to correct any impression given by the pamphlet that the fungi lived on the common material in the gut, rather than the specific, 'perfected juices' of the host.

[3] Budd, *Malignant Cholera*, pp.21 ff.

otherwise expressing 'extreme satisfaction': 'the conclusions he arrives at, and the practical deductions from them, with one or two exceptions, my own investigations confirm'. This, however, hardly amounts to a commitment to Budd's whole view, and Brittan never did so commit himself. After the first stage of the controversy he retired, and the Bristol side of things was managed entirely by Swayne. Brittan's one ambition for his work was that 'through it there might be obtained at least one common ascertained fact on which the profession may be agreed'. In all his papers he 'studiously avoided giving any opinion at all' on the facts, and made only such statements as could be proved true or false by anyone who took the trouble.[1] He did not deny having formed opinions, but reserved them for publication at a later time. It is possible that he was deterred from doing so by the repressive treatment meted out to Budd.

It is obvious, even from his own paper, that Brittan's distinction between 'fact and mere opinion' was more nominal than real, but the support he received prior to publication, and the comments made thereafter, show the extent to which his contemporaries shared his ideal of 'fixed and demonstrated truth'.[2] The current medical fear of theory or speculation was naturally, though paradoxically, aggravated by the conditions of the epidemic. Consequently, Budd's baldly presented conclusions were met with reserve or condemnation. *The London Medical Gazette* welcomed the (contingent) contagionism of the fungus theory, but in its review of Budd confined itself to exposition because the matter was *sub judice*. More significantly, the *Provincial Medical and Surgical Journal* received the work, but never reviewed it. Elsewhere the *Journal* (like many others) remarked on Budd's discovery of the organisms in water supplies but otherwise mentioned him only to point a contrast with the 'wise reserve' of Brittan. The anonymous article in *The Times* accused Budd of speculating with results not his own. The *Morning Chronicle*, while eager to believe that Brittan's fungi were the cause of cholera,

---

[1] Brittan, *The Times*, 27 Sept. 1849; idem, 'Report of a Series of Microscopical Investigations', pp.541, 530.

[2] On mid-Victorian methodological philosophy, see Ellegård, *Darwin and the General Reader*, Ch. 9.

criticized Budd for attempting to explain all the phenomena of the disease. Brittan, in contrast with Budd, was universally approved, and it was assumed on all sides that the matter could and would be decided on observational grounds. *The Lancet*, which had described Budd's views as 'clever but uncertain', stated confidently that 'the whole profession is roused upon the subject, and the truth can hardly elude the thousand eyes of the profession . . .'[1]

A modern reader might also believe in this kind of verification, and yet consider the whole exercise doomed because of the technical limitations involved. Although contemporary microscopes were more than capable of the range required, there were at this time no 'isolation procedures', and the means by which small objects might be described objectively were very limited.[2] These disabilities, however, must be admitted of the whole of the period preceding the technical innovations of Koch. Given a likelihood of subsequent negative or indefinite results, what matters is the observer's reactions; whether he perseveres, or publishes, is a question of judgement depending upon the view he already has of the significance of the phenomena. This relativity of observation was not appreciated by Budd's contemporaries at least.[3] With their notion of fact they made very literal use of 'presence —absence' criteria. If the discovery of the cholera-bodies had been predicted by a generally accepted theory, these criteria might unconsciously have been relaxed. Without this motive for acceptance, they were applied as if to ideal conditions; consequently the criteria laid down as having to be fulfilled before the bodies could be accepted as the cause of cholera,

---

[1] *Lond. Med. Gaz.* 9 (1849), 724–5; *Prov. Med. Surg. J.* 13 (1849), 572. *The Times*, 5 Oct. 1849; *Morning Chronicle*, 26 Sept. 1849; *Lancet*, 1849, ii. 406.

[2] Present-day optical microscopes will resolve objects of the order of 0·25 micrometres. The instrument most widely used in 1849 was a Ross with an object glass of $\frac{1}{8}$in., which in practice resolved objects of 0·9 micrometres. A Ross's $\frac{1}{12}$ which could resolve objects of 0·4 micrometres was also used, e.g. by Brittan and by contributors to the Royal College of Physicians' report (see below). The smallest bodies described during the controversy had a diameter of $\frac{1}{10,000}$ in., which is equivalent to 2·5 micrometres. The Bristol findings were not globulist illusions; nor is there any likelihood of their having had any relation to the known causative agents in cholera.

[3] For some attempt to amend this lack of appreciation, see J.W. Griffith and A. Henfrey, *The Micrographic Dictionary* (1855).

were impossible: '[The bodies] must be found coincident with cholera in all districts; not there before or after the disease. They must be found in every body affected with disease, or in the [evacuations] as they come from the body ...' Similarly, disproof was easy because negative evidence was taken at face value: '... if it is possible to be proved indisputably in only one instance, that a case of cholera may occur at the same time as these cells are absent both from the water and from the air, it is evident that we must look in some other direction for the *fons et origo mali ...*' Naturally, these views, though shared by Brittan and Swayne, worked to their disadvantage. Budd, having a fully developed view of the causal relationship, did not himself feel that he was similarly affected by single counter-instances. Since the important point for him was that the cholera-bodies were present in large numbers, it did not matter if a few 'stray bodies of similar character' were found associated with other diseases.[1] However, negative results with cholera products or environments could damage his theory; no opponent would allow him to plead the practical difficulties involved.[2]

In the event, no member of the profession produced a piece of research comparable with Brittan's. Instead, the problem broadened to become that of epi- and endo-phytes in general.[3] It was George Busk, president of the Microscopical Society of London, who at last dealt directly with the Bristol investigations.[4] By this time (mid-October), Brittan's account had

[1] *Lancet*, 1849, ii. 482; T. Herapath, *Lond. Med. Gaz.* 9 (1849), 846; Budd, *Malignant Cholera*, pp.8, 29.

[2] For Budd on these difficulties, see *Malignant Cholera*, p.30.

[3] See e.g. 'Nemo', *Morning Chronicle*, 5 Oct. 1849; W.R Basham, *Lond. Med. Gaz.* 9 (1849), 686; N. Parker, ibid., p.668.

[4] Busk (1807–86), M.R.C.S. 1830, F.R.C.S. 1843, F. Linnaean Soc. 1846. Asst. surgeon, 1832, to *Grampus* Hospital Ship; then *Dreadnought*. President of Royal College of Surgeons, 1871. Founder member of the (Royal) Microscopical Society; its President, 1848–9; editor, with Lankester, of its *Journal*, 1853–68. Known for systematic work on marine Polyzoa etc. See *Plarr*; *DNB*; R.M. MacLeod, 'The X-Club: A Scientific Network in Late Victorian England', *Notes Rec. R. Soc. Lond.* 24 (1970), 305–22. Busk was an associate of George Budd's at the Royal Medical and Chirurgical Society as well as on the *Dreadnought*, and had supplied William Budd with specimens (e.g. 'cancer cells', *c.* 1842), and case histories. The latter was himself briefly connected with the *Dreadnought*, possibly as a trial replacement for George. William left the ship, and London, on account of illness. See Budd Letters, 1837–40.

been superseded by that of Swayne.[1] Swayne published his more detailed account a week later than Brittan and Budd, and it is his descriptions and handsome woodcuts which are reproduced in the report of the Bristol Subcommittee. Swayne saw a variety of different 'cells', and like his colleagues (and Quekett) regarded them as different stages of a single development. He defined three types: small, medium, and large. The small were found in the atmosphere and the vomit, and also in the lower gut in the company of the large cells. If, as seemed justified by their structure, the large cells were regarded as parent cells, these observations defined a cycle.[2] In a few cases Swayne had found an intact 'parent cell', like a mulberry, which he put forward as the 'perfect cholera cell'. He sent samples of this cell to observers in Exeter, Liverpool, and Edinburgh, and also submitted samples to E.O. Spooner in Blandford, Carpenter, Edwin Lankester, Arthur Hassall, and Charles Daubeny in Oxford.[3] Daubeny displayed his sample to the local Ashmolean Society.[4] Swayne added to his paper a third table of results (seventeen positive specimens from seventeen patients), and defined the chemical as well as microscopical properties of normal and choleraic evacuations.

Busk had long been an active member of the London-based Microscopical Society, and was a recognized authority on multicellular organisms and other objects. In the 1840s he

[1] Swayne, 'Account of Certain Organic Cells'. On 18 Oct. Brittan was appointed a Board of Health inspector with an initial tenure of two months: *Farley's Bristol Journal*, 20 Oct. 1849. He is next heard of acting in his official capacity in Bridgewater, near Bristol; he may have supplied Swayne with samples from this town. He was apparently enjoined by the Board to 'continue the prosecution of his microscopic inquiries touching the fungoid origin of cholera', but there is no evidence of his having done so. He was employed under the same conditions as Parkes. During the third epidemic he prepared a report on the water supply of Sandgate.

[2] 'Report of Microscopical Subcommittee', pp.600 ff. Given his emphasis on reproductive continuity, Swayne is more likely to have had in mind independent organisms, than the cells of current cell theory.

[3] Of these, Carpenter and (to a lesser extent) Hassall gave timely support: *Farley's Bristol Journal*, 15 Dec. 1849; Swayne, *Lond. Med. Gaz.* 9 (1849), 861, 950. For Lankester, Hassall, and Spooner see also below. Daubeny recorded his reaction later: 'Influence of the Lower Vegetable Organisms in Epidemic Diseases', *Edinb. Phil. J.* 2 (1855), 102–3.

[4] R.J. Morris, 'Religion and Medicine: The Cholera Pamphlets of Oxford, 1832, 1849, and 1854', *Med. Hist.* 19 (1975), 256–70: 261. Note the reaction of Henry Acland.

had contributed to the growing literature on the incidence of minute organisms in the body, while implying that he thought these were nothing other than *ad hoc* occurrences. As surgeon to the *Dreadnought* Hospital Ship he had had clinical experience of cholera, and according to his friend Lankester had examined cholera evacuations, always with negative results. [1] Between them Busk and Lankester now divided the alleged cholera-bodies into two classes, definite and indefinite. In the latter class, and dismissed as consisting of 'various organic and inorganic matters', were included all the bodies found in the water or the atmosphere, and the smallest of those found in the evacuations and vomit. The definite forms were those which most resembled the specimens then being exhibited and supplied to interested parties by Swayne, and these Busk thought could be divided into three types. On 17 October, at a meeting of the Microscopical Society, he demonstrated the presence of all three forms in a loaf of bread purchased in Greenwich. [2]

Or so went one of the many published accounts of the meeting. In fact, Busk had identified two of the forms with starch grains and wheat husk or bran respectively; the third, Swayne's 'perfect cholera cell', he stated to be spores of a uredo of the same genus, though not of the same species, as the smut of grain. [3] Three days later Lankester, though not entirely abandoning his own opinion that the bodies were altered (human) epithelial cells, expounded and endorsed Busk's views to the Westminster Medical Society. The weekly and emergency meetings of this society had provided Snow, as well as Swayne, with an opportunity of airing their views. [4]

Busk's contribution was widely taken as showing that the cholera cells were in no way peculiar in themselves or related

---

[1] See Busk, *Microscopic Journal*, 1842, pp.321–3; idem, 'Observations on Parasitical Growths in Living Animals', ibid. 1841, pp.145–52. *Lancet*, 1849, i. 293; ibid. 1849, ii. 404.

[2] *Lond. Med. Gaz.* 9 (1849), 692. A fuller, but no more accurate account, reprinted from the *Athenaeum*, appeared in the *Bristol Mirror*, 27 Oct. 1849. *The Times*, on 24 Oct., reprinted an account from the *Globe*.

[3] For further details see Swayne, *Lond. Med. Gaz.* 9 (1849), 861. Busk himself corrected the errors in the first reports: ibid., p.732. None the less they reappeared in the Royal College of Physicians' report.

[4] *Lancet*, 1849, ii. 459 ff.

to each other. This conclusion persisted, even when in the Royal College of Physicians' report Busk's became included in a range of possible identifications. As is shown most clearly in the case of the uredo, it was enough for Swayne's opponents to have established a *general* resemblance between the cholera-bodies and familiar bodies of known and innocuous origin. Given that there was no motive for regarding the bodies as incongruous, it was of no use for Swayne to prove that his cholera cells were distinguishable not only from the uredo of smut but from all other uredos hitherto described. [1] Similarly, with the other bodies, there was no onus on Swayne's opponents to fix their exact nature.

Experience is something in such matters, but there is no reason for the modern reader to suppose that Busk's role was that of *deus ex machina*. His previous reactions to lesser propositions of the same type make him a participant, and disqualify him for the role of objective authority.[2] One can, however, say (with the defenders of the cholera fungus) that Busk's reputation was a major factor in determining the response to his statements. Swayne's supporters further suspected that Busk, under the inevitable delusions as to the amateurishness of provincial microscopy, had made only the most perfunctory investigation of their claims. *The Lancet*, partly by way of reforming zeal, was enough in sympathy with this to see the situation as one man's word against another's, and therefore no solution. When doctors disagree, it stated, 'doctors shall decide, and under the sanction of government authority'. It then called for a Royal Commission, to consist of men whose minds were known to be 'uncramped by the prejudices of the day'.[3]

Mention has already been made of the lack of precedent for investigations other than those of the consensus type. In 1849 there were three institutions which could be envisaged as sponsoring an 'official inquiry': the Government, the new

---

[1] Swayne, *Lond. Med. Gaz.* 9 (1849), 861. This opinion was also held by the Revd. Miles Berkeley: ibid., pp.1035 ff.

[2] One of Busk's identifications was later contradicted by J.W. Griffith: *Lond. Med. Gaz.* 9 (1849), 760.

[3] See a letter, 'The Bristol Microscopical Society *versus* the President of the Microscopical Society of London', by a member of the former, *Lancet*, 1849, ii. 460; ibid., p.462.

General Board of Health, and the Royal College of Physicians.[1] In the first two cases it was assumed that the inquiry would be manned by persons approved by the profession. No medical man, of course, was satisfied with the composition of the Board itself. The *Morning Chronicle* early in the controversy made the suggestion that the Board conduct an inquiry, as part of a general demand that it concern itself with the actual causes of disease.[2] However, this suggestion and others like it made by the profession should be taken as expressing criticism of the Board, rather than definite notions of its properly having a research role. With respect to government in general, medical men presumably conformed to the contemporary taste for Royal Commissions; but only those with as much reforming zeal as *The Lancet* would have advocated a Commission in the present case, rather than the more obvious alternative of adjudication by the College of Physicians.

As it happened, the College had machinery already in existence, and had taken up the option even before it was offered — or rather, two of its members had. Its Cholera Committee had been set up in October of the previous year, and consisted of 'physicians of the great metropolitan hospitals and certain other eminent persons'. Besides the President (John Ayrton Paris), Censors, and Registrar, these included Sir William Burnett (of 'Burnett's Disinfecting Fluid'), Thomas Watson, William Guy, Richard Bright, and George Budd.[3] At the second meeting there were added William Baly, George Roupell (attached to the *Dreadnought* and therefore like George Budd a colleague of Busk), and Southwood Smith. William Gull joined them in the following January. Of this committee (described by Clark as 'strong, or at least ... large'), it can be said that the well-known names are those of clinicians (Watson, Latham, Burrows, Bright, Budd), or of sanitarians and medical administrators (Southwood Smith,

---

[1] It had already been suggested that 'the Government' conduct investigations to test the ozone theory of cholera: 'M.D.', *Morning Chronicle*, 12 Sept. 1849.

[2] Ibid., 26 and 27 Sept. 1849.

[3] College Cholera MSS., Minute Book, 21 Oct. 1848: Copy of letter by J.A. Paris to Sir George Grey. The remaining members were Peter Latham, George Burrows, Sir James McGrigor, C.J.B. Williams, Benjamin Guy Babington, Henry Roots, Charles Forbes, Thomas Mayo, W.E. Page, P.N. Kingston, H. Burton, A. Frampton, and J.A. Wilson; for all of whom see *Munk*.

Burnett), and that the lesser-known names belong to faithful servants of the College.[1] The first concern of this Committee had been to put out their own list of precautions as a reply to those published by Chadwick's General Board of Health. This was drawn up by Babington, Burrows, and Budd on condition that the other Committee members submitted their opinions in writing.[2] As Finer points out, the apparent disagreement between the College and the Board was of little or no significance in medical terms. At the end of the correspondence between Paris and Sir George Grey, the Fellows of the Committee passed a resolution praising their President's prudence and concern for the public and the honour of the College.[3]

Three months later, in January, Baly and Gull were asked to draw up a report on cholera based on the best literature and experience available. Circulars requesting information on treatment were sent out to hospital physicians and other members of the College. This proceeding was welcomed by the *London Medical Gazette*, but (like the similar efforts of the Provincial Medical and Surgical Association) it proved unproductive.[4] Baly and Gull were then transformed into a paid subcommittee and directed to take 'more active' measures. A second circular was sent out early in September, asking for the results of post-mortems, analyses of the blood, and similar information; seemingly this, too, met with little response, since in a letter of 13 October Baly and Gull requested members of the College to hand out copies of it to *non*-members with experience of cholera. At the same

---

[1] Clark, *College of Physicians*, ii. 700. As a faithful servant see e.g. Henry Roots. It is relevant to note here that George Budd's views on epidemic disease were in opposition to his brother's: see G. Budd (with Busk), 'Report of Cases of Cholera on the Dreadnought, 1837', *Med. Chir. Trans.* 21 (1838), 152–86; G. Budd, 'Statistical Account of Cholera in the Seamen's Hospital in 1832', ibid. 22 (1839), 110–23. William assisted George with the preparation of one of these papers: Budd Letters, William to Richard, November 1837. For George Budd (1808–82), B.A. Cantab. 1831, M.D. Cantab. 1840, F.R.C.P. 1841, F.R.S. 1836, attached to King's College London 1840–67, author of standard works on the liver and the stomach, see Budd Letters (1836–46); *DNB*; *Venn*; R.E. Hughes, 'George Budd (1808–1882) and Nutritional Deficiency Diseases', *Med. Hist.* 17 (1973), 127–35.

[2] College Cholera MSS., Minute Book, 7 Oct. 1848. For the statement issued, see *The Times*, 3. Nov. 1848, and above, p.147.

[3] Finer, *Life of Chadwick*, p.341; College Cholera MSS., Minute Book, 21 Oct. 1848. The correspondence is recorded in this book.

[4] Ibid., 7 Jan. 1849; 7 Oct. 1848. *Lond. Med. Gaz.* 9(1849), 298.

time they enlisted the co-operation of members in a 'special enquiry respecting the origin and mode of propagation of cholera'. A questionnaire was sent out, which related not to pathology but to the circumstances of epidemic diffusion, and especially to the first cases in a given area. The belated result of these efforts was the *Reports on Cholera* published by the College in 1854. Clark sees a decision of the Committee in October 1849 not to publish at that time as evidence of a great improvement since 1832 in public sanitary arrangements: 'There was no longer any need for help from the College, and the public authorities did not ask for it.' The authorities did not ask, but not for that reason, and many writers did ask the College to assume a positive role. It is more likely that nothing was published firstly, because of the dilatoriness of contributors, and secondly, because Baly and Gull were otherwise occupied.[1]

This is enough to indicate the College's main concerns: its investigations were clearly of the consensus variety.[2] In the meantime Baly and Gull were acting in a rather different manner, and apparently on their own initiative.[3] As early as 19 September (after Brittan's paper had gone to print but three days before it was first announced) they had begun examining samples of matters condensed from the atmosphere and of water obtained in so-called cholera districts. Some of these samples were also examined by Brittan, and some of the specimens of water were provided by John Snow.

Baly and Gull's report offers no means of ascertaining the respective contributions of its authors.[4] Gull does not appear in the controversy in any other connection, and one is tempted to regard him as the sleeping partner, except that this was not his reputation.[5] Gull's training was clinical, and

[1] College Cholera MSS., Minute Book, 29 Aug. 1849; *Lond. Med. Gaz.* 9 (1849), 497, 735; Clark, *College of Physicians*, ii. 700.

[2] According to Clark the College had abandoned its chance of being other than a 'mere spectator of the rise of the public health services' as early as 1831: *College of Physicians*, ii. 658, 674.

[3] There is no mention of their activities until the presentation of their report: College Cholera MSS., Minute Book, 17 Oct. 1849.

[4] W. Baly and W.W. Gull, *Report on the Nature and Import of Certain Microscopic Bodies* (1849).

[5] (Sir) William Withey Gull (1816–90), M.D. London 1846, F.R.C.P. 1848, F.R.S. 1858. Connected with Guy's Hospital from 1837; built up large London

his interests lay with physiology and with the management of the patient. He favoured an expectant mode of treatment, and was known for such maxims as, 'not a typhoid fever, but a typhoid *man*'. It is unlikely that he would have thought the single-factor fungus theory in any way a solution to the problem of cholera, especially since that theory was at its most deficient in accounting for effects on the body. Gull's contribution to the *Reports* of 1854 was entirely clinical and pathological. There is no evidence of a special interest in microscopy.[1]

Of Baly it was said that 'his intellectual strength was not in any one of his mental powers, but in the fair proportions of them all. He had . . . very clear observant power; great caution and sobriety in thinking.' After becoming physician to the Millbank Prison in 1841, Baly established himself as an authority on dysentery and prison hygiene, in which capacity he was consulted by a succession of governments.[2] His views on epidemic disease were fairly typical, with a definite sanitarian emphasis.[3] He was in complexion a clinician; Brittan would have consulted him not primarily as a microscopist, but for his experience, which included clinical microscopy, of diseases affecting the gut. It seems likely that it was this consultation which led to the College's report on the fungus theory. At least at the outset Baly did not regard the question of whether lower organisms could cause disease as not worth discussing. When first shown the cholera-bodies he was struck by their resemblance to peculiar structures he had observed (after much application) several years earlier in the discharges of

---

practice. Published original descriptions of myxoedema, anorexia nervosa, etc. Intimate with F.D. Maurice. See *DNB*; *Collection of the Published Writings of W.W. Gull* (1894, 1896).

[1] Ibid. ii, pp.xv, xxi, xxiii. Gull published on skin diseases after 1851, but it seems that his personal skill in microscopy was, typically, developed in the 1850s rather than the 1840s. His later position was akin to that of Busk. See ibid., especially i. 562, 564–5.

[2] *Med. Times Gaz.* 1861, i. 151. William Baly (1814–61), L.S.A., M.R.C.S., M.D. Berlin 1836, F.R.C.P. 1846, F.R.S. 1847, educated University College, then Paris, Heidelberg, and Berlin. Appointed a Royal Physician, 1859. See *DNB*. Baly's early career was successfully directed by his clinical teachers, Latham and Burrows, both of whom were also members of the College's Cholera Committee.

[3] See Baly, *Lond. Med. Gaz.* 4 (1847), 529, where he stated that dysentery like cholera was 'produced by a poison . . . generated mostly by the decomposition of matters contained in the soil'.

epidemic dysentery.[1] At the time he had been inclined to think them bodily products; now he thought that if Brittan's bodies were fungi his were also. After further study he decided that they were not identical but similar, having the 'same endogenous mode of multiplication, the same gradual development' and both being 'evidently of extraneous origin'. He had not found his bodies in other diseases, and he raised the question of their relation with dysentery, and of the relevance of this relation to the fungoid theory of cholera. Baly was actually engaged in investigating the Bristol claims at the time of writing this paper; he did not attempt to answer his own questions. He did, however, specify conditions amounting to strict 'presence–absence' criteria. His specifications are interesting because (at least in the earlier paper) he envisaged their effect with respect to explanations of a class of diseases, rather than of a single disease; that is, he was prepared tentatively to envisage broad theoretical generalizations in which analogy led from the explanation of one disease to that of another. These presence–absence criteria preoccupy the College report; none of the awareness shown by Baly in his earlier contribution reappeared, and there was no trace of his ever having thought about development and 'endogenous multiplication'. This was partly due to the 'chalk and cheese' pronouncements of Busk, but it is obvious that the authors of the report believed that their decision was one which should be taken on the simplest observational grounds without reference to the fungus theory itself. Budd is not mentioned, except in connection with his discovery of the cholera-bodies in drinking water.

By mid-October, Baly and Gull had completed seven sets of examinations of water condensed from 'cholera atmospheres', and seventeen of drinking water from cholera districts. In all cases the results were negative. They had decided from their own observations (of what is not specified), that 'objects totally different had been regarded as similar', but had come to no conclusion as to the nature of the most distinctive of these objects. At this point they received the unsolicited and

---

[1] Baly, 'Note on Peculiar Microscopic Bodies in Dysentery', *Lond. Med. Gaz.* 9 (1849), 580.

decisive assistance of John Marshall, then assistant surgeon at University College Hospital, and demonstrator of anatomy at University' College.[1] Marshall was evidently already engaged in a fairly systematic inquiry into various aspects of cholera, which involved a series of experiments on the communicability of the disease; these became well known after Marshall published an account of them in 1853. He was prompted to do so not by any conviction as to the conclusiveness of his findings, but by the forwardness of other investigators.[2] His intervention in the cholera-fungus controversy may be regarded as similarly occasioned.

Marshall's identifications, based on chemical criteria and comparisons with forms produced artificially from ordinary substances (like cheese), dominated the College's report. Baly and Gull also received contributions from William Jenner,[3] the clinician, and from J.W. Griffith, author of a manual on the microscope and of works on the chemistry of the blood and urine.[4] Both Griffith and Marshall joined Baly and Gull in later examinations. Griffith was responsible for identifying the smallest fungi as 'chalky bodies', on the grounds that they polarized light and reacted with acids. Griffith and Swayne later clashed over this point, the former accusing the latter of 'an insufficient combination of chemistry with microscopy'.[5] Like Busk, Griffith had examined cholera evacuations prior to the controversy without result. Jenner had found bodies like the cholera fungi in the products of typhoid, and was inclined to attribute their presence (or advent) to the alkalinity of both cholera and typhoid evacu-

---

[1] For Marshall (1818–91), M.R.C.S. 1844, L.S.A. 1846, F.R.C.S. 1849, F.R.S. 1857, educated University College, professor of anatomy at Royal Academy 1873, see *DNB*; Hale-Bellot, *University College*, p.348 and *passim*.

[2] Marshall, 'The Communicability of Cholera to Animals', *Br. For. Med. Chir. Rev.* 11 (1853), 409.

[3] (Sir) William Jenner (1815–98), L.S.A., M.R.C.S., M.D. London 1844, M.R.C.P. 1848, F.R.C.P. 1852, F.R.S. 1864, of University College, a pupil of Parkes. Remembered as settling the distinction between typhoid and typhus fevers, according to clinical and pathological criteria. See *DNB*; Hale-Bellot, *University College*, pp.275–6 and *passim*. Jenner also made an unsolicited contribution to the Committee for Scientific Enquiries' Report of 1854.

[4] For John William Griffith, M.D. St. Andrews, M.R.C.P., M.R.C.S. 1841, F. Linnaean Soc., physician to Finsbury dispensary, first Medical Officer of Health for Clerkenwell, 1856, see *Medical Directory; Surgeon-General's Catalogue*.

[5] For an attacking letter by Griffith, see *Lond. Med. Gaz.* 9 (1849), 1034 ff.

ations. Baly's early specifications are relevant here: in a different theoretical context these findings might have been interpreted on the principle of 'like effects, like causes', to the benefit of the fungus theory of cholera.

On 17 October, at a meeting of the College's Cholera Committee, 'the Secretaries reported the results of experiments made by themselves as a subcommittee to determine the question of the existence of Brittan and Swayne's bodies in the atmosphere and water, also observations by themselves, Dr. Jenner and Mr. Marshall on the nature of the bodies'. Baly and Gull were authorized to circulate their report among members of the College, as the epidemic was rapidly declining and 'it seemed desirable to make the results known before the opportunity of verifying them should be lost'. To this, the 'substance' of the report as later published, were added the conclusions of Busk and of Griffith, and further observations by Marshall. At the next meeting of the Committee it was decided that the report should be published, and that it should appear with the explicit sanction of the Committee and therefore of the College.[1]

Many persons had known beforehand of the report, and newspapers in particular contented themselves with reproducing its list of conclusions, which was probably distributed as a communiqué by the College.[2] Particularly striking is the case of the *Morning Chronicle*, which first noticed the report by reprinting a laudatory account of it from the *Medical Times*. This paper's initial enthusiasm for the fungus theory had been opportunist: by 9 October, while allowing the theory to be the most probable of a lengthy list, it had returned to the themes of social concern and sanitary solutions. *The Times*, ever informative, printed the main text of the report in full, again without comment. There was some local protest: the *Bristol Gazette* referred approvingly to the earlier suggestion by *The Lancet* of a Royal Commission. Generally, however, the mood was one of acceptance, the only extremists

---

[1] College Cholera MSS., Minute Book, 17 and 31 Oct. 1849; Baly and Gull, *Report on Certain Microscopic Bodies*, Preface. Busk's conclusions were communicated to the Microscopical Society of London on 17 Oct.

[2] e.g. Golding Bird: *Lancet*, 1849, ii. 458. Baly and Gull's report was also widely reprinted in America.

being *The Lancet* and the *London Medical Gazette*. The *Gazette* stated flatly that the cholera-fungoid theory had now 'no substantial existence', and declined printing a letter of Swayne's until the latter had had an opportunity of studying the College's report. *The Lancet*, on the other hand, found the report 'lengthy, somewhat twaddling . . . and rather unintelligible'. As usual, it was attacking the College itself. Brittan and Swayne, it stated,

should have been invited (as would have been done in the French Academy of Medicine) to submit the facts which they proposed to exhibit to a competent committee, which would report on the subject submitted. In place of which we find a gentleman 'collecting cobwebs' or 'scraping broken and dirty glass' in St. Giles's . . .[1]

Swayne made his attack on the report locally, at a meeting of the Bristol Medico-Chirurgical Society held on 10 November. He was armed for the occasion with more of the perfect cholera cells, and with specimens of the uredo, supplied to him by Busk.[2] The meeting decided with Swayne that these objects were dissimilar, and expressed the opinion that the positive evidence of Brittan and Swayne was worth more than the merely negative evidence of the report. Members reported that the wide circulation given to the report had led people in London to consider the matter settled, and it was agreed that Swayne should give as much publicity as possible to his counter-statement.

This obtained full coverage locally, and in the *Provincial Medical and Surgical Journal*, and was also entrusted by Swayne to *The Lancet*, because, he said, of the 'independent tone' which this journal had adopted during the controversy. The ensuing events were few. Both Griffith and Swayne invoked the Revd. Miles Berkeley, Swayne in order to prove for all time that his cholera-bodies were not identical with any uredo, and also 'to absolve my colleagues and myself from the charge of having brought forward what is neither new

---

[1] *Morning Chronicle*, 29 Oct. 1849; *The Times*, 29 Oct. 1849; *Bristol Gazette*, 1 Nov. 1849; *Lond. Med. Gaz.* 9 (1849), 761, 780; *Lancet*, 1849, ii. 487.

[2] For a full account of this meeting, see *Farley's Bristol Journal*, 15 Dec. 1849. The cholera cells were from Bridgewater, one of the few places where cholera still lingered.

nor true'.[1] An epilogue was spoken by another mycologist, Henry Stephens of Bristol, and the *Edinburgh Medical and Surgical Journal* conducted a post-mortem.[2]

It may appear then, as it did to most of Swayne's contemporaries, that the College's report had directly and successfully contradicted the facts of the Bristol fungus theory. In fact, this describes only the outcome of the matter. The report itself is not, upon analysis, an impressive document. More importantly, it did not need to be, for in spite of what was thought at the time the issue turned on probabilities. Hence the report had only to produce a cumulative effect; there was no need for Baly and Gull to make out an incontestable case for any one point or one point rather than another. The only defence available to Swayne was that of contesting each point in turn; so that although he was able to produce contradictory evidence piecemeal, and to show that the report was in places inconsistent and even unfair, he could do little to dispel the over-all impression.

The proposition which the report chose to disprove was that the cholera-bodies constituted a single species of fungus, which was invariably present in cholera situations and invariably absent in all others. In so doing the authors involved themselves in an inconsistency. In order to demonstrate absence in some situations and presence in others, the report

---

[1] *Prov. Med. Surg. J.* 13 (1849), 659, 657; Swayne, *Lancet*, 1849, ii. 532. Griffith, *Lond. Med. Gaz.* 9 (1849), 1034; Swayne, ibid., p.950. Berkeley's contribution appeared in the same number as Griffith's: ibid., p.1035. Miles Joseph Berkeley (1803–89), M.A. Cantab. 1828, F. Linnaean Soc. 1876, F.R.S. 1879, was regarded as the ultimate authority in England on fungi and algae from about 1836 to 1870: *DNB*; Green, *History of British Botany*, pp.446 ff.

[2] Stephens, *Lancet*, 1849, ii. 688. Henry Oxley Stephens, L.S.A. 1830, M.R.C.S. 1831, surgeon to St. Peter's Hospital, Bristol, was in 1849 Vice-President of the Bristol Microscopical Society; he had been consulted at a late stage by Swayne as an expert on uredos (see *Lond. Med. Gaz.* 9 (1849), 861), and had himself applied for help to Berkeley. A second sample of fungi, supplied by W.B. Herapath, evidently decided him to publish the rather negative contribution just cited. 'Documents on the Cholera Fungus Hypothesis', *Edinb. Med. Surg. J.* 73 (1850), 81–118. The Bristol claims were investigated by W. Robertson and J. Hughes Bennett as members of the Edinburgh Medico-Chirurgical Society. These experienced observers recognized the peculiarity of the bodies, but denied that they had any specific relation to cholera: *Mon. J. Med. Sci.* 9, Pt. 3 (1849), 1232. This reaction could however have been predicted of Bennett at least. For Edinburgh opinion on the cholera fungus see also 'A Surgeon', *Bristol Mirror*, 20 Oct. 1849.

made use of a concept of 'the characteristic cholera body', and yet the other part of its intention was to prove 'how various are the bodies which have been confounded together'. When considering the nature of the cholera-bodies the authors of the report defined 'four principal forms' by the somewhat dubious procedure of averaging out the drawings published by Brittan, Budd, and Swayne, and then discussed the identity of the body or bodies which they found to fill these categories.[1] In this they were greatly assisted by Marshall, although the latter's chemical classification, even more than their own, depended on his having had under survey nothing but the cholera-bodies. The points made against the 'cholera-fungus' were, in fact, made severally of the various objects alleged to have been mistakenly brought together under this heading. This was not legitimate if those objects included any of the neutral items (spores, bran cells) also recognized in their own samples by the Bristolians.

The alleged presence of the cholera-bodies in air and water would be as difficult to verify as to disprove, but in a theoretically neutral (ideal and impossible) context, the advantage must lie with the observer who has positive results. The negative results of Baly and Gull in cholera areas were, as they themselves recognized, frequently questionable because of the length of time which had elapsed since the disease last occurred. This, however, did not matter; the report argued typically as follows:

A much larger amount of evidence would have been required to disprove the statements to which our observations refer, had those statements been unassailable from other points. But the facts to be detailed . . . will show that the bodies found in the ricewater dejections have no particular relation to cholera; and that, if they should occasionally be present in the atmosphere, or impure water, this will not happen exclusively, or even especially, in districts infected with the epidemic.[2]

Swayne might justifiably argue that the report presented nothing to match his and Brittan's record of seventy positive results. Baly and Gull's reply was that the diversity of origin,

---

[1] Baly and Gull, *Report on Certain Microscopic Bodies*, pp.20–1. One of the four forms was taken as 'the type of the bodies discovered by Messrs. Brittan and Swayne': ibid., p.12.

[2] Ibid., pp.2–3. 'Will not happen', that is, on the supposition that the bodies were bran cells etc.; ibid., p.19.

and frequency of incidence of one or another of the forms in other circumstances, would readily explain so many occurrences; and in any case, they themselves had not observed them to occur so regularly.

Thus, though based on observation, the report was not a trial of the kind envisaged by Brittan. Its effect was simply to reduce the probability, already made minimal by an unsympathetic theoretical context, of there being any relation between the different cholera-bodies, or between the bodies and the disease. Therefore it hardly mattered that, as Swayne pointed out, the report had frequently asserted identity where Busk and Marshall had spoken only of similarities; that it made no reference to a form which Marshall described and could not account for; and that the identification of Swayne's cells as uredos was later contradicted by both Stephens and Berkeley.

Although some account has been given of the institutional and other conditions that helped to produce the cholera-fungus theory, it has so far been implied that the theoretical context in which the hypothesis originated was unsympathetic to its further development. In retrospect, there are few grounds for resisting this implication, but elements did exist in the contemporary situation which were sufficient to allow some critics to form, at the time, a very different impression. The *Morning Chronicle*, for instance, stated its belief that 'It is by far the most prevalent opinion . . . in the present day, that [the fungoid] hypothesis more completely accounts for all the peculiar phenomena [of cholera] than any other'. Later the *Chronicle* described the reaction to Brittan's discovery as one of 'astonishment and interest, rather than incredulity', and gave an account of recent developments by which the minds of medical men had been 'prepared' for the event. It is not wonderful that the *Chronicle* should so endorse the fungus theory, or that the theory should arouse general interest, because theories involving agents of this kind were then and always, as one critic put it, 'admirably fitted for popular apprehension'. Many practitioners who took part in the controversy might fairly be equated with the general public in this respect. None the less, the *Chronicle's* remarks were echoed in professional quarters, and there is enough substance in its account of recent developments to justify the conclusion that the fungus theory had more than popular appeal.[1]

The obvious course is to consider those theories which were said to have 'predicted' Brittan's findings. In this connection John Grove, a germ theorist, went so far as to make a comparison between the cholera fungus, and the prediction and subsequent discovery of the planet Neptune, this being an enviable achievement of the physical sciences. The theories to be considered here, had much in common; it is also noticeable that their exponents were often, though in different ways, cut off from the body of the profession. The authors under consideration are Henry Holland, Jacob Henle, Charles Cowdell, and John Grove.[2] Of secondary interest are the theories of Charles Daubeny, Edward Long Fox of Bristol,[3] and John Kearsley Mitchell of Philadelphia.[4]

The most obvious feature of all these theories is their dependence upon analogy. In this manner they employed not only the properties of larger organisms and biological interpretations of fermentations, but also the growing knowledge of parasites and the inferred characteristics of smallpox. The rest of what they have in common arises from this usage. In

[1] *Morning Chronicle*, 21, and 26 Sept. 1849; 'Scrutator', *Prov. Med. Surg. J.* 13 (1849), 585; *Lancet*, 1849, ii. 406.

[2] Grove, *Mon. J. Med. Sci.* 11 (1859), 438. See H. Holland, *Medical Notes* (1839, 1840); Henle, *Miasms and Contagions*; Cowdell, *Disquisition on Pestilential Cholera* (1848); Grove, *Epidemics Examined and Explained* (1850).

[3] Daubeny, 'Influence of Lower Vegetable Organisms in Epidemic Diseases'; Fox, *Surmises Respecting the Cause and Nature of Cholera* (1831). Fox (1761–1835) is to be distinguished from a better-known grandson of the same name, also of Bristol. The elder, M.D. Edinburgh 1786, L.R.C.P. 1787, physician to Bristol Infirmary 1786–1816, moved to Bristol when the death of a local quaker physician seemed to offer an opening. Interested in mesmerism and the non-restraint system in lunacy; called in on the case of George III. His son Henry Hawes Fox (1788–1851), a more exact contemporary of J.C. Prichard, was also interested in lunacy. The eldest Fox is treated as a precursor of Pasteur by local studies, e.g. Smith, *Bristol Royal Infirmary*, pp.475–6.

[4] Mitchell, *On the Cryptogamous Origin of Malarious and Epidemic Fevers* (Philadelphia, 1849). Mitchell (1793–1858), father of S. Weir Mitchell the neurologist, is mentioned because his speculations were included in discussions in England. For reviews, see *Edinb. Med. Surg. J.* 73 (1850), 473; *Lancet*, 1849, ii. 482. See also P. Allen, 'Early American Animalcular Hypotheses', *Bull. Hist. Med.* 21 (1947), 734–43; R.N. Doetsch, 'Mitchell on the Cause of Fevers', ibid. 38 (1964), 241–59.

all of them the *contagium animatum* was arrived at only after a process in which other theories were eliminated. This was done to justify both the use of analogy (which was and is, at least by repute, a vulgar mode of reasoning), and the resumption of a kind of theory which many regarded as pre-scientific. Most thought of it as an old 'exploded' theory without knowing much about earlier authors; only Athanasius Kircher (1598–1680) and Linnaeus were frequently mentioned. Not much later, it was possible to envisage a modern theory of *contagium animatum*, dissociated from the earlier, primitive, version, in a development parallel to that of the doctrine of spontaneous generation. It is an indication of the contemporary commitment to the methods of natural philosophy, if not to reductionism, that none of the authors under consideration except Grove would willingly have been called a vitalist.[1] They were aware that in using such analogies they laid themselves open to this charge, levelled by others as well as Liebig. Daubeny and Cowdell both combined the agency of living organisms with processes (fermentation, catalysis), which could be described in physical and chemical terms.

Another common feature was the time spent in explaining the behaviour of diseases in the field. This was the most obtrusive aspect of the problem of cholera, and cholera was the chief concern of all except Henle. It was in this particularly inscrutable, but well-documented, area that the analogy with living organisms was put to most use. Holland thought the agent was animalcular because animalcules had their own powers of locomotion, and the 'capricious' distribution of the disease could then be explained in terms of instincts like those which caused swarming and migration in insects. Mitchell rejected animalcules because of their lack of resistance to extremes of temperature, and because they were not known to be poisonous. He decided on the lower plant forms because they showed an 'inherent power of extension' which operated independently of meteorological conditions. The analogy here is principally with blights like the 'red snow' (*Pseudomonas nivalis*). The caprices of cholera required no further expla-

---

[1] See Grove's arguments against Liebig's 'chemical theory of epidemics': *Epidemics Examined*, pp.108 ff.

nation: the disease spread 'accidentally', just as the distribution of fungi was subject to accident or chance. The rise and fall of epidemics was further explained by the ability of germs or spores to remain dormant when conditions were unfavourable, and by their great fecundity in suitable soil. Notions of the fixity of species (admittedly derived from higher animals and plants) were used to account for the constant appearances presented by a disease over an extended period involving long absences as well as epidemics.[1]

These arguments show the advantages and disadvantages of using analogies, for while it was encouraging to observe the similarities between disease plagues and plagues of organisms (organisms being a 'known and natural agency'), the reasons why either kind of eruption occurred at a particular time and place remained as mysterious as before.[2]

Obviously, the sources of analogy were much enriched in the 1840s by the increased use of the microscope, and by the concomitant increase in knowledge of the lower forms of life. The theorists we are considering made extensive use of this often rather mixed information. It is worth noting here that Budd did not. Apart from fermentation, the case most widely used was that of muscardine, the fungus disease of silkworms, in which Agostino Bassi and Jean Victor Audouin had established a cause-and-effect relation experimentally.[3] There were almost no other successful experimental studies, but a great many observations had been made of 'minute vegetable parasites or their germs' in association with abnormal states of man as well as of other animals and living plants.[4]

Like Budd, most of the authors being discussed stressed that the substances and processes most widely used in the treatment of cholera or of other epidemic diseases were also

---

[1] See Sachs, *History of Botany*, pp.108 ff.; 207.

[2] As admitted by Cowdell, *Disquisition*, p.183.

[3] See R.A. Major, 'Agostino Bassi and the Parasitic Theory of Disease', *Bull. Hist. Med.* 16 (1944), 97–107.

[4] Cowdell added the experimental work of Berg on thrush in children: *Disquisition*, pp. 121 ff. N. Parker gave forty-three references for observational work for the years 1837–48: *Lond. Med. Gaz.* 9 (1849), 669–70. See J.H. Swartz, *Elements of Medical Mycology* (1944), p.13; F.M. Keddie, 'Medical Mycology, 1841–1870', *Medicine and Science in the 1860s*, ed. F.N.L. Poynter (1968), pp.137–49. This work was done chiefly on the continent.

destructive of organic life. Fox's belief in the animalcular origin of contagious diseases stemmed from his own experience of the efficacy of such substances in the treatment of glanders in horses. He recommended essential oils (for example camphor), sulphur (a specific in scabies), and mercury. Nearly twenty years later Grove made similar recommendations with a special emphasis on sulphur. Henle made capital of the fact that the same agents inhibited fermentation as putrefaction.[1]

As individuals and as medical men these authors were more disparate. Sir Henry Holland, that 'much travelled tuft-hunter', was a man somewhat resented by his professional colleagues, and his intellectual capacity has probably been underestimated.[2] He had had some of his education at Dr. Estlin's school in Bristol, and was initially apprenticed to a merchant. Abandoning commerce for the professions, he studied medicine at Glasgow and then at Edinburgh, where he joined the Whig circle which included Brougham, Stewart, and Sydney Smith (later his father-in-law). He became travelling physician to Caroline of Brunswick, and won fame for his defence of her at her trial. After 1816, Holland built up an extensive practice in aristocratic circles. However, he spent only part of each year in the pursuit of his profession; he had independent means, and was addicted to travel. He acted for many years as President of the Royal Institution, and was the associate of Davy, Faraday, Wollaston, and Herschel.

Holland 'did not', as one medical journal put it, 'attain eminence by such means as are commonly held to be the necessary steps to success in our profession'. He was never attached to a hospital, and 'took no active part in, and was rarely ever seen at' any of the medical societies. Nor did he teach or lecture. His detachment from the profession limited the nature of his influence; *Medical Notes & Reflections* went to at least three editions, but his contemporaries chose to

---

[1] Fox, *Surmises Respecting Cholera*, pp.15 ff.; Grove, *On Sulphur as a Remedy in Cholera* (1848); Henle, *Miasms and Contagions*, p.929.

[2] Clark, *College of Physicians*, ii. 663. Holland (1788–1873), M.D. Edinburgh 1811, F.R.S. 1816, F.R.C.P. 1828, was first appointed to the Royal Household 1837. See *DNB*.

regard it, at least overtly, as a collection of elegant and speculative essays, rather than as a serious contribution to medicine.
However, it is unjust, as well as incorrect, to say as Futcher
does that Holland 'probably did little more than voice a now
quite general dissatisfaction with the age old miasm theory'. [1]
His essay was not of the same stature as Henle's, but had some
of the same validity as an analysis of a given problem. William
Budd thought highly of Holland, and when *Medical Notes*
was published recommended it as a whole to his brother as
'quite new and a very clever and philosophical book'.[2] In
essence, Holland's theory of animalcules was an extrapolation
of the known properties of insects. It was cited by Farr in his
justification of analogy. Later editions of *Medical Notes*
showed few changes, although the second edition (1840) had
a reference to yeast fermentation and a note on Henle, and
the third (1855), notes on Schwann, La Tour, Liebig, and
Daubeny. In a work of 1872, Holland described his theory
as 'a hypothesis which fully satisfies my own mind'. He still
regarded the detailed history of the migration of cholera as
the 'most conclusive proof' of his view, and thought that its
deficiencies, in that it stopped short of minute pathology and
therapeutics, could reasonably be discounted because they
were shared by all other theories.[3]

Jacob Henle is the most substantial of the figures we are
considering, but his influence in England was severely limited
by the fact that his *Pathologische Untersuchungen* was not
translated.[4] Many of the participants in the cholera-fungus
controversy knew of his work on miasms and contagions, but

[1] *Med. Times Gaz.* 1873, ii. 498; P.H. Futcher, 'Notes on Insect Contagion',
Bull. Inst. Hist. Med. 4 (1936), 536–58: 554.

[2] Budd Letters, William to Richard, 13 May 1839 [Tagged, '1839. Catalogue
of Medical Books']. Budd was impressed by Holland in general, and as much by
his essay 'on diseases which occur only once in life', as by his theory of cholera:
Budd, 'Observations on Typhoid', *Br. Med. J.* 1861, ii. 549 n.; p.605. Holland in
his turn was impressed by Budd's paper on symmetry in disease, which related to
his own 'On the brain as a double organ': Budd Letters, William to Richard,
November 1842 [Tagged, '1842'].

[3] Farr, *Report on Cholera Mortality*, p.lxxiv; H. Holland, *Recollections of
Past Life* (1872), pp.325–6.

[4] Friedrich Gustav Jacob Henle (1809–85), son of a Jewish merchant. Drawn
to medicine by J. Müller; later his prosector. To Zurich as professor of anatomy,
1840; later at Heidelberg and Göttingen. Chief works: *Pathologische Untersuchungen* (1840); *Allgemeine Anatomie* (1841); *Handbuch der rationellen*

most, like William Farr, knew it only at second hand.[1] A proof of this limited acquaintance is that none of the participants mentioned Henle's specific references to cholera and to the 'cholera-fungus' of Ludwig Boehm.[2] One secondary source was Liebig's *Animal Chemistry*, where Liebig argued against Henle and the 'parasitic theory'.[3] More often, however, he argued against 'some physiologists' and mentioned 'the celebrated Henle' by name in different connections.[4] Rosen has observed (largely on the basis of some remarks in the *British and Foreign Medical Review*) that Henle had an excellent reputation in England even before 1840, 'at least among those who kept in touch with medical literature'. With respect to a somewhat later period one might agree with this without having to consider the magnitude of the qualification. By 1849, Henle was regarded as a major figure by journals other than those that dealt specifically with foreign literature.[5] None the less, there is no evidence that his reputation as a pathologist and anatomist led to a better acquaintance with his theories of contagia, even in the case of Farr.[6]

Charles Cowdell is something of an opposite case, being a provincial physician well known to some of his contemporaries, but ultimately obscure.[7] A graduate of London, he was a member of the Provincial Medical and Surgical Associ-

---

Pathologie (1846-53); *Systematische Anatomie* (1871-9). Founded *Zeitschrifte für rationelle Medizin*, 1844. See *DSB*; J.B.S. [John Burdon Sanderson?], 'F.G.J. Henle', *Proc. R. Soc. Lond.* 39 (1885), iii-viii; G. Rosen, 'Social Aspects of Jacob Henle's Medical Thought', *Bull. Inst. Hist. Med.* 5 (1937), 509-37.

[1] For a possible exception see N. Parker: *Lond. Med. Gaz.* 9 (1849), 669.

[2] Henle, *Miasms and Contagions*, p.947. Boehm (1811–69) of Berlin, soon left micro-anatomy for ophthalmology: *Biog. Lexicon*. His contention that the chief pathological change in cholera was desquamation of the epithelium of the gut was the main basis for the controversy over this point. English writers knew of his work through an account by Henle in *Müllers Archiv*, translated in *Lond. Med. Gaz.* 1839-40, i. 333-6. See also an account by Parkes in his 'On the Intestinal Discharges in Cholera', *Lond. J. Med.* 1 (1849), 134-52.

[3] See especially *Animal Chemistry* (1846), pp.208 ff.

[4] e.g. on irritation: ibid., p.171.

[5] See e.g. *Mon. J. Med. Sci.* 11 (1850), 438.

[6] Cf. Rosen, 'Henle and Farr', pp.588-9.

[7] Cowdell (1815–71), M.R.C.S. 1837, M.B. London 1846, M.D. London 1852, published several papers, one of them on a novel treatment for neuralgia: *Med. Times Gaz.* 1871, ii. 785. Apparently 'beloved and esteemed' in Dorchester for his skill and Christian piety, nothing is known of him there today.

ation, and for nearly twenty-two years physician to Dorset County Hospital. His *Disquisition* was almost his only claim to fame, yet it was remembered and acknowledged when beliefs changed, and again at his death.[1] When it appeared, just before the epidemic, it was reviewed by at least four medical journals, and was widely noticed during the controversy itself. The *Morning Chronicle* described it as 'most to the purpose'. It must have achieved some circulation, since it reached Mitchell in Philadelphia and prompted him to publish his own ideas on the subject.[2] Cowdell himself had worked in almost complete isolation, claiming to have spent the previous ten years 'shut within the walls' of Oundle, 'not supplied with a medical institution of any kind'. His only resources were to be found on his own bookshelves. Under these circumstances it is not surprising to find him a member of the Sydenham Society. He knew of Holland's theory and sent him a copy of the *Disquisition*, but he knew nothing of Henle, or of Mitchell, until the latter sent Cowdell his work. On Cowdell's own account the history of the *Disquisition* was that he had been struck, while revising his literature on cholera, with 'the analogy apparently existing between the origin and phenomena attending the course of cholera, and some other natural phenomena constantly before us'.[3]

The *Disquisition* was an extremely conscientious, and therefore popular, study covering the nature, history, and symptomology of cholera as well as its aetiology. Notwithstanding its author's geographical isolation, it was, of the works being considered, the most representative of its theoretical context. Unlike Holland or Henle, Cowdell felt it necessary to revise the debate as to the contagiousness of cholera, which he did by taking James Copland and George Budd as representative of the two extremes of opinion.[4] Cowdell's own conclusion

---

[1] See *Med. Times Gaz.* 1871, ii. 785; *Lancet*, 1872, i. 63. One reason for his being remembered was the revival of the cholera-fungus theory by Ernst Hallier: see Appendices to *9th Rep. of Med. Officer of Privy Council*, PP, 1867, XXXVII. 514 ff.

[2] *Morning Chronicle*, 21 Sept. 1849; *Lancet*, 1849, ii. 482. See Doetsch, 'Mitchell on Fevers', pp.255–8.

[3] Cowdell, *Prov. Med. Surg. J.* 13 (1849), 585; idem, *Disquisition*, Preface.

[4] Ibid., pp.52 ff. Copland (1791–1870), M.D. Edinburgh 1815, F.R.S. 1833, F.R.C.P. 1837, prolific author of the famous *Dictionary of Practical Medicine*

was that the debate should be subsumed under the question of the nature of the *materies morbi*, which he decided must be animate and fungoid. Much of his book was concerned with showing that fungi were capable of producing cholera. Cowdell was notably more interested in the capabilities than in the classification of fungi. These were demonstrated for him (and others) not only by fermentation, but by diseases of plants and of food plants in particular. This was a well-established field of inquiry.[1] Cowdell chiefly depended upon Carpenter's *Principles of Physiology*, Liebig's *Organic Chemistry*, Graham's *Elements of Chemistry*, John Lindley's *Introduction to the Natural System of Botany* (1830), and G.E. Day's translation for the Sydenham Society of Johann Franz Simon's *Animal Chemistry* (1845-6). His general position was that: persons were predisposed to disease by the same agents (electricity, moisture, and heat) which favoured the propagation of the fungi; the fungi were inhaled and entered the blood; in the blood they acted both parasitically and catalytically, first by robbing the blood of some of its nutritious properties, and secondly by altering its chemical condition and probably producing in it some 'deleterious new ingredients'. These actions were analogous to those effected in vegetable substances by ferments. Cowdell adopted the compromise description of fermentation given by Carpenter in 1841, and criticized Liebig ('with whom we scarcely dare to differ') for denying that yeast consisted in any sense of organisms. None the less, Liebig had 'anticipated, as it were, our view of pestilential diseases being communicated by means of ferments'. Other indications of an indebtedness to both Schwann and Liebig may be found elsewhere in Cowdell's work.[2] His stress on the blood as the site of diseased action, in the context of a biological theory of cholera, is a strong indication of the current emphasis on this type of pathology.

(1832-58), was a true, and notorious, contagionist: *Examiner*, 27 Nov. 1831 (account of meeting of Westminster Medical Society).

   [1] Cowdell, *Disquisition*, pp.114, 102; E.C. Large, *The Advance of the Fungi* (1940); G.L. Carefoot and E.R. Sprott, *Famine on the Wind* (1969).

   [2] *Disquisition*, pp.100-1, 132-3, 129, 133 ff., 101 ff., 115; Carpenter, *Principles of Physiology*, p.74 n. For a summary of Cowdell's position, see *Edinb. Med. Surg. J.* 73 (1850), 82 ff.

John Grove[1] was not a man who was taken seriously by his contemporaries, although *The Lancet* was for some reason indulgent towards him, and his claims were later advanced by Benjamin Richardson.[2] He and Richardson were both members of the Epidemiological Society, and Grove was well known there for his enthusiastic exposition of the 'vital germ' hypothesis. *The Lancet* described him as 'indefatigable in searching for the remote causes which underlie and lead up to the phenomena of disease'. He had, as well, definite clinical and microscopical interests. Grove entered the cholera-fungus controversy with a series of articles entitled, 'The vitality of the choleraic fungi demonstrated', the first of which described fungi he had found in the urine of cholera patients. He had watched these undergo further development, and also increased his supply by transplantation to fresh urine. These observations ultimately damaged the cholera-fungus theory, as W.B. Herapath among others was able to point out that Grove's fungi were torula or yeast, a common incident in urine.[3] For the first time in the controversy, the possibility of contamination was raised, and other writers had no trouble in attributing the advent of the torula in urine to the presence of sugar.[4]

It was Grove's contention that epidemic diseases could be explained only in terms of powers belonging exclusively to living organisms. His theory was truly a germ theory, for the analogy on which he laid most stress was that between putative disease agents, and spores, seeds, and ova. By assuming that the ova of parasites and the spores of fungi commonly circulated in the blood, he could explain the appearance of developed forms in otherwise anomalous situations, such as the yolk of hermetically sealed eggs. His work showed a generalized interest in the origin and distribution of species.

[1] Grove (1816–95), M.R.C.S., L.S.A. 1840; M.D. St. Andrews, 1862. Of French extraction. Fellow of Royal Medical and Chirurgical Society of London. Medical Officer to Wandsworth Board of Guardians; active as a general practitioner in Wandsworth 1840–60: *Lancet*, 1895, ii. 903.

[2] See e.g. Richardson, *Trans. Epidem. Soc.* 2 (1862–6), 123. Grove was taken very seriously by a Mr. Dolan, in 1881: see *Lancet*, 1895, i. 903.

[3] Ibid.; Grove, 'Vitality of Choleraic Fungi Demonstrated', *Lancet*, 1849, ii. 427; W.B. Herapath, ibid., p.453.

[4] See e.g. F. Branson, *Prov. Med. Surg. J.* 13 (1849), 614.

By way of analogy with the spread of epidemic disease he gave an account (based on J.C. Prichard) of the geographical distribution of plants, and in another place he speculated on the geological origin of disease germs.[1]

Those reviews of the works of Henle, Holland, Cowdell, and Mitchell which appeared before the epidemic, were not usually hostile or even facetious.[2] The review of Henle already cited could even be described as expressing assent. None the less, there were special limits to this approval, signified by the almost invariable use of the term 'ingenious'. This expressed appreciation only of the author's self-consistency; so that, even though an author might also be complimented on his 'facts', the question of the impingement of his theory on current doctrine, let alone practice, was not raised at all — pending, it was maintained, 'ocular demonstration'.[3] The review of Henle mentioned two defects in his theory: first, the remoteness of the analogy between diseases of worms (i.e. muscardine) and of men, and second, 'the absence of any actual observation of such parasites as are supposed to constitute contagion in the bodies of the higher animals'. The *Monthly Journal of Medical Science* ended its review of Cowdell by saying:

We must however inform him that the idea is not new, and that he will find a masterly exposition of it . . . by Professor Henle, in his *Pathologische Untersuchungen*, published in 1840. But, notwithstanding all the talent and research which have been lavished on this speculation, Dr. Cowdell has failed to exhibit greater proofs of its correctness now, than when Henle wrote eight years ago. It is true that the blight among plants, the muscardine of silkworms . . . tinea favosa . . . and other diseases in man, may spread by the propagation and development of fungus germs. In all these cases, the microscope furnishes us with ocular proof . . .

---

[1] Grove, 'Vitality of Choleraic Fungi Demonstrated', pp.556–7, 451–12; idem, *Epidemics Examined*, pp.64–8. For a reaction to the latter, see *Mon. J. Med. Sci.* 11 (1850), 439 ff.

[2] A possible exception to this was *The Lancet's* review of the animalcular theory of cholera of Thomas Henry Starr, M.D. in which 'the great Liebig' was quoted against both Starr and Cowdell: *Lancet*, 1848, ii. 69–71.

[3] Consistency with his own premisses was the main ground on which his friends could defend Snow: see Richardson in *Snow on Chloroform* (1858), pp.xxvi–xxvii. The review of Henle singled out his essay on contagion for praise, in the context of criticism of what was regarded as Henle's new habit of speculation, in important physiological and pathological areas: *Br. For. Med. Rev.* 9 (1840), 398, 404–10.

Farr made a similar demand: 'Henle has proved the existence of this cause, and the truth of the theory in every way but one: he has never seen the epidemic infusoria. The omission is, no doubt, important; and the more so on the part of Henle, who is justly considered one of the best microscopic observers in Germany.' The point is further underlined by the opportunism of Liebig, who stated, in connection with the particular example of putrefaction in urine, that 'if, in only one such case, the absence of vegetable or animal organisms can be demonstrated, this one fact is quite sufficient to dissipate every doubt concerning the true cause of its putrefaction'. [1] This is, of course, reminiscent of the impossible criteria imposed against the proponents of the cholera-fungus theory. Among the authors themselves, Holland was careful to point out the obstacles in the way of 'actual proof' of the existence of his animalcules; Cowdell being somewhat later was more sanguine; but of authors and critics alike, only Henle saw that 'in order for the experiences to develop they need the light of a reasonable theory'. [2] He might have said, the light of a general commitment to a (reasonable) theory.

Sachs gives a sufficient account of the state of mycology at this time and of its relevance to larger questions. In 1849, after little more than ten intensive years of study, the field was expanding rather than well defined. This is almost enough to account for the occurrence of the cholera-fungus controversy. At the outset, all the recent developments (the product of French and German rather than British research) were rehearsed, and it was claimed that no hypothesis came recommended by a 'stronger body of plausible analogies'. [3] However, it soon became clear that although the question of whether fungi represented cause or effect was much debated, it was generally thought, even in the case of fermentation, that their role was only secondary. In its review of Starr, *The Lancet* called the process of fermentation 'the great "cheval de bataille" of our theorists'. By the end of the 1840s, it was

---

[1] *Br. For. Med. Rev.* 9 (1840), 403; *Mon. J. Med. Sci.* 8 (1847–8), 679. Farr, *Appendix 1840*, p.18 n.; Liebig, *Animal Chemistry*, p.219. See also pp.209 ff.

[2] Holland, *Medical Notes*, pp.565 ff.; Cowdell, *Disquisition*, pp.2–3; Henle, *Miasms and Contagions*, p.981.

[3] Sachs, *History of Botany*, pp.203 ff.; *The Times*, 5 Oct. 1849.

accepted that yeast consisted wholly or in part of fungi, but the nature of the relationship between the organism and the process of fermentation was still in doubt. As the 'appointed executioners and and nimble scavengers of nature', the presence of fungi was generally seen as retribution for some personal or sanitary neglect. Even to an enthusiast like J. Stuart Wilkinson, the 'essential part of the malady' was the 'conditions producing the soil'. Carpenter had already stated that where fungi appeared unequivocally on living bodies, there was reason to believe that they were 'generally the indications of a state of previous disease'.[1]

Analogies offer only prospective knowledge, and when they are used it is open to anyone to claim that they provide no explanation of the facts. During the cholera-fungus controversy there were some who repudiated the analogy with blights and similar phenomena, and demanded to know the origin of the fungi and the reasons for their sudden increase; but for the most part, as in the potato-fungus debate, criticism centred on the lack of explanation of the disease process.[2] Henle alone made a real attempt to explain the pathology of diseases caused by living organisms. The reviewer of 1840 rewarded this venture by stating that it was 'unnecessary', and that Henle had 'weakened his case by throwing this burden upon it'. In 1849, however, after the publication of *Organic Chemistry* and *Animal Chemistry*, the *London Medical Gazette* in its review of Budd stated that the point of 'paramount importance' to be determined in respect of the cholera-bodies was how they related to the symptoms of cholera. It was in this respect that the analogies used offered least. Something was known of the conditions in which fungi (and animalculae) appeared, but almost nothing could be said of their action on the body. With the exception of Henle and perhaps Cowdell, the authors we are concerned with contented themselves with pointing to the general capabilities of organ-

---

[1] *Lancet*, 1848, ii. 69; *The Times*, 5 Oct. 1849; J. Stuart Wilkinson, 'Some Remarks on Epiphytes', *Lancet*, 1849, ii. 449; Carpenter, *Principles of Physiology* (1839), p.61.

[2] See e.g. A.B. Granville, *The Times*, 28 Sept. 1849. The suggestion that the potato blight was caused by a fungus came from Berkeley; see Large, *Advance of the Fungi*, pp.17, 28.

isms. It is not surprising that most readers agreed with Nicholas Parker when he stated baldly that 'the presence of a few fungi does not serve in any way to explain the terrible symptoms of cholera'.[1] This, of course, was the attitude taken by Liebig. His attack did not include a denial of living agency in scabies and muscardine; instead he concentrated on denying such agency in putrefaction and fermentation, knowing the importance of these as the only useful analogues of the disease process.

None of the authors discussed above was anything but serious in his intentions. Several (Budd, Holland, Henle) were men of consistently high intellectual achievement. Their *contagium vivum* theories were, therefore, neither frivolous nor trivial. None the less, the impression made by these theories was very fleeting, and it was not cumulative, unless the initial enthusiastic reaction to the cholera-fungus theory can be regarded as evidence of this. In the two outstanding cases of Holland and Henle, the *contagium vivum* theory was only a small and comparatively insignificant part of the work of each taken as a whole;[2] in Holland's case, much of this other work was also speculative in quality. The contributions of Cowdell and Mitchell seem to have dominated their thoughts because they otherwise published so little. In every instance, however, the writer concerned was simply modifying, according to his own resources and what was available to him at the time, a hypothesis which was always accessible at need. The theory of *contagium vivum* appears at all periods: 'again and again it has presented itself anew in an improved form, since the manifestations in the course of the contagious diseases must at all times . . . have led to it.'[3] It is unnecessary to suppose any continuity between the different versions. Each is more likely to reflect not its precursors but its own context. Obviously, all versions of this hypothesis may with more or often less legitimacy be taken together and compared;

---

[1] *Br. For. Med. Rev.* 9 (1840), 404; *Lond. Med. Gaz.* 9 (1849), 725; Parker, *Lond. Med. Gaz.* 9 (1849), 671.

[2] The same could be said of Fox, about whom less is known, and of Daubeny.

[3] Henle, *Miasms and Contagions*, p.923. Or, from another point of view, 'when authors are at fault for a theory, fungi and animalculae are at hand, to enable them to proceed': *Lancet*, 1843, ii. 70.

but this does not allow the conclusion that they should be combined to represent a major element in mid-nineteenth-century epidemiological theory.

6

EXCLUSIVE AND INCLUSIVE: JOHN SNOW AND THE COMMITTEE FOR SCIENTIFIC ENQUIRIES

I

There are three main procedures in epidemiology: induction from effects, manipulation of an alleged cause, and isolation of the alleged cause. The previous chapter was primarily concerned with the last of these; the present one, in dealing with John Snow and the context in which his ideas were put forward, will be concerned with the first and then with the second. Snow's reputation as an epidemiologist is well established. After his early death in 1858, his claims were taken care of by friends (notably Benjamin Richardson, William Farr, Edwin Lankester, J. Netten Radcliffe, and the Revd. Henry Whitehead) who, while establishing the priority of his discovery that cholera was waterborne, also created the various legends of his life and work. For the modern student, as P.E. Brown has pointed out, Snow's work on cholera in the field serves as an epitome of epidemiological method, and Snow himself appears as a tutelary deity to teachers and pupils alike.[1] He is also commonly regarded as a voice crying in the wilderness for the germ theory. As some writers have discovered, the conventional view in many respects requires correction. It is not proposed now to go over ground already covered elsewhere.[2] Less attention, for example, will be given

---

[1] Brown, 'Another Look at John Snow', *Anaesth. and Analg ... Current Researches*, 43 (1964), 652-61: 652. For different styles of modern textbook with references to Snow, see B. MacMahon, T.F. Pugh, and J. Ipsen, *Epidemiologic Methods* (1960), pp.33, 42-4, and *passim*; M. Susser, *Causal Thinking in the Health Sciences* (1973), pp.54-9.

[2] The best critical pieces on Snow are by P.E. Brown: 'John Snow — the Autumn Loiterer', *Bull. Hist. Med.* 35 (1961), 519-28; idem, 'Another Look at Snow'. See also S.P.W. Chave, 'Henry Whitehead and Cholera on Broad Street', *Med. Hist.* 2 (1958), 92-108. The most useful appreciation is by W. Hampton Frost in *Snow on Cholera*, which reprints *On Continuous Molecular Changes* and *On the Mode of Communication of Cholera* (1855). Snow's work on anaesthesia

to the details of Snow's fieldwork. The present interest is to examine more closely his notions of the nature and mode of action of the disease agent, to place him in a context continous with that already described, and to draw attention to the coincidence of his work with the development of governmental research and investigation.

In 1858, John Simon summarized Snow's 'peculiar doctrine' of cholera in the following terms:

This doctrine is, that cholera propagates itself by a 'morbid matter' which, passing from one patient in his evacuations, is accidentally swallowed by other persons as a pollution of food or water; that an increase of the swallowed germ of the disease takes place in the interior of the stomach and bowels, giving rise to the essential actions of cholera, as at first a local derangement; and that 'the morbid matter of cholera having the property of reproducing its own kind must necessarily have some sort of structure, most likely that of a cell'.

This is a fair summary, and may serve as such for the purposes of this chapter. Brown claims that Snow was ill-equipped for his work on cholera, and that he arrived at the above conclusions 'almost intuitively', or by a 'haphazard process of reasoning which no later rationalization could ever turn into a convincing argument'. Brown is clearly tired of both the perpetual emphasis on Snow's fieldwork and the usual uncritical response to it, and consequently overstates his case.[1] He also questions Snow's account of the derivation of his views (although Snow's tone is hardly autobiographical), and criticizes his 'failure' to defend his views by describing how he arrived at them. It is perhaps unwise so freely to equate 'intuitive' with 'irrational', and 'impossible to prove' with 'indefensible', and certainly injudicious to expect anything impressive of the way in which theories are first formulated. However, Brown's aims are clear enough. On this particular point, it

will not be dealt with here although it should be pointed out that it may have been of higher intellectual quality than his work on cholera, and tended to contain his thoughts on major physiological topics. It had also a high experimental content. See *Snow on Cholera*, p.xxxiii; N.A. Bergman, 'The Legacy of John Snow', *Anaesthesiology*, 19 (1958), 595–606; W.W. Mushin, 'Craft and Intellect. The John Snow Memorial Lecture, 1964', *Br. J. Anaesth.* 37 (1965), 520–7.

[1] Simon, *Public Health Reports*, i. 443 n.; Brown, 'Another Look at Snow', p.646; idem, 'Snow, the Autumn Loiterer', p.527. The only reply to Brown is conventional and does not deal in detail with his arguments: Lord Cohen of Birkenhead, 'John Snow – "The Autumn Loiterer"?', *Proc. R. Soc. Med.* 62 (1969), 99–106.

seems that Snow's 'own account' may be accepted, that he reached his conclusions from a consideration of the pathology of the disease *and* from a conviction, based on cholera's predilection for lines of human intercourse and on consecutive cases in the one household, that the disease was communicable person to person.

Brown suggests that Snow was led from an interest in temperance to toxicology, and thence to his study of the physiology of respiration and to his own peculiar views on cholera. [1] It is quite possible that Snow approached cholera from a vaguely toxicological point of view, but this in itself does not explain the peculiarity of his opinions since, as we have seen, many others did the same without arriving at the same conclusions. If Snow had made any protracted use of the poison analogy he would have been forced to conclude that the poison of cholera circulated in the blood. As we shall see, Snow used several analogies. He was at an early stage in his reasoning prevented from making much use of the poison analogy by the requirement that the disease agent be particulate.

Brown's opinion appears to be that Snow first derived his ideas from pathological views which were neither sound nor novel, and then, after a process of elimination more or less forced upon him, defended them solely on epidemiological grounds. Whatever Snow's merits as a pathologist, it is unjust to criticize him for this deficiency in the context of his theory of cholera because (partly due to the lack of marked post-mortem appearances) no one was in a position to argue with any greater security from the pathology of the disease.[2] Snow was, in fact, little concerned to claim priority for any of his pathological views. This is not to say that he was free to prove his case to his contemporaries independently of its pathological component, as he claimed he could, and as he naturally wished to do. Here as elsewhere Snow was criticized not because he held certain views, but because he held them to the exclusion of all others. He allowed only one mode of entry for the poison, and denied any essential affection of the blood; this

[1] Brown, 'Another Look at Snow', pp.648–50.
[2] See e.g. W. Lauder Lindsay, 'Clinical Notes on Cholera', *Ass. Med. J.* 2 (1854), 530 ff.

purely localist interpretation (though not unprecedented)[1] ran counter to the current revival of humoralism, as well as to most sources of analogy. Snow never changed this view in spite of later considering that diseases like typhoid in which the blood was affected might spread in the same way as cholera.

The unreasonableness of Snow's views in the contemporary context may be brought out by examining his use of the smallpox analogy. On the one hand, Snow stated that in origin and specificity cholera was analagous to smallpox; that, as in smallpox, there was in the course of the disease a dormant period in which the agent multiplied (there was palpable proof of this in smallpox, and in other diseases this increase could be inferred from the fact of their extension); and that, since in smallpox the agent defied analysis, no stress could be placed on the negative results of microscopic and similar investigations in cholera. The 'exclusiveness' of Snow's view of cholera was a condition which, if it could be asserted of any disease, properly belonged to smallpox. Snow put it most succinctly in 1853 when he stated that 'to be of the human species, and to receive the morbid poison in a suitable manner, is most likely all that is required'.[2] Elsewhere he dispensed explicitly with the necessity for predisposition or predisposing causes, or even causes of sudden epidemic extension, as well as with the possibility that cholera might be contagious in some circumstances and not in others. He also argued that if specifically contaminated water was admitted to be a factor at all, or on any one occasion, it must be admitted as a sufficient cause; this amounted to regarding such water as equivalent to the fluid vehicle (serum, from the pustules) of the smallpox poison.

On the other hand, Snow was just as concerned to make negative use of the analogy, in order to establish that cholera was by definition a disease transmitted by water contaminated with alvine discharge. As he was well aware, smallpox and its pathology provided the only firm definitions of contagiousness and communicability. Snow wished to establish different criteria, and consequently argued that cholera had a pathology

---

[1] See e.g. *Br. For. Med. Chir. Rev.* 14 (1854), 142.
[2] *Snow on Cholera*, pp.15, 161.

different from that of smallpox. There was no primary reaction involving the whole constitution, such as fever, but rather a local affection of the bowels. Furthermore, while smallpox and similar diseases had to run their full course, an attack of cholera could be cut short in the early stages.

This examination shows the mutual dependency of the pathological and epidemiological parts of Snow's argument, a point of which Brown takes insufficient account. Together the parts form a narrow set of propositions having every justification for the modern reader and none for Snow's contemporaries. In the next chapter this exclusiveness will be seen to provide a contrast with the flexibility of Budd.

Snow's claims to being considered an exponent of the germ theory require examination in detail. As was pointed out in the last chapter, it is misguided to assume that relations must necessarily exist between persons advocating a biological explanation of disease, and it is therefore not requisite, for example, that Snow should have been influenced by Henle.[1] Snow differed from the theorists already considered in that he attributed to his agent only such properties as followed directly from his views on pathology and propagation. He claimed that it was cellular, and, according to Richardson, persisted with this claim as much as with his views on propagation. This insistence is, however, best ascribed to its being essential to these views on propagation that the agent be particulate (or 'indivisible') and thus distributed like tapeworm eggs, rather than dissipated evenly like soluble chemical substances.[2] Snow's scattered remarks as to the nature of the agent and its mode of operation occasionally go beyond the dictates of necessity, but never in such a way as to imply that he held a single developed view. His first publications on cholera in general, as well as in relation to the cholera-fungus controversy, showed no particular commitment. Brown, although not making much of Liebig's influence on Snow, claims that Snow's earliest views on the nature of contagion were derived from Liebig. It is true that Snow, like most

[1] Frost seems to think that it is, although Snow never mentioned Henle: ibid., p.xvi.
[2] Richardson, 'On Cholera', pp.430–1; Snow, 'Cholera in the Baltic Fleet', *Med. Times Gaz.* 1854, ii. 170.

of his contemporaries, was influenced by ideas on organic chemistry of the kind advocated by Liebig, and in particular by his application to organic processes of the law of Berthollet and La Place. This, as we shall see, was combined with an equally typical interest in forces and the basic properties of matter. However, Snow was at no time a single-minded adherent.[1] His few speculative remarks show a variety of influences. In August 1849, he wrote of 'some matter' which multiplied itself in the gut 'by the appropriation of surrounding matter, in virtue of molecular changes going on within it, or capable of going on, as soon as it is placed in congenial circumstances'. Then, after finding a precedent for the mode of communication of cholera matter in that of the ova of intestinal worms, he stated that he did not 'wish to be misunderstood as making this comparison so closely as to imply that cholera depends on veritable animals or even animalcules but rather to appeal to that general tendency to the continuity of molecular changes, by which combustion, putrefaction, fermentation and the various processes in organised beings are kept up'.[2] At the same time he argued briefly for the non-involvement of the blood in cholera by reference to the analogous properties of irritant poisons.

In a paper given in October 1849, Snow stated by way of reply to possible objections to his theory of water-carriage, that a poison capable of multiplication in the body must be organized and therefore insoluble; or, 'if the poison be really a chemical compound . . . it might yet be imbibed by minute cells, such as mucous globules or epithelial cells, and be thus conveyed without being much diluted'. This last suggestion had the merit of clarity, but it did not occur again. With unusual and perhaps significant disinterest Snow credited the idea to Lankester, who in his turn thought it was Snow's. Before Busk's investigations of the cholera fungus, Lankester had given it as his opinion that any 'cholera-bodies' in the discharges were altered epithelial cells. After the publication

---

[1] Brown, 'Snow, the Autumn Loiterer', pp.521–2. Brown gives no indication until his second paper that many of Snow's references to Liebig were critical: 'Another Look at John Snow', p.649. See e.g. Snow, *Lancet*, 1842–3, ii. 130. For Snow on zymosis see *Snow on Cholera*, p.156.

[2] Snow, *Mode of Communication of Cholera* (1849), p.8.

of Snow's polite note, priority for the suggestion was seized by a third party, E.O. Spooner of Blandford, who held views similar to Budd's. In January, Spooner had quoted Boehm's description of desquamation of the gut in cholera in order to show the affinity of that disease to exanthemata, especially smallpox. He then suggested that the morbid epithelial cells cast off, 'generated' the specific poison of cholera. Whether these cells were shed in the gut in cholera as a result of specific morbid changes was a much debated question from the time of the first epidemic onwards, and is a good example of the difficulties experienced in deciding even well-defined pathological questions.[1]

In 1854, Snow spoke rather obscurely of 'a low form of organic action going on upon the interior surface of the stomach and intestines', and then made a further suggestion:

The morbid poison so multiplying or reproducing itself probably acts as an irritant, and causes the great effusion of watery fluid . . . or, what is still more probable, if the *materies morbi* have a cellular structure, is, that it withdraws the fluid from the blood circulating in the capillaries by a power analogous to that by which the epithelial cells of various organs abstract the various secretions in the healthy body.

A similar use of the supposed powers of epithelial cells had been made in 1849 by Francis Plomley. Plomley, however, was thinking in terms of secretion, rather than assimilation. Like Lankester, he thought the cholera-bodies were modified epithelial cells.[2] Snow repeated his own version of the activity of these cells in the same words in his major work (1855). Apart from this not uninteresting suggestion, his remarks on the nature of the agent are in that work so far reduced in number as to allow the modern student to believe that he never entertained any but 'modern' ideas on the subject. He stated merely (and far too concisely) that the question was one of natural history, not of chemistry; and that the agent, having the property of self multiplication, must be organized

---

[1] Snow, 'On the Pathology and Mode of Communication of Cholera', *Lond. Med. Gaz.* 9 (1849), 928 and note; *Lancet*, 1849, ii. 404; Spooner, *Lond. Med. Gaz.* 9 (1849), 1078; idem, 'Contagion of Asiatic Cholera', p.37. It is presently accepted that epithelium is lost in cholera, but that this is a post-mortem effect: Barua and Burrows, *Cholera*, p.170.

[2] Snow, 'Principles on which the Treatment of Cholera should be Based', *Med. Times Gaz.* 1854, i. 180; *Prov. Med. Surg. J.* 13 (1849), 615. Presumed to be Francis Plomley, Extra-L.R.C.P., F. Linnaean Soc., of Maidstone, Kent: *Medical Directory*.

(and therefore insoluble). Later papers merely repeated these points.[1]

Snow's only major speculative excursion was the *Continuous Molecular Changes* of 1853. This address is referred to disparagingly, in brief, or not at all by modern writers.[2] This is not surprising, since it has none of the apparent, anachronistic simplicity of Snow's other writings, and suggests instead the problems of the contemporary context. The influence of Liebig seems obvious merely from the title, but the address reflected a climate of opinion brought about by Liebig's work rather than any more personal indebtedness. The drift of the argument was away from rather than towards Liebig's point of view. This drift was detectable even in the remarks of 1849 quoted above. Snow, none the less, illustrates the contemporary habit of going to Liebig for notions of process, among which may be included his views on respiration.[3] Snow considered under his title a range of phenomena of transference or continuity, stretching from combustion, fermentation, and heredity, to crowd behaviour and the education of the child by the parent — that is, he went well beyond events which could be called chemical, even by Liebig. Eventually it becomes apparent that Snow was interested not so much in processes as in reproduction and heredity.

His intention was, as he put it, 'to make a few remarks on the chief phenomena of living beings', and he began by adopting an exemplary position as to the impossibility of separating so-called vital and chemical phenomena. The word 'molecular', he said, was chosen as a general term covering 'physical', 'chemical', and 'vital', in order to avoid disputes such as those in which 'such authors as Humboldt, Liebig and [William] Alison' were engaged.[4] Using the example of

[1] *Snow on Cholera*, pp.15, 113; Snow, 'Outbreak of Cholera at Abbey Row', *Med. Times Gaz.* 1857, ii. 417 ff.

[2] See e.g. 'M.G.', 'John Snow, 1813–58, A Painstaking Statistician', *Brit. Med. J.* 1937, ii. 595–6: 595. P.E. Brown does not mention the address itself. It is briefly commented upon in *Snow on Cholera*, p.xiv. Snow spent 'nearly twelve months' in its preparation: ibid., p.xxxvii.

[3] See e.g. Snow, 'On Narcotism by the Inhalation of Vapours', *Lond. Med. Gaz.* 10 (1850), 622.

[4] *Snow on Cholera*, p.145. Cf. Snow, 'On the Circulation in the Capillary Blood Vessels', *Lond. Med. Gaz.* 1843, i. 813.

fermentation, he suggested a possible distribution of the terms vital and chemical, but stressed that the formation of the yeast sporules and the chemical changes were interdependent. Here Snow noted from Schleiden's *Principles of Scientific Botany* (translated by Lankester), the author's opinion that yeast cells originated without the influence of a living plant. 'If it be so,' Snow commented, 'their formation may be looked on as a natural link between the vital and non-vital — between ordinary chemistry and physiology.' He also noticed Schleiden's opinion that the whole process of cell formation could be considered a chemical act. This 'blending together of what we call vital and what we call chemical' was not surprising , since 'all changes of composition . . . whether taking place within the living body or not, are alike the result of the attraction or affinity which exists among the ultimate atoms or molecules of matters'. Snow did, however, derive a criterion by which to recognize vital action. After referring to 'changes of a more complicated nature — those to which plants and animals owe their development and continuance — that have never commenced anew within the experience of man' he stated that

The most characteristic property . . . of vital actions probably is, that they are always caused by similar processes which have preceded them, whilst all other molecular changes may arise, occasionally at least, from other causes. A species of plant or animal consists, in fact, of a number or collection of continuous molecular actions.

The higher the organism the more continuity or 'points of contact' — hence the references to education or the learning process among human beings. Here Snow appears to have become metaphorical, although there is some reason to believe that he thought a material kind of transfer, or rather, a transfer of action as a property in material, was responsible for all forms of heredity. Sexual reproduction he thought had the effect of 'preventing deviations from the form and character of the species'. Earlier he stated as a general principle that 'the quantity of matter in which any molecular change or group of changes is taking place may diminish to a very small amount without the continuity of action being broken', and that, in particular, 'at the point at which new individuals commence the molecular actions are often confined to a minute quantity of substance'. He thought, however, that there was reason to believe 'that this substance contains all the chief elementary and proximate principles of the mature being, as well as the power of communicating all those changes to suitable materials, by which they are assimilated, and made to form part of the individual.' In seeds or ova the changes were arrested, but the 'continuity by contact of material' was not interrupted. Thus Snow was able to use the Liebigian emphasis on the state of action of matter, rather than the diversity of matter itself which modern chemistry had shown to be far less than might have been supposed, to suggest a solution to the problem of how the contents of a single cell or seed could adequately represent and reproduce the characteristics of the full-grown individual. Snow (who was probably not acquainted with a wide range of such literature) here referred to Richard Owen's *On Parthenogenesis, or the Successive Production of Procreating Individuals from a Single Ovum* (1849). Owen coined the word 'parthenogenesis' for the phenomena of asexual or vegetative reproduction. He considered that sexual reproduction was primary and normal, and that asexual reproduction could only take place because of the 'presence, in the proliferating region, of unchanged descendants of the primitive spermatized cells of the embryo' — that is, there was a retention of 'spermatic force' after the first, sexual proliferation.[1]

Snow subsequently passed on to molecular changes having for their result not the preservation of the individual and the species, but the reverse. These 'divert part of the substance of the individual from the actions which are natural to the species to another kind of action, in consequence of which this substance is employed in the multiplication and increase of the materies morbi of communicable disease'. This sentence might have been written by Liebig; but Snow went on to state that 'the material cause of every communicable disease resembles a species of living being in this , that both one and the other depend on, and in fact consist of, a series of continuous molecular changes, occurring in suitable materials'.[2]

---

[1] *Snow on Cholera*, pp.150–4. Owen was influenced by both *Naturphilosopnie* and English Platonism. See a critical account by T.H. Huxley in Owen, *Life of Owen*, ii. 321–30.

[2] *Snow on Cholera*, p.156.

By taking Liebig and the modern chemists at their word as to the power of chemistry to define the properties of living beings, Snow was able both to use their explanations and to maintain his own proposition, that the agents of disease were themselves living according to the terms of current definitions. This compromise, as Snow himself indicated, was reminiscent of if not suggested by that effected between the different explanations of fermentation.

Thus for Snow, communicable diseases were fixed species, species in all senses of the term; and the question of the origin of smallpox became, as for Southwood Smith and Budd, equivalent to that of the origin of 'the first tiger or upas tree'.[1] However, in spite of the emphasis thus placed on 'continuous', Snow did feel obliged to admit the possibility of spontaneous generation in the 'putrefactive' diseases like erysipelas, because of their ubiquity; he could not imagine that the morbid material of such diseases could be as widespread as the spores of fungi or moulds. According to Snow, the reason why Sydenham thought no disease communicable except the plague was his understandable ignorance of natural history: he was aware of the resemblance between the material cause of an epidemic disease and a species of animal or plant, but 'he was not aware that animals and plants proceed only from procreation by their own kind'. Elsewhere Snow drew a more definite parallel between the disease agent and parasites, applying to the latter the 'general principle, "omne vivum ex ovo"'.[2] If Snow had applied this aphorism of Harvey to cells, he would, of course, have been accepting a cell theory in advance of that of Schleiden, who postulated the production of cells by an unorganized matrix or blastema.

It is clear that Snow's notion of 'continuous molecular change' was extremely broad. Ultimately, one is tempted to reduce his discussion to the statement that the one definitively vital action was the multiplication of kind, with (at some

---

[1] Ibid., p.171 and, as an anecdote by Richardson, p.xlv. Cf. a comment made by him in Snow's lifetime: *J. Publ. Hlth Sanit. Rev.* 1 (1855), 131–2.

[2] *Snow on Cholera*, pp.170–1, 158, 166. Snow gave no indication that Sydenham might have been aware of the principle behind this contemporary aphorism; the demands he made on Sydenham are, otherwise, historically unreasonable. He was further at fault in regarding natural history as having been 'little cultivated' in the seventeenth century.

distance) the proviso that all actions depended eventually on the basic properties of atoms or molecules. Certainly Snow took little account, except by implication, of Liebig's arguments for purely chemical forms of increase, and it is significant that he referred to Grove, the only writer considered in Chapter 5 above who was avowedly a vitalist.[1] He had, of course, every motive for turning his discussion in this direction, in terms of his theory if not of its possible reception.

The argument of *Continuous Molecular Changes* does not confirm the conviction of the modern reader that Snow was a germ theorist 'out of his time'. A closer examination of his views shows that he belongs, as one should expect, to the group already discussed, rather than to the true germ theorists of the period just before Koch.

II

In 1849, Snow was thirty-six years old, and, having attended assiduously for ten years, had just been re-elected a vice-president of the Westminster Medical Society, later the Medical Society of London. He had been born in York, the son of a farmer, and was educated locally.[2] Apparently, he was at school especially fond of arithmetic. At the age of fourteen he was apprenticed to a surgeon in Newcastle upon Tyne, and until 1836 worked in the north as a surgeon's assistant, without formal qualifications. As a youth he became a vegetarian and total abstainer, and retained an interest in the temperance cause which he shared with his friend Benjamin

---

[1] *Snow on Cholera*, p.156.

[2] Snow (1813–58), M.R.C.S.., L.S.A., 1838; M.D. London 1844. Fellow of Royal Medical and Chirurgical Society, 1845. Medical Society of London's orator, 1853; its President, 1855. Also a member of the Pathological and Epidemiological Societies, and the British Medical Association, taking a particular interest in the second. Circumstances not good intil *c.* 1850. Consulted as anaesthetist but not called in, for the birth of Prince Arthur, 1850; called in for Prince Leopold, 1853, and Princess Beatrice, 1857. The obvious biographical source is B.W. Richardson, preferably his memoir in *Snow on Chloroform*, which is fuller, more critical and more feeling than the version of it in the *Asclepiad* (1887) and in *Snow on Cholera*. For some corrections to Richardson, see G. Edwards, 'John Snow M.D., 1813-1858', *Anaesthesia*, 14 (1959), 113–26. On surviving manuscripts, see R.S. Atkinson, 'The "Lost" Diaries of John Snow', *Progress in Anaesthesiology*, Excerpta Medica International Congress Series no. 200 (1968), pp.197-9; and below, p.275, n. 1.

Richardson. As a young man he also walked the country, gathering information which might have been intended for a medical topography of the local districts. Between 1836 and 1838, apparently unassisted but under circumstances which remain obscure, Snow migrated to London, attended the Windmill Street school of medicine and the wards of Westminster Hospital, and passed the examinations for M.R.C.S. and L.S.A. He bought no practice, merely putting up a plate; eventually he established a hospital connection and some foothold in local medical societies. Like Budd, but more collectedly, Snow was fully aware of what needed to be done to make a creditable living in professional life; his 'getting into an ether practice' must be seen in economic terms, as well as a practical reflection of his already developed interest in the physiology of respiration. He had since 1847 spent most of his time in acquiring an expert knowledge of anaesthesia; before that he had at a modest level published and spoken on current topics as they arose.[1]

Snow had had some experience of cholera as an apprentice in Newcastle, though he never claimed to have formed his ideas at that period.[2] Instead, he dated them from late 1848, at which time he confided in A.B. Garrod, Edmund Parkes, and several other medical men who remained unnamed. Garrod was also a member of the Westminster Medical Society; Parkes became one of Snow's most discerning critics, and in his turn accepted corrections from Snow to his study of the first London cholera cases.[3] He and Garrod were colleagues at University College London and had in common considerable experience in the analysis of the body fluids in

[1] See Richardson in *Snow on Chloroform*. Snow, being without influence, had difficulty in attracting fee-paying patients. He saw much practice, being 'encumbered with four sick clubs', and acting as an outpatients physician: ibid., p.xii. In such situations the expedient normally adopted was that of trying for some original observation suitable for publication. Frost's bibliography of 'principal writings' lists one or two papers a year from 1841 until 1847: *Snow on Cholera*, p.187.

[2] Richardson's claims lack detail and seem retrospective: *Snow on Chloroform*, p.xxvi. For a brief reference to this experience by Snow, see ibid., p.20.

[3] Snow, *Mode of Communication of Cholera* (1849), p.12; *Snow on Cholera*, p.125. Brown, 'Another Look at Snow', p.651; Parkes, *Lond. Med. Gaz.* 10 (1850), 41 ff.

cholera.[1] Snow used their results to support his pathological views.[2] Motives of friendship apart, he may (realizing the extent to which current trends were against him) have taken these two into his confidence originally to discover how far the most advanced haematological research might be thought compatible with the different pathology he wanted to establish for cholera. Parkes (who, as we have seen, had his own opinions) at no time worked to establish Snow's theory, but when it had become accepted he helped to defend the latter's priority.[3]

Snow's first statement on cholera appeared in August 1849, somewhat prematurely as Snow himself admitted, but, as Budd pointed out, Snow by so doing acquired priority rights to the suggestion that cholera was chiefly caused by contaminated water. By the time the cholera-fungus controversy began his views were fairly well known; indeed, such was Snow's persistence that it cannot be said his work ever suffered neglect for lack of an audience.[4] It is unnecessary to suppose, as does Brown, that Snow was dependent for his publicity upon that given to the cholera-fungus theory. In October he gave a long paper to the Westminster Medical Society which, as will be recalled, was one of the few societies in session during the epidemic. This is doubtless the only reason why on 13 October Swayne, as well as Snow, is found speaking there. Snow had already made cautious reference to the Bristol findings on 4 October in a lecture to the Western Literary Institution, but on this occasion he was more definite, stating that if the cholera-bodies were to be generally found in the atmosphere they could not be the real cause of cholera.[5] Swayne for his part briefly expressed himself as in agreement with Snow's pathology, but passed on immediately to an account of his own concerns.

Brown suggests that since demonstration of the agent was

---

[1] For (Sir) Alfred Baring Garrod (1819–1907), M.D. London 1843, L.R.C.P. 1851, F.R.C.P. 1856, F.R.S. 1858, see *DNB*.

[2] See e.g. *Snow on Cholera*, pp.10 ff.

[3] For a review of Snow by Parkes, see *Br. For. Med. Chir. Rev.* 15 (1855), 449–63.

[4] Budd, *Malignant Cholera*, p.19 n.

[5] Brown, 'Snow, the Autumn Loiterer', p.522; *Lancet*, 1849, ii. 431–2; ibid., p.413.

the nearest way of proving his theory, Snow would have wished to join with the Bristolians, and was deterred from doing so by the thought that he might thereby endanger his claim to priority. It is fair to point to Snow's concern for his own claims, as it was always pronounced; but, given the nature of his remarks on the agent of cholera, it seems doubtful whether he would at any point have agreed with Budd either that 'the detection of the actual cause of the disease and the determination of its nature were all that was wanting to convert his [Snow's] views into a real discovery', or that a fungus was that actual cause.[1] Because the cholera-fungus controversy and the first emergence of Snow's views on cholera occurred at the same time, it is difficult to tell to what extent his later policies might have been determined by the unfavourable outcome of that controversy. However, it seems likely, given the necessity of his assuming an unequal distribution, that Snow would always have been cautious enough to predict negative results from the analysis of contaminated water. Again, Snow's refusal to admit air as a vehicle in the communication of cholera was one of the chief differences between his view and that of the Bristolians. Later he suggested, as some kind of equivalent, contamination through the agency of flies and other insects, or (a suggestion attended with greater risk to his exclusive view) that the evacuations could, when dry, be 'wafted as a fine dust'. These hypotheses helped to account for some anomalies, without absolutely implying a different mode of entry for the poison, or any kind of regularity in its distribution: both of which were features of the contemporary hypothesis that an agent of disease might be carried by the molecules of gases in the atmosphere.[2] Allowing that the poison could be inhaled as well as swallowed would require a different pathology, including, perhaps, other modes of egress of the poison; and since most cases occurred in already infected areas, it would weaken in any one case the supposition that the disease was caused by the water that the victim had drunk. It was this supposition which Snow was always most anxious to claim as his own,

---

[1] Brown, 'Another Look at Snow', p.650; Budd, *Malignant Cholera*, p.19 n.
[2] Snow was of course taking advantage of the behaviour of insects in the same way as e.g. Holland.

rather than an elaborated theory of cholera. Apart from these considerations, there is the fact that as early as 26 September Snow had provided samples for Baly and Gull, and he was doubtless aware of the tenor of these investigations and of their possible outcome.

The events of 1849 foreshadowed all developments in relation to Snow's theory. His claim to the generalization that bad water affected the incidence of cholera was allowed; he established contact with Farr; the most substantial review of his pamphlet, after describing it as a 'modest contribution to medical literature on the subject', examined his evidence from the field and found his case not proved; and a colleague at the Westminster Medical Society stated that he 'could not but regard [Snow's] water theory as far too exclusive . . . we must not take a circumscribed or merely *microscopic* view of the recent epidemic, but rather a telescopic range of the subject, in all its vastness'.[1] Finally, Dr. P.H. Williams, in summarizing the results of the Provincial Medical and Surgical Association's consensus inquiry into cholera, concluded that 'the aggregate of evidence supplied by members of the Association decidedly preponderates in favour of contagion, infection or any other term which expresses the transmission of the disease from person to person and from place to place', and cited Snow's work as doing most to bring about this result.[2]

The set pieces of Snow's epidemiology are the Broad Street pump epidemic and the South London water-supply comparison, both of which investigations took place during the third cholera epidemic in 1854. The second of these was a large-scale statistical exercise methodologically much in keeping with the period, which is one reason why the idea of conducting a comparison of the effects of different water supplies had occurred to others besides Snow.[3] Another is that although agitation over water supply apparently began in

---

[1] *Lond. Med. Gaz.* 9 (1849), 470; *Lond. J. Med.* 1 (1849), 1083. For Snow's response, see *Snow on Cholera*, pp.16 ff.

[2] *Prov. Med. Surg. J.* 14 (1850), 507.

[3] See e.g. 'Oenophilus', *Morning Chronicle*, 19 Oct. 1849. The General Board of Health gave directions for this type of enquiry to be carried out in Newcastle in 1853: *Snow on Cholera*, pp.107–8.

earnest about 1850, this had little to do with Snow, whose interest was as much a product of the climate of gradually gathering concern as was the agitation itself.[1] As Brown points out, Snow could not have carried out his investigations had not some improvements already been made. Medical men were aware before 1849 that polluted water was one factor in epidemic disease.[2] Again, it is the specificity of Snow's views that distinguished him from his contemporaries; this guided his actions and (in a variety of ways) gave him the determination to carry out his plan.

The results of water analyses affected the acceptance of Snow's theory in that, as in 1849, negative findings were taken at face value.[3] The techniques of water analysis changed little between 1850 and 1870.[4] Considerable conflict between expert witnesses took place in the 1850s; but while this was, in part, a reflection of the limitations of analysis, it was also owing to the absence of conventions regulating the employment of such witnesses. The sudden adoption of chemists as persons fit to make official judgements on public-health matters was much resented by the medical men.[5] It is assumed that the rise of organic chemistry must have led to a finer differentiation in analysis , but what was established by 1850 as the condition most indicative of dangerous contamination of water, was the presence of very simple nitrogenous compounds which were the end product of decomposition in general. This test came into prominence through the analyses of R. Angus Smith in Manchester from 1846, and of R.D. Thomson in Glasgow in 1845. Thomson stated that it was

[1] For a history of London water, see H.C. Richards and W.H.C. Payne, *London Water Supply* (1899). Protest and official investigation were both in evidence in 1821: D.L. Emblen, *Peter Mark Roget: The Word and The Man* (1970), pp.212 ff. 1850 was marked by the *Report of the General Board of Health on the Supply of Water to the Metropolis:* PP, 1850, XXII. 1. On this 'revolutionary' report, see Finer, *Life of Chadwick*, p.394.

[2] Brown, 'Snow, the Autumn Loiterer', p.526; see e.g. *Lancet*, 1848, i. 103.

[3] See e.g. Simon in *Report to the Local Board of Health of Croydon* (1853), p.5; cf. his testimony in 1869, when Snow's findings had become acceptable, that too much stress was sometimes laid on the chemical analysis of water, and that the real test of its poisonousness 'has been in the killing of the people': *First Report of Royal Sanitary Commission*, PP, 1868–9, XXXII. 408.

[4] For the later methods see A. Shadwell, *London Water Supply* (1899).

[5] See R.A. Smith, 'Science in our Courts of Law', *J. Soc. Arts.* 8 (1860), 133–42; *Ass. Med. J.* 2 (1854), 961.

Liebig who, in 1845, suggested that he test for nitric acid. Leibig had 'directed much attention to the subject' as early as 1825, when he had confirmed experiments made over seventy years before, and had traced the nitric acid found to the organic matter of towns. Thomson subsequently discovered nitric acid in city, but not in country, wells. In 1850, however, Hofmann gave it as his opinion that 'on the Continent, the water question has been discussed far less than in this country and I am not aware of any results which would be worth the notice of the Board'.[1] Water which tended to preserve the putrefiable matters which entered it, was thought as undesirable as water in which putrefaction was actively taking place; the ideal (given that water could not be absolutely pure) seemed to be water in which this process ran through its (unknown) stages as rapidly as possible to produce the harmless end-products. A little later, under the influence of the 'Munich chemists', it began to appear as if there were a dangerous stage preceding 'ordinary' putrefaction.[2]

After 1850, Arthur Hill Hassall began to press the rival claims of microscopy, which he said was essential in determining the *quality* of waters.[3] The significance of the presence in water of muscle fibre and undigested vegetable matters was plain enough, but controversy arose over that of animalcules. This was a legitimate controversy in spite of the part taken in it by *The Lancet*, the water companies, and Chadwick, who took evidence from Hassall in 1850. Hassall inclined towards a biological explanation of epidemic disease, and found the suggestion that organisms were present in the body under normal conditions, 'disgusting'.[4] However, there was an obvious absence of evidence showing whether or not the

---

[1] *Scientific Enquiries Report*, pp.351 ff.; *Metropolitan Water Supply Report*, p.857.

[2] See e.g. W.T. Gairdner, *Public Health in Relation to Air and Water* (1862), pp.73–4.

[3] See evidence by Hassall in Minutes of Evidence taken before the Select Committee on the Metropolitan Water Bill, PP, 1851, XV. 230 ff. See also *Q. Jl. Microsc. Sci.* 1 (1853), 60. For Hassall's contribution as a whole, see E.G. Clayton, *A Memoir of the late Dr. A.H. Hassall* (1908), pp.5 ff.

[4] Ibid., p.5; Hassall, 'Memoir on Organic or Microscopic Analysis of London Water', *Lancet*, 1850, i. 230; *Metropolitan Water Supply Report*, pp.697 ff.; *Metropolis Water Bill Committee*, pp.229 ff. Hassall, Appendix to *Scientific Enquiries Report*, p.378.

animalcules themselves were harmful, and debate centred rather on the question of whether their increase in the water indicated the presence of harmful organic matters. In 1851, Hassall found himself placed in opposition to Liebig on this point, but in spite of Liebig's authority, and of occasional attempts at ridicule, it became the general view that, while nothing very precise could be inferred, the presence of animalcules in water indicated an undesirable degree of organic pollution.[1]

In very many cases however, consumers and experts alike relied upon their unaided senses. When it came to proving that bad water caused disease, most arguments rested on what Simon called the 'common principles of taste', rather than on 'inferences deducible from medicine', though few stated as clearly as did Simon that this was their mode of reasoning. The validity of principles of taste, as inculcated by years of sanitary propaganda, was rarely challenged by the knowledgeable. When it was, as by Snow in 1855 (in relation to the atmosphere), and to a lesser extent by the chemists Graham, William Allen Miller, and Hofmann in 1851, other scientists reacted by temporarily abandoning what they knew of the inefficacy of gases given off by putrefaction, and what they knew they did not know about organic decomposition.[2]

Important analytic work was done for the Medical Council

---

[1] *Metropolis Water Bill Committee*, pp.701 ff. For Liebig on animalcules, see *Familiar Letters on Chemistry* (1844), p.211. To the modern reader Liebig appears to be talking of algae, but Hassall does not question his terminology. On the presence of animalcules, see *Scientific Enquiries Report*, p.43. For an actual investigation, and significant reservations as to interpretation, see Brittan and Etheridge's report on the waters of Sandgate, *Report by T.E. Blackwell on Sandgate*, PP, 1854–5, XLV. 244 ff. Criteria had changed little two decades later: see J.D. Macdonald, *Guide to the Microscopical Examination of Drinking Water* (1883), pp.ix–x.

[2] Lambert, *John Simon*, p.166. Progress in the analysis of the atmosphere resembled that of water. Again R.D. Thomson and R. Angus Smith were involved. See e.g. Thomson, 'Chemical Researches on Cholera', *Lancet*, 1850, i. 154–5; idem, 'Chemical Conditions of Cholera Atmospheres', ibid. 1856, i. 63–4. For Smith, see *DNB*; A. Gibson and W.V. Farrar, 'Robert Angus Smith, F.R.S. and "Sanitary Science" ', *Notes Rec. R. Soc. Lond.* 28 (1974), 241–62. The later history of atmospheric analysis is perhaps more interesting: see J.K. Crellin, 'Airborne Particles and the Germ Theory', *Ann. Sci.* 22 (1966), 49–60. Snow, evidence before Select Committee on Public Health and Nuisances Bills, PP, 1854–5, XIII. 430 ff; *Report of Commission on Chemical Quality of Water*, PP, 1851, XXIII. 8 ff.; *Lancet*, 1855, i. 634–5.

set up by the temporary Board of Health under Sir Benjamin Hall, which succeeded Chadwick's General Board. Hall's Board was constituted in August 1854, and its most pressing problem was obviously the cholera of that year. The Council consisted of thirteen medical men and scientists officially nominated by Hall and by the Colleges, and it was led by Paris, President of the Royal College of Physicians. For the purposes of tackling the problem of cholera, it divided itself into three Committees: Scientific Enquiries (Arnott, Baly, Farr, Owen, and Simon); Treatment (Nathaniel Bagshaw Ward, (Sir) James Alderson, Tweedie, Paris, and a third member of the College of Physicians' Cholera Committee, Babington); and Foreign Correspondence (Babington, John Bacot, Sir James Clark, and Sir William Lawrence). When he reported on the Council's behalf in July 1855, Paris hoped that its members might be allowed 'to express their satisfaction at Science having at length been recognised by the State as the ally of civil jurisprudence and as the guide to a more enlightened code of medical police'.[1] As well as establishing a precedent (though of degree, rather than of kind) for the involvement of the profession in the formulation of official doctrine, the work of the Council constituted (for the nineteenth century) the first occasion on which the health department of government had 'directly promoted and financed scientific research of a "combined and systematic nature" and of the highest possible calibre'. This description must be assumed to exclude pieces of research carried out in 1832 or 'instigated' by Chadwick's Board rather later, as well as all work aimed at an official settlement of claims. As Lambert himself points out, the creation of the Council superseded a request from the new Epidemiological Society for public money to be used in cholera research.[2]

As Lambert also admits, the importance of this Council lay not so much in its work as in its very existence. The chief disadvantage under which it laboured was lack of time; the

---

[1] Lambert, *John Simon*, pp. 222 ff. Lawrence represented the Royal College of Surgeons; Ward and Bacot the Apothecaries' Society. *Report of the Medical Council*, PP, 1854–5, XLV. 3.

[2] Lambert, *John Simon*, p.228 and note. Compare the involvement of Arnott, Kay, and Southwood Smith in 1838.

cholera died away at the end of the year. None the less, the Council attempted in the spirit of Snow's critic to take 'a telescopic range of the subject, in all its vastness'. The Treatment Committee reported that although gathering information had proved very difficult, and the end result of largely negative value, 'the science of statistics, for the first time, has been applied on a large scale to medical treatment'.[1] The Committee for Scientific Enquiries put together a vast amount of meteorological data, and further encouraged R.D. Thomson, George Rainey, Hassall, and G.W. Callender of St. Bartholomew's Hospital to carry out investigations of waters, atmospheres, bodily fluids, and post-mortem appearances. This research was perhaps rather less than 'commissioned'. The Committee's report, after deploring the state of pathological knowledge, said that it was thought 'it might be conducive to good if this state of the case should be represented to persons who were likely to undertake scientific investigations'. Apparently the response was, in general, poor. The reports 'received' from Thomson, Hassall, and Rainey were printed 'entire or in part', and were considered in the report of the Committee in relation to its pathological questionnaire, which was sent out to all practitioners appearing in the *Medical Directory* of 1854. These proceedings would indicate that the methods of the Committee were little removed from those of the consensus type of inquiry conducted by largely the same personnel as members of societies and the Colleges. Accordingly, it is not surprising that this Committee's conclusions were either general or provisional, and that it found in favour of a statistical generalization, that is, Farr's formula for the influence of elevation. Later, however, exceptions to Farr's rule were noted, and it was suggested that there was an underlying constant factor, that is, 'excess of organic impurity'. The report ended with pleas for more research; the problem, it stated, was ignorance not of what factors were involved, but of the normal working of these factors. In particular, the Committee thought that a better knowledge of the 'chemistry of organic decomposition

---

[1] *Medical Council Report*, p.7. The Council gave other testimony of its faith in the 'numerical method': see e.g. *Scientific Enquiries Report*, pp.21–2.

especially successive transformations of animal refuse' might be 'all revealing', for there were 'reasons for believing, in respect not only of cholera, but of many kindred diseases, that the means and agencies of morbid infection stand in intimate relation to decaying animal products within and without the body'. The Council then made its excursion into 'doctrine', with its 'wandering ferment'. With some justification, it concluded that 'taking this as a hypothesis, and testing it by the facts before us, we find that it would include and explain them'.[1]

Before arriving at this conclusion, the Committee passed definite judgement on Snow. In connection with the Broad Street outbreak it stated that it saw 'no reason' to adopt the specific explanation of Snow:

We do not find it established that the water was contaminated in the manner alleged; nor is there before us any sufficient evidence to show whether inhabitants of the districts drinking from that well, suffered in proportion more than other inhabitants of the district who drank from other sources.[2]

The Committee did not fail to appreciate the exceptional nature of the case of the Hampstead widow, which fulfilled the definition of 'a crucial experiment' laid down by the *London Medical Gazette* in its review of Snow's first work on cholera. 'The Hampstead widow' had acquired a taste for the water of the Broad Street well, and a large bottle of it was delivered to her regularly by relatives still living in the area. At the time of the outbreak in Soho, she had not been in the neighbourhood of Broad Street for many months, and there was no cholera where she lived in Hampstead. She died, and a niece who visited her, and who lived in a 'high and healthy' part of Islington, also died of cholera. In view of Snow's description of this case as 'perhaps the most conclusive of all in proving the connexion between the Broad Street pump and the outbreak of cholera', Brown's opinion, that he did not appreciate its full significance, requires amplification.

[1] Ibid., pp.52 ff., 15, 49, 66, 48.

[2] Ibid., p.52. The Committee presumably did not have before it the *Report on the Cholera Outbreak in the Parish of St. James Westminster*, of July 1855, which contained Whitehead's demonstration of the contamination of the pump: Chave, 'Whitehead and Cholera on Broad Street', pp.97 ff. Whether this contamination was at the requisite moment specific, remained a matter of dispute.

Brown also states that because of its scale this 'experiment' made no impact on those who observed it. However this may be, it is clear that persons who knew of it at second hand were fully aware of its exceptional nature. Parkes spoke of it as a 'most extraordinary case, which, if there is not some fallacy, is certainly unanswerable'. That neither he nor the Committee changed their view accordingly, indicates the limits of 'crucial experiments'. The Committee were led by this case not to adopt Snow's views, but to contrive other explanations of the phenomena. It was probable, they admitted, that the water of the well did act as the vehicle of the cholera infection, but this did not mean that infection depended on the specific material alleged. The Broad Street pump caused cholera in persons dwelling at a distance because its water had participated in the atmospheric infection of the district. The same influence which converted organic matter in air to poison, could do so for water. In addition, nothing particular was found by Hassall in an analysis of two samples of Broad Street water.[1]

Snow, who predicted such negative results, also recorded an analysis by Hassall of Broad Street water. His interest was simply to establish the probability of contamination by ordinary sewage, since where ordinary sewage went, specially contaminated sewage could go also.[2]

In his comparison of cholera incidence among persons supplied by different London water companies, the probabilities were more in Snow's favour. Because the populations were so large it was safe to assume that a sufficient number of persons actually drank the water supplied, and that all other factors (which Snow was apt to ignore) were evenly distributed.[3] Very consistently, John Sutherland found it 'difficult to resist' the large-scale statistical terms of Snow's results, and concluded that 'the use of . . . water has aggravated the severity of the late epidemic, especially in the districts south of the Thames'. Like the Committee, he felt in no way

---

[1] *Lond. Med. Gaz.* 9 (1849), 468; *Snow on Cholera*, pp.44–5; Brown, 'Snow, the Autumn Loiterer', p.525; Parkes, *Br. For. Med. Chir. Rev.* 15 (1855), 456; *Scientific Enquiries Report*, p.52 and Appendix, p.241.

[2] *Snow on Cholera*, p.52.

[3] For a criticism of Snow's argument at this point, see Brown, 'Another Look at Snow', pp.651 ff. On Snow's omission of other factors, see e.g. Parkes, *Br. For. Med. Chir. Rev.* 15 (1855), 453, 459; Richardson in *Snow on Chloroform*, p.xxvi.

pressed to accept Snow's further contention that the water was specifically contaminated and therefore constituted a sufficient cause of cholera. In a similar way the Committee rejected the exclusiveness of Snow's pathology.[1]

The task of the Council was to arrive at a theory sufficient to dictate practical action, and on this depended the most significant factor in the official rejection of Snow. After referring to the differences between Snow and his opponents, Sutherland's report stated that 'the matter in dispute is really of no great practical value, for if it be a fact that the use of impure water is dangerous to public health, the manner of its action is of very secondary importance'.[2] Thus, if the authorities took steps to ensure the purity of water supplies, the desired effect would follow without need of further theoretical justification.

It is likely that Baly, Farr, and Simon were the most influential members of the Committee for Scientific Enquiries. Baly jointly with Gull had just published the other of what Budd called 'the two most considerable investigations yet undertaken, in this country at least, into the causes of Cholera' — the *Reports on Epidemic Cholera* of 1854.[3] This was, of course, the culmination of the project begun by the Royal College of Physicians in 1849. Over 400 replies to the circulars sent out that year had eventually been received, and the labour of collating and supplementing these was one of the reasons Baly gave for the delay in completion of the project. His other reason was that he had wanted, firstly, to have the benefit of consulting Farr's report (1852), and secondly, to be able to take full advantage of the returns which Farr had not had published. Not surprisingly, the *Reports* immediately became a standard reference. Parkes, in a review, applauded the broad base of the work and its method, which was that of 'getting generalisations to follow out of the facts', and of these prompting further questions, until eventually conclusions were arrived at 'as certain as any in what are rather ostentatiously

---

[1] 'Letter to Palmerston with Report on Cholera by Sutherland', PP, 1854–5, XLV. 114, 116; *Scientific Enquiries Report*, p.57.

[2] *Letter with Report by Sutherland*, p.108.

[3] The one being, of course, the *Scientific Enquiries Report*: Budd, 'Mode of Propagation of Cholera', *Ass. Med. J.* 4 (1856), 259.

called the exact sciences'. These conclusions were not novel; in a 'great number of cases' they agreed with opinions previously held, but instead there was provided 'confirmatory testimony of the best description, — testimony which we should regard in the same light as when one chemist repeats the experiments and confirms the conclusions of another'. There is something in Greenwood's remark that the *Reports* was 'strictly orthodox, as the official report of a professional body is sure to be', but considering the independence of Baly and Gull, it is perhaps more accurate to attribute the orthodoxy of the *Reports*, like its popularity, to its methodology.[1] It is fair to say that, irrespective of differences in scale, the *Reports* is a more impressive piece of work than the report on the cholera-fungus theory of 1849.

Like the Committee for Scientific Enquiries, Baly took the inclusive view, and considered all factors alleged to have an influence on the origin and distribution of cholera. However, his investigation was further organized by his considering these factors in relation to six theories of cholera isolated by him from the current literature. The object of his report was 'to inquire into the facts, and to learn which of these theories is most in accordance with them'.

Baly had, evidently, intended from the beginning of the project in 1849 to test the 'water theory', and he gave it a good deal of attention. 'Dr. Baly', said Snow later, ' . . . has done me the honour of giving a very full and impartial account of my views.'[2] Nevertheless, the replies to the circulars, 'in all their variety', evinced 'very decidedly the feeling of the profession that an *exclusive* theory of the mode of propagation . . . of cholera cannot be maintained', and Baly himself found that 'this theory, as a whole . . . is untenable', although it 'directed attention to circumstances which may be hereafter shown to bear a part in the production or increase of this as well as other epidemics; and the enquiries it suggests must

---

[1] Baly and Gull, *Reports on Epidemic Cholera* (1854), Preface; Parkes, *Br. For. Med. Chir. Rev.* 14 (1854), 130. M. Greenwood, 'A Cholera Centenary', *Br. Med. J.* 1949, ii. 797.

[2] Baly and Gull, *Reports on Epidemic Cholera*, pp.4–5, 121 ff., 195–213; *Snow on Cholera*, p.20. Baly signed his Preface in December 1853, and therefore could not have considered either of the 'set pieces' of the epidemic of 1854.

not be neglected'. Baly's criticisms of the 'water theory' need not be considered in detail; they were diffuse, and consisted principally in showing that for all Snow's positive instances, as many negative counter-instances might be found, and that for many of his positive instances there were alternative explanations. The only arguments of Snow's for which Baly found 'a wide basis in facts', 'might be used in favour of any theory which should regard the cause of cholera as a poison partially distributed — not diffused as a gas — through the air, having a connection . . . with poverty and dirt, and capable of being conveyed from place to place by human means'. Baly had decided that the only well-supported theory was that which regarded the cause of cholera as 'a matter increasing by some process, whether chemical or organic, in damp air', and which assumed that, although the cause was diffused by the air, it was also distributed (and perhaps occasionally produced) by human means. But the arguments having reference to the reproduction or increase of the poison in the alimentary canal, and to its diffusion by means of the admixture of the intestinal discharges with food and especially with drinking water, were 'exceedingly defective in facts of a conclusive nature'.[1] Baly concentrated on effects, and modes of propagation in particular, and did not speculate on the nature of the 'poison'.[2]

Snow had the opportunity of replying to these criticisms in the book which came before Baly and the other members of the Council, but he made little use of it, partly perhaps because of the diffuseness of the criticism, and partly because he may have hoped that the evidence from the 1854 epidemic placed his theory on a new footing.[3]

It is a little more difficult to decide what Farr's part in the judgement against Snow might have been. Snow clearly found him very helpful; although preoccupied in 1852 with the overriding effects of elevation, he was careful to note the

---

[1] *Reports on Epidemic Cholera*, pp.3, 213, 223, 210 (my italics).

[2] But see ibid., pp.216, 218.

[3] Snow made some reply (*Snow on Cholera*, pp.20, 65), and also tried to imply that Baly's own practice belied his critical theoretical position: ibid., p.95; see also *Committee on Public Health and Nuisances Bills*, pp.433 ff.

influence of different water supplies, and stated of Snow's theory that it was 'in many respects the most important theory that has yet been propounded'. After 1852, Farr made several moves aimed at collecting the sort of evidence used by Snow, and in 1854 he conducted the last ten weeks of the water-comparison inquiry. He was also destined 'to play the principal role in proving that the next epidemic of cholera in London (1866) was waterborne'.[1] By 1866, he had combined Liebig with Darwin and Pasteur, and had consequently arrived at an idea of the disease agent similar to Snow's (although more closely related to that of germ theorists of that period). He remarked, for example, that 'disease development is evidently associated with the life development of species and has with it some analogies'.[2] However, one may say that in 1854 Farr, though taken with the style of Snow's investigations, was still Liebigian in his faith. One can say, too, that Farr saw most clearly the defects in Snow's evidence, and that he apparently suggested the wider inquiry into the influence of London water supply made by Simon in 1856.[3]

John Simon is a necessarily important figure in the present context.[4] Of Huguenot descent, his father was an increasingly prosperous stockbroker, and a member of the Stock Exchange's Committee from 1835. The family retained many of its continental connections. At sixteen, John Simon was sent abroad for a year to learn foreign languages and consolidate his character. Before this it had been decided that he would

---

[1] Farr, *Report on Cholera Mortality*, p.lxxvi; idem, *Vital Statistics*, pp.357 ff.; Snow, 'Cholera and the Water Supply in the South Districts of London in 1854', *J. Publ. Hlth Sanit. Rev.* 2 (1856), 240, 242 ff.; *Snow on Cholera*, p.xviii.

[2] Farr, *Appendix 1868-9*, p.299.

[3] Simon, *Sanitary Institutions*, p.261 n.; *Report on the Last Two Cholera Epidemics of London, as affected by the Consumption of Impure Water*, PP, 1856, LII. 357.

[4] Simon (1816-1904), M.R.C.S. 1838, F.R.C.S. 1844. Senior asst. surgeon at King's College Hospital, 1840-7; lecturer in pathology at St. Thomas's Hospital, 1847-70; full surgeon at St. Thomas's, 1853-76. F.R.S. 1845: see J.B. Sanderson, 'John Simon', *Proc. R. Soc. Lond.* 75 (1905), 341. On Council of Royal College of Surgeons, 1868-80; President, 1878-9. First Medical Officer of Health to City of London, 1848; Medical Officer of Health to Central Board of Health, 1855; to Privy Council, 1858; to Local Government Board, 1871. Retired 1876. K.C.B. 1897. For a selection from his official and other writings, see *Public Health Reports*. The obvious biographical source is Lambert's study: *John Simon*. See also *DNB*.

become an apprentice of Joseph Henry Green, professor of surgery at King's College, London, and the friend and literary executor of Coleridge. Simon was influenced by Green to the extent of forming a society for the study of German metaphysics.[1] He married a woman of literary and artistic interests as strong as his own, and they were in later life on intimate terms with William Morris and the Pre-Raphaelite circle, especially John Ruskin.

The paucity of material makes it difficult to account for Simon's entry into one of the very few, comparatively unremunerative posts in public medicine. Although unaccountably on the central committee of the Health of Towns Association (1844), he apparently played no active role in the public health agitation of the 1840s. He had some degree of acquaintance with Utilitarianism, which his biographer is disposed to depreciate in favour of the influence of continental philosophies; he also wrote for the *Penny Cyclopaedia*.[2] His connections with King's College were not exclusive, since in 1839, aged twenty-three, he appears as a student of University College.[3] His hospital, St. Thomas's, was, of the metropolitan general hospitals, the most closely associated with both the Benthamite circle and the public health movement (University College Hospital was not founded until 1834). Simon became the first Medical Officer of Health for the City of London in 1848. This post was only the second of its kind in England, the first having been created by Liverpool in 1846. It was doubly significant in that the City had successfully resisted, and continued to evade, outside attempts to reform its administration in the interests of health. The City's Act, which it put forward to forestall a worse threat to its independence, was closely modelled on that of Liverpool, but its Medical Officership, not surprisingly, proved of greater importance on the national level. The City, from a variety of motives, looked for a young man, 'possessing the necessary talent, who would be glad of the opportunity this appointment

---

[1] Lambert, *John Simon*, p.24.

[2] Ibid., pp.64, 104, 33. Lambert places his main stress on Simon's 'empiricism' and 'professionalism'. *Penny Cyclopaedia*, xxvii (1843), pp.v–vii; C. Knight, *Passages of a Working Life* (1864–5), ii. 230.

[3] Hale Bellot, *University College*, p.187.

would give [him] of rising in [his] profession', and who could be encouraged to continue partly to support himself by medical practice. It is likely that his family's City connections were effectively used to promote Simon's candidature. Among his referees were Thomas Watson, Richard Owen, and Sir Benjamin Brodie.[1] There were nineteen losing candidates, including Henry Letheby (Simon's eventual successor in the post), Hector Gavin, Alfred Smee, and J.W. Griffith.[2] Farr submitted his name, but later withdrew it.[3]

Simon made the most of his opportunities and, with the aid of the national press, was able to achieve a good deal. His 'theoretical' basis was simply the sanitary generalizations already established. Lambert sees the 'supreme accomplishment' of Simon's seven years in the City as his sanitary organization, which 'pushed the Corporation into unexplored areas of interference with an impetus never wholly to be lost'. This organization had as its centre the post of Medical Officer, for which Simon 'first realised its potentiality, established its character and ensured it an enduring and prominent place in English local administration'. In 1855, the appointment of Medical Officers was made compulsory for every other district of the metropolis; these Metropolitan Officers formed, in 1856, a professional association which complemented others of the same period, such as the Epidemiological Society.[4]

As Medical Officer of Health to the Privy Council, Simon was responsible for official doctrine from 1855 to 1876; one of his achievements was to eliminate the gap between that doctrine and the opinions of the profession as a whole. In that he was medically qualified, his appointment was consistent with the change in policy evident in the setting up of the new Board of Health's Medical Council in 1854, and any medical man in his position would have reaped the benefit of the profession's approval of this change, whatever its real effects might have been. However, Simon was not only well qualified as a medical scientist and as a critic of medical science, but

---

[1] Lambert, *John Simon*, pp.99–100.
[2] Lambert gives the last named as 'I. Griffith': ibid., p.105 n.
[3] Ibid., p.104.
[4] Ibid., pp.214, 217; R. Dudfield, 'History of the Society of Medical Officers of Health', *Public Health*, Jubilee Number (1906), 1–207.

also defined his task in terms of these qualifications. His aim was 'to develop a scientific basis for the progress of sanitary law and administration', and for him the first step was to investigate with different kinds of experiment the causes of disease. 'Disease can only be prevented by those who have knowledge of its causes.' This the profession regarded as a truism (however they might have interpreted it, or however little they may have acted upon it), which had been violated by the lack of respect for specificity in disease shown by Chadwick's Board of Health. The new Medical Officer's peculiar virtues were 'caution, flexibility, and an ability to wait upon certitude'.[1] The difference between Simon and other 'objective assessors' was that he needed to admit, and felt himself justified in admitting, only that degree of theory which was required to dictate practical action. Because of this, his later official pronouncements occasionally give an appearance of undue conservatism; but this aspect of his work was complemented by his encouragement of 'pure' research, and his critical awareness of European developments. In any event, Simon was merely maintaining the dichotomy between theory and sanitary practice, which was characteristic of the profession before 1850.

Simon's first and most lasting commitment was to the chemical explanation of infectious disease.[2] In later years he became increasingly 'objective', or non-committal, but as late as 1865 he was to be found saying that 'more and more the once chaotic phenomenology of contagion is tending to become an intelligible and consistent section in the great science of organic chemistry'. His fullest personal statement was the *General Pathology* of 1850. These lectures are, among Simon's published statements, of the same importance as the *Continuous Molecular Changes* in the work of Snow, and similarly repay the attention of the modern reader. In *General Pathology*, Simon distinguished morbid from ordinary poisons but took as the closest analogue of the disease process, the simple one of chemical conversion:

---

[1] Simon, *Sanitary Institutions*, p.287; idem, *Public Health Reports*, ii. 593; Lambert, *John Simon*, p.56.

[2] For Lambert's description of Simon's views and their theoretical context, see ibid., pp.48 ff.

A certain organic material A, soluble and partially volatile affects [*sic*] particular relations with B, an ingredient (apparently a normal ingredient) of the blood: the results of their coming together are (1) the utter destruction of the latter, B; and (2) the immense increase of the former (A); not, indeed at the spot of infection but elsewhere.

This sounds Liebigian, but at this time Simon objected strongly to Liebig's views, on the grounds of their dependence upon the latter's interpretation of yeast fermentation, as well as on pathological grounds. For Simon, the increase of yeast was not an example of a result which was in principle possible in all forms of fermentation. Instead it was a primary phenomenon, which was owing not to yeast's being a ferment, but to yeast's being an organized vegetable production which was also an agent of fermentation. Simon himself conjectured that the disease process could be classed as a new species of catalytic action, but no more than Liebig was he able to explain the increase in morbid material. This, he admitted, was an 'almost overwhelming difficulty. What is there like it in chemistry, or in physics, or in any operation of brute matter on the living body?' One might imagine from Simon's notion of yeast fermentation that he would be tempted to give a solution to this difficulty in biological terms. He was, however, convinced that all known relations of parasitic agents with the body were of an entirely different nature. Parasitic diseases, he stated, were essentially local, even the muscardine of silkworms cited by Henle in support of his views on living contagia.

... all that we know of parasitic influence on the health (and I may observe that a great deal is known) ... is referable to these two heads: local inconvenience from pressure or from irritation; general inconvenience, either febricular — from that local irritation becoming inflammatory — or anaemiative, by draining and impoverishment of the blood ... their effects on life are in direct proportion to their manifestness in parts.

It followed from this quantitative mode of action that parasites, if present, were conspicuous. Simon concluded with what he considered to be his 'best argument': no parasite formation had been observed in connection with the contagious diseases. Of cholera Simon was at this time prepared to say little. He thought it a humoral disease, caused (like marsh ague) by a paludal rather than a true morbid poison. It was not primarily communicable person to person: 'the power of infection may be considered an appurtenance of the district rather than a property of the sufferers'.[1]

By 1853, it appears that for the sake of 'generalisations which would be popularly understood and popularly applied', Simon was prepared to tolerate Liebigian terminology, and even Liebigian ideas, if these were not applied too directly to pathology. He wrote of cholera that 'in all human probability, the poison arises in specific changes impressed by some migratory agent upon certain refuse elements of life . . . . Just as the infective ferment acts on men, so appears the epidemic ferment to act on locality.'[2] In this Simon was, of course, conforming to current trends. That Liebig was so readily 'popularly understood' was a measure not only of the compatibility of his views with contemporary interests, but also of the attention he had paid to the popular reception of his theories.

Lambert states that Simon's 'private persuasion and public example' were instrumental in the setting up of the Medical Council of 1854, and that he was its most active member. There is nothing in the Council's reports which conflicts with Simon's views; and the negative use of the parasite analogy, which appeared as an argument against Hassall's vibriones and against organisms in general, was undoubtedly the same as that quoted above.[3] The 'intelligible and practical' doctrine of the wandering ferment (which was reiterated in Simon's Report of 1856) is as likely to have been dictated by Simon as anyone.[4]

His report of 1856 was presented as a continuation of the work of the Medical Council and as a necessary official inquiry into the allegations made against the water companies. Snow's name was not mentioned, and the work did much to increase

---

[1] Simon, *Public Health Reports*, ii. 237; idem, Lecture XII, *Lancet*, 1850, ii. 228–32. Simon had tested the 'fermentability' of the blood with negative results.

[2] Simon, *Public Health Reports*, i. 113–14.

[3] Lambert, *John Simon*, pp.227, 230. *Scientific Enquiries Report*, p.46. Vibriones were organisms commonly associated with putrefaction. They aroused a fleeting interest in 1854 reminiscent of the cholera-fungus issue. Hassall himself and Hassall's biographer later made claims for these organisms at the expense of the Bristol investigators: Clayton, *Memoir of Hassall*, pp.6–10. See also De, *Cholera: its Pathology and Pathogenesis*, p.15. All conclusions in 1854–5 were against the vibriones' having any specific relation to cholera.

[4] *Report on the Last Two Cholera Epidemics by the Medical Officer*, pp.14–15.

Simon's reputation.[1] In conception, the two investigations were identical, but they are not strictly comparable because of differences in scale and sources.[2] Simon arrived at a ratio for mortality among those supplied by the two water companies of 3:1 for the epidemic period 1853 to 1854; Snow's figure for the epidemic as a whole was 6:1.[3] The higher the ratio the less the likelihood of causes other than the water being involved; but although Snow implied as much, acceptance of his result would not have hastened acceptance of the specific terms of his theory. His contemporaries would still have had no motive for accepting his specific version of pollution. It did not exceed their views in explaining power, required them to follow exactly the same practical procedures, and entailed what to them were improbabilities, such as a drastic variation in the effects of measures, including filtration, carried out by both companies for the purification of their supplies. Parkes also criticized Snow's test for sodium chloride, which he used to distinguish one supply from another. For Simon, there was also counter-evidence: the negative results obtained by Pettenkofer in a large-scale inquiry into the influence of water supply on the Munich cholera.

Simon considered that the positive value of the results of what he as well as Snow thought of as a 'grand experiment', was beyond dispute; the statistics obtained constituted 'the final solution of any existing uncertainty as to the dangerousness of putrefiable drinking water during visitations of epidemic cholera'. This solution clearly could not have been arrived at by any other means (for example analysis). The limits of the inquiry were equally clear; it was aimed 'only at giving a more exact knowledge of one cause'.[4]

---

[1] Lambert, *John Simon*, p.249. For [Richardson's] protest at the neglect of Snow, see *J. Publ. Hlth Sanit. Rev.* 2 (1856), 192. Snow himself protested to the *British Medical Journal*: see *Br. Med. J.* 1857, ii. 864.

[2] This is Frost's comment. He is however prepared to give Snow's figures the edge: *Snow on Cholera*, p.184.

[3] Snow, 'Cholera, and the Water Supply in the South Districts of London', *Br. Med. J.* 1857, ii. 864. In another paper, 'Cholera and the Water Supply in the South Districts of London in 1854', Snow amended his earlier analysis using figures obtained for Simon 'by order' and only made available in the latter's report: ibid., p.248.

[4] Parkes, *Br. For. Med. Chir. Rev.* 15 (1855), 459–62; *Report on the Last Two Cholera Epidemics by the Medical Officer*, pp.11, 9, 14.

Simon was eventually convinced of the communicability of cholera not by any induction from effects, but by manipulation of an alleged agent — or, as he later put it, by the 'scientific' rather than the 'popular' experiment (that is, 'the experiments which accident does for us'). As an example of the popular experiment he gave (in 1881) 'that performed on half a million human beings in South London, by the commercial water companies'; as an example of the 'scientific', the experiments of Karl Thiersch.[1] In 1876, Simon justified Thiersch's work in these terms:

Till these experiments were performed in Germany, and had been repeated here, I may confess for myself that I did not consider it to be proved that cholera spread in that way. It had been suspected; it was a theory of cholera which began in 1849 in the teaching of John Snow; and that theory has been converted by experiments into such a degree of certainty, as can properly be held to justify the advice of a Government department.

Thiersch's experiments had been repeated at Simon's direction by John Burdon Sanderson in 1866, at which time Simon himself repeated and confirmed the experiments of Jean-Antoine Villemin on the communicability of tubercle.[2] They had, however, been carried out as early as 1854, and were considered by the Committee for Scientific Enquiries.[3] In accounting for this delay some weight has to be given to questions of opportunity and timing. Between 1855 and 1866 cholera was absent from England, and no material was available for experi-

---

[1] Simon, *Experiments on Life* (1881), in *Public Health Reports*, ii, 595. Karl Thiersch (1822-95), b. Munich, son of the philologist Friedrich Thiersch. Studied in Berlin, Vienna, Paris; Ph. D. Munich. Distinguished service as army surgeon (1850). Prosector at Munich Pathological Institute, 1848-54. Professor of surgery at Erlangen, 1854. Known for work on wounds, and on the pathology of cancer (1865). An 'earnest follower' of Listerian methods; see *Clinical Lectures . . . by various German Authors*, New Sydenham Society (London, 1877). Obituaries in English journals did not mention his work on cholera, which was doubtless by then overshadowed by his Listerism: *Lancet,* 1895, i. 1156; *Br. Med. J.* 1895, i. 1360.

[2] Simon, evidence to Vivisection Commission, PP, 1876, XLI. 372. 'Report by Dr. J. Burdon Sanderson on the Experimental Communicability of Cholera', Appendix IX to *9th Rep. of Med. Officer of Privy Council*, PP, 1867, XXXVII. 434; Simon, 'Results of Inoculation with Tubercular Matter', *Trans. Path. Soc.* 18 (1867), 290-3. On Villemin (1827-92), see S.L. Cummins, *Tuberculosis in History* (1949), pp.133-46.

[3] Thiersch, *Infectionsversuche an Thieren mit dem Inhalte des Choleradarmes* (Munich, 1856). See also *Haupt-Berichtüber die Cholera Epidemie des Jahres 1854 im Bayern* (Munich, 1857). *Scientific Enquiries Report*, p.59.

ment. During that time Simon, as Medical Officer, conducted a series of inquiries of the 'popular experiment' variety, collectively entitled 'The distribution of disease in England, and the circumstances by which it is regulated'. In 1865, he told the Lords of the Privy Council (and the taxpayer) that 'enquiries of the same type would only extend, not really strengthen for practical purposes, the evidence already at hand'. Further progress required 'improved methods of aetiological observation'; and 'scientific researches must first have created a far more intimate knowledge than is yet current as to the nature of the morbid processes which are to be prevented, and as to the physical and chemical conditions of their development'. Very likely Simon had had it in mind to institute such researches, especially those of a chemical nature, well before 1865; he had been, after all, primarily interested in pathology. At the later date, however, as well as having completed the survey already mentioned, he had the advantage of the precedent just established by the commissioners of inquiry into the cattle plague, who, in response to the clamour of threatened interests, had ordered government-financed research on a scale never before seen.[1]

Apart from these more contingent circumstances, it is possible that Simon was inspired to repeat Thiersch's experiments in particular, by Villemin's recent successful experiments on animals, and by Sanderson's work on cattle plague, which showed 'for the first time' that disease could be artificially induced in an animal, and its blood used to produce the same effect in another.[2] It would appear, however, from earlier favourable references, that Simon did not need this encouragement. The reactions of the Committee in 1855, and Simon's subsequent caution, must be referred to the different ways in which the experiments could be interpreted.

Until about 1860, experiments on the communicability of

---

[1] Lambert, *John Simon*, pp.331 ff.; Simon, *Public Health Reports*, ii. 216, 217.

[2] *Third Report of Royal Commission on the Cattle Plague*, PP, 1866, XXII. 324. The blood of affected subjects had been used in inoculation experiments by a number of previous investigators. See e.g. Holland, *Medical Notes*, pp.70–1, 602; Henle, *Miasms and Contagions*, pp.918–19. These mainly involved human diseases.

disease were few and poor.[1] The only disease of man to have associated with it a persistent tradition of experimentation was smallpox. The relation established between smallpox and cowpox at the end of the eighteenth century was naturally a source of inspiration, and encouraged some experimentation on lower animals and on other, apparently similar diseases (such as glanders of the horse). Much of this was carried out by one man, Robert Ceely of Aylesbury.[2] Ceely, a prominent medical reformer and member of the Provincial Medical and Surgical Association, was praised for his experimental work, but not emulated by his contemporaries. As a reformer, he took a particular interest in the medical services planned for the new Poor Law, and in campaigns for the eradication of smallpox, in both of which State-run endeavours professional interests were thought to be at stake. He later worked for Simon as one of the Privy Council Medical Department's 'inspectors', or advisers, on cattle diseases and vaccination. Ceely (among English experimenters) demonstrated, in Farr's terms, that 'varioline' was converted to 'vaccinine' in the cow; that is, that the poisons of smallpox and cowpox were modifications of one another, as originally claimed by Jenner. Because of the long-continued practices of inoculation and vaccination, even human subjects could be used in experiments of this type. Hopes were held out for the influence of cowpox vaccine on diseases other than smallpox, and these were sometimes put to the test. Because it was known that a person who had not had smallpox or cowpox almost invariably developed it if exposed to it, experiments could be devised to determine the effects on the poison of heat, dilution or 'disinfection'. Such experiments were carried out by George Fordyce (who had been a pupil of Hunter), by Faraday (for the Central Board of Health of 1832), and by William Henry, but they were very few in number; Henry's, in particular,

---

[1] Some history of this form of experimentation is given by J. Burdon Sanderson (Appendix to *9th Rep. of Med. Officer of Privy Council*, pp.434 ff.), by Lauder Lindsay ('Clinical Notes on Cholera', pp.1111 ff.) and by Hirsch (*Handbook of Geographical Pathology*, i. 476 ff.).

[2] For Ceely (1797–1880), M.R.C.S. 1819, F.R.C.S. 1843, L.S.A. 1849, see *Plarr*.

were universally depended upon, rather than followed up by other experimenters.[1]

Obviously, if the impulse to experiment existed at all, one would expect most rapid progress in respect of diseases which were also epizootics, and the case of anthrax fulfils these expectations.[2] In England, however, the diseases of lower animals appear to have attracted very little scientific interest, and there was as little exchange between farmers and others with direct experience of animal diseases, and persons who might be interested in veterinary medicine for its own sake or as a source of analogy. Comparative studies were therefore few. The investigation of epizootics did not appear in the inaugural programme of the Provincial Medical and Surgical Association, except as a part of medical topography, an order of priorities which may be contrasted with that of the Epidemiological Society, founded eighteen years later in 1850. A Veterinary Department of the Privy Council was nominally established after the cattle plague of 1865; other institutions concerned with veterinary medicine grew or reformed themselves with even greater slowness.[3]

In the case of cholera, the first epidemic left a legacy of some scattered observations of effects on animals, and the negative results of some heroic experiments, chiefly those performed on themselves by French medical men in Warsaw.[4]

[1] See Williams, *Morbid Poisons*, i. 13. Henry published his results in the *Philosophical Magazine* in 1831 and 1832; see also his 'Report on the State of our Knowledge of the Laws of Contagion', *Rep. of 4th Meeting of British Association* (1835), pp. 67–94. Henry's experiments were less forgotten, than allowed to stagnate; they were mentioned (e.g.) by Michael Ryan (1836), by Holland (1839, 1840, 1855), by Thomas Graham (1842), by Thomas Watson (1843), by Farr (1843), and by Snow (1851). A 'committee' at York extended the experiments in the 1860s, as did William Budd: Budd, 'Investigation of Epidemic and Epizootic Diseases', *Br. Med. J.* 1864, ii. 356.

[2] See the work of Rayer (1850), Casimir Davaine (1812–82), and others, including Budd, Pasteur, and Koch: Bulloch, *History of Bacteriology*. For Davaine, see *DSB*.

[3] Budd, 'Variola Ovina, Sheep's Smallpox', *Br. Med. J.* 1863, ii. 142 and note. The chief obstacles to development were institutional and social: see F. Smith, *The Early History of Veterinary Literature* (1919-33). The earliest British attempt at a comprehensive survey of epizootic epidemics was probably G. Fleming, *Animal Plagues* (1871–82). See also idem, *Manual of Veterinary Sanitary Science* (1875).

[4] *Lancet*, 1830-1, ii. 422; Ackerknecht, 'Anticontagionism 1821-1867', pp.567-8. In most cases there was no definite result.

These latter were long remembered, in spite of some recognition of their defects; they were, for example, quoted against the cholera-fungus theory and against Snow. Snow himself felt obliged to account for the results of these experiments, seeing them as offering the only 'material opposition' to his theories. Baly and Parkes, in particular, criticized Snow for 'giving no facts to prove that the evacuations have the power he attributes to them'. Obviously the onus was on Snow to provide these facts, and it is not surprising that Baly and Parkes were content to rest their criticism on rather meagre negative findings, especially since cholera showed few signs of being contagious in 'natural' situations, such as the dissecting room. Nevertheless, the lack of experimental activity on the part of Snow's compatriots is rather striking.[1] John Marshall of London, and William Lauder Lindsay of Edinburgh, produced perhaps the only sustained work of this kind, and their experiments may serve as a contrast to those of Thiersch.

Marshall's experiments were performed in 1849, and he used mainly dogs.[2] The number of his experiments was unusually large; many other studies involved single animals, especially in the case of dogs and cats. In seven cases, Marshall injected diluted 'defibrinized' blood from patients who had died in the collapse stage of cholera. In six further cases, he used defibrinized blood from living patients; in five he injected massive amounts of filtered choleraic discharges; and in nine, considerable quantities of alvine liquid were introduced into the stomach. The third of these series was described by John Burdon Sanderson as 'the only exact experiments' involving the injection of alvine liquid.[3] The over-all results, Marshall thought, were 'not unfavourable to the notion of a certain susceptibility in the dog and perhaps in the cat'. However, he

---

[1] *Lancet*, 1830-1, ii. 422; *The Times*, 5 Oct. 1849, *Lancet*, 1849, ii. 433. Snow, 'On the Pathology and Mode of Communication of Cholera' (1849), pp.927-8; in 1855 Snow gave another possible explanation for a similarly negative (accidental) experiment: *Snow on Cholera*, pp.111-12. Baly and Gull, *Reports on Epidemic Cholera*, p.121; Parkes, *Manual of Practical Hygiene*, p.57. John Marshall gave some reasons why, in the prevailing climate, communicability experiments might be thought useless by each shade of opinion: 'Communicability of Cholera to Animals', p.391.

[2] 'Communicability of Cholera', pp.398 ff. Marshall knew of much of the continental work and this account presented his own experiments comparatively.

[3] Sanderson, Appendix to *9th Rep. of Med. Officer of Privy Council*, p.435.

attributed the 'state of indisposition' induced in the first series to the blood's being 'charged with the products of its own decomposition', and thought that more experiments of the second type should be made, using large quantities of blood taken from patients in all stages of the disease. The results of the third series led him to find it 'abundantly proved' that the evacuations contained some 'deleterious agent', but not that this agent was specific. He did not think that either the *flocculi* or the inorganic constituents of the evacuations were responsible. To determine the latter point he had, in a manner reminiscent of his proceedings in 1849, 'imitated' the inorganic constituents, and injected them, with no results. Marshall's conclusions were honest, but it is not surprising that at the time they were quoted in some quarters as for communicability, and as against it in others.[1] Lauder Lindsay praised Marshall's experiments highly, stating at the end of a comparative account that Marshall had 'not only repeated many of the experiments of continental observers', but had 'varied them in accordance with improved views in zoochemistry, pathology, histology, etc., arising from modern discoveries in science'. In general, like Parkes, Marshall found it 'impossible to rid oneself of the conviction that cholera has some definite agent self-itinerant or conveyed, as its constant effective cause'; the conclusions reached in his much praised report on the Broad Street epidemic were also representative, in that he held water supply to have been perhaps the most important factor, without deciding on its mode of operation. [2]

William Lauder Lindsay obtained the highest honours in the course of his medical studies, but is remembered primarily as a botanist.[3] Among his numerous publications the most impressive were those on lichens and his last work, *Mind in the Lower Animals in Health and Disease* (1879), in which he argued for the proximity of lower animals and man. During

---

[1] See e.g. J.W. Begbie, *Edinb. Med. Surg. J.* 82 (1855), 90; Baly and Gull, *Reports on Epidemic Cholera*, p.121.

[2] Lindsay, 'Clinical Notes on Cholera', p.1114; Marshall, 'Communicability of Cholera to Animals', p.391; [idem *et al.*], *Report on Cholera in St. James*, pp.81 ff., 91.

[3] For Lauder Lindsay (1829–80), b. and educated Edinburgh, M.D. Edinburgh 1852, Medical Officer to Murray's Royal Institution for the Insane at Perth, see *DNB*.

the third cholera epidemic, he acted as resident physician of the City Cholera Hospital in Edinburgh. In 1854, he published a comprehensive survey of all aspects of cholera, with a view to defining subjects for future research. Among the subjects he thought 'specially worthy of research' were the 'epidemic diseases of plants' and 'epizootic diseases of the lower animals'. In the course of his survey he gave details of a wide range of continental (especially Italian) 'transmissibility experiments', and while not thinking highly of these, lamented the inactivity of the English. No positive conclusion could, he thought, be extracted from the experiments done anywhere so far. While pointing to many sources of error which the modern reader might appreciate, Lauder Lindsay also considered the failure of these experiments to have been owing to the 'non-production of a sufficient predisposition' and 'inaccurate imitation of the whole conditions in which the human subject is placed prior to and during his seizure'. In his own experiments, his subjects (seven dogs and a cat) were confined for periods 'varying from a few days to nearly two months' in a damp close room, and fed on the evacuations of living cholera patients and on the blood and viscera removed after death in various stages of the disease. The only result was a non-specific diarrhoea, until the animals were exposed to the 'concentrated virus of cholera' in the shape of effluvia from the bodies of patients as collected on their bodies or bedclothes; then, because the animals were predisposed, they were attacked with 'symptoms and pathological appearances exactly resembling those met with in man'. Two of the dogs died.[1] In general, these were accepted as positive results by Lindsay's contemporaries, and his experiments noted for the prominence they gave to airborne effluvia.[2] In their inclusiveness of alleged factors they correspond in method to the approach of Snow's critics, and demonstrate that this methodology was operative on what would now be called the experimental level, rather than being merely a function of a lack of experimentation itself.

The unusual feature of Karl Thiersch's experiments was their particularity, just as the unusual feature of Simon and

---

[1] Lindsay, 'Clinical Notes on Cholera', pp.1110, 1113 ff., 837.
[2] See e.g. Richardson, *J. Publ. Hlth San. Rev.* 1 (1855), 133; Parkes, *Br. For. Med. Chir. Rev.* 15 (1855), 463.

Sanderson's repetitions of the same experiments was that they observed Thiersch's conditions in every detail, even to the coat colour of the subjects.[1] Thiersch chose mice, because of the resemblance of their alimentary system and eating habits to those of man; secondly, he administered very small quantities of substance, because only then would the mode of infection be comparable with that occurring in man (in this his experiments were unique); thirdly, he concentrated on a single (and that the least disturbing) mode of entry, that is, ingestion; fourthly, he used a large number of animals (110, on which were performed fifty-five experiments). His method was to allow fresh intestinal liquid to decompose spontaneously in the presence of air, to steep in this liquid at the end of each day strips of filter paper, which were weighed before and after steeping and drying to determine the quantity of solid matter taken up; and to give each of these different kinds of paper to a pair of mice on four consecutive days.[2] Thiersch found that papers steeped in fresh discharges gave no result; that of fifty-six mice fed 'middle-aged' discharges, forty-four were 'more or less disordered' and fourteen died; and that papers steeped in liquids still more advanced in decomposition again had no effect. He concluded:

That in spontaneous decomposition of the intestinal liquid in cholera, a substance is formed in from two to six days which is possessed of specific activity. That this substance is not volatile, and has the property, when introduced even in the smallest quantity into the alimentary canal of animals, of inducing a disease which agrees with cholera in the character of the alvine discharges and in the spasmodic affection of the muscular system . . .

Sanderson obtained similar results, the 'liability to attack' being greatest with papers steeped in liquids three to four days old. He further improved on Thiersch by using, with the same results, liquids obtained from animals which had been 'infected' during earlier experiments. B.W. Richardson was possibly the only English writer before Sanderson to experiment according to this postulate of Koch (and Henle). Richardson, of course, thought his agent was purely chemical.[3]

---

[1] For criticism by Simon of other repetitions see his Note to Sanderson's Appendix to *9th Rep. of Med. Officer of Privy Council*, pp.458 ff.

[2] Ibid., pp.438 ff. Sanderson improved on this method by also steeping the papers in bacon fat, to ensure that the mice ate them.

[3] Ibid., pp.439, 452; Richardson, *On the Poisons of Spreading Diseases* (1867).

Thiersch had carried out his studies as one of the commissioners for scientific researches appointed by the government of Bavaria, and his account of them was not translated. It was, however, publicized, but in a context different from that we have been considering. The agent involved was Liebig. It seemed to him that the work both of Thiersch, and of his own pupil Pettenkofer, supported his views on the role of fermentative processes in the production of disease poisons. He sent an open letter to this effect to Hofmann, and followed it up with an account of an official discussion held in Munich on the subject of cholera, in which both Thiersch and Pettenkofer (but not Liebig himself) took part. Liebig naturally stressed the process taking place in the evacuations (which he and Thiersch both regarded as nitrogenous matters transuded from the blood) outside the body under the influence of oxygen and a certain degree of temperature. It was left to the reader to decide when specificity entered in. Liebig stated, in conclusion, that 'the blood-producing substances, in the condition of their normal metamorphoses, are essential to nutrition and health. The same substances and their products, in a state of abnormal decomposition, give rise in the healthy organism to disease and death.'[1]

Although there is little doubt that he was active in discussion, it does not appear that Liebig published anything on cholera, or that he conducted experiments like Thiersch's. They were sometimes attributed to him, for example by the Report of the Committee for Scientific Enquiries. In 1849, during the second epidemic, he was ill; in 1854, during the severe epidemic in Munich, he was ill again, this time (in his own opinion) with cholera. On recovery, probably just after writing to Hofmann, he wrote also to his friend Wöhler, mentioning the relation of the 'merkwurdigen Entdeckungen' of Thiersch and Pettenkofer to his own views:

Other things have surprised me more, than that my theory of contagion should triumph on this occasion, as I was wholly convinced that these diseases are generated and propagated by means of a kind of ferment.

---

[1] J. Leibig (and A.W. Hofmann), 'Etiology of Cholera', *Med. Times Gaz.* 1854, ii. 515; 'Munich: Discussion on Cholera', ibid., pp. 550–1. See also ibid., p.575.

It is nonetheless particularly gratifying, when one has participated in the emergence of a doctrine.[1]

Liebig's open letter to Hofmann may have been written with the Committee for Scientific Enquiries in mind. It began by suggesting that Sir James Clark as well as Hofmann might be interested in its contents; Clark, being a close and influential friend of both Liebig and Hofmann, would possibly have been approached in any case, but he was also at this time a member of the Medical Council's Foreign Correspondence Committee. Hofmann sent the letter to Clark, and received the following reply:

I have read the paper on cholera . . . I must say that I scarcely think it fit for the *Times*. The conclusions of Pettenkofer are well known, and have been acted on in this country for a *long time*, and their only use would be to add confirmation to the views entertained in this country — the antiseptics recommended are also used here — the only new part of the paper is contained in the observations of Thiersch, and they are on a limited scale — still they are interesting and may lead to some useful results, if the experiments on animals were further prosecuted — my advice would be to give the paper to one of our medical weekly journals, the *Medical Times*, and from that it could be transferred to the *Times*. I am jealous of any thing appearing in the papers from Leibig [*sic*], which is not of real importance, as all his writings are sure to attract much attention and remark.[2]

This letter is interesting as an indication not only of the view taken of the work of the 'Munich chemists', and the role played by Clark, but also of the different values placed on the lay and medical press on such occasions. These recall the action taken by some of the participants in the cholera-fungus controversy. The letter further implies that Liebig showed some discernment in directing his views as much at the laity as at the medical profession. The more detailed and technical 'account of discussions' was always intended by Liebig for the *Medical Times and Gazette*.

The achievement of the 1850s was to narrow down Chadwick's large indictment of all filth to one kind in particular: that produced by human beings. A reviewer of 1857

---

[1] *Scientific Enquiries Report*, p.59. *Aus J. Liebigs und F. Wöhlers Briefwechsel* (1888), ii. 20–1: 31 Oct. 1854.

[2] Munich, Bayerische Staatsbibliothek, Liebigiana 58 (Clark): J. Clark to A.W. Hofmann, 2 Nov. 1854. I am grateful to the Director of the Staatsbibliothek for a copy of this letter and for permission to quote from it.

found some reference to faecal impurity to be the common factor in a list of works that incorporated the report of the Committee for Scientific Enquiries, various of Simon's reports including that of 1856, Henry Acland's report on Oxford, the *Report on the Cholera Outbreak in the Parish of St. James's, Westminster* (Marshall's official account of Snow's Broad Street epidemic), and Pettenkofer's work of 1855.[1] Presumed local causes were first reduced by the reviewer to 'impure water, lowness of site, and the emanations arising from the decomposition of animal refuse'; and he eventually found his view confirmed, that 'an atmosphere impregnated with the products of fermenting excrement is at once the most obvious and most constant concomitant of cholera'. There was no proof, he added, of the poisonous character of *fresh* cholera evacuations. Earlier, the reviewer described Thiersch and Pettenkofer as borrowing and then 'essentially modifying' the ideas of Snow, and defended Snow's priority while expressing disbelief in his ideas.[2]

Because of the emphasis on faecal impurity, most writers found no difficulty in circumventing the notion either that Thiersch's experiments proved the communicability of cholera person to person, or that these experiments in any way enforced the theories of Snow. The Committee for Scientific Enquiries dealt with the German claims rather than with other communicability experiments because it was specifically considering Snow, and the German experiments had like Snow's theory pointed to a certain class of 'ingesta'. The Committee gave as its opinion that there were insufficient grounds for believing that the lower animals were susceptible to cholera, and that any indisposition in the subjects of such experiments showed that the discharges were noxious because they were putrescent. It reported that Thomson had experimented in a similar manner with negative (but to Thomson, inconclusive) results. Thomson had been forced

---

[1] Acland, *Memoir on the Cholera in Oxford* (1856). Pettenkofer's work — *Untersuchungen und Beobachtungen über die Verbreitungsart der Cholera* (Munich, 1855) — was not translated, but, although Pettenkofer was always more aware of the English than they were of him, his theories did become well known in England.

[2] *Br. For. Med. Chir. Rev.* 19 (1857), 84, 68. My italics.

to obtain cholera fluid outside London. Residues were fed to a single mouse which had already been the subject of experiment.[1]

Snow himself did not regard Thiersch's experiments as providing support for his own views. His conclusion, with reference to Thiersch's opinion that 'cholera evacuations are not at first capable of generating the disease', was, not surprisingly, the same as that of the Committee, although he thought it 'not contrary to all analogy that some change or development should take place in the cholera poison in the interval between its leaving one person and entering another'. He may have been thinking here of the different phases in the life-cycles of parasites and other organisms, the scattered, but increasing, knowledge of which had been gathered together by Steenstrup in 1842 under the heading 'alternation of generations', and used by Owen in his *On Parthenogenesis*. Later, Snow referred to 'the opinion of Drs. Thiersch and Pettenkofer, that some kind of change or fermentation is necessary in the peculiar excretions of cholera to enable them to propagate the disease', and stated that 'this is a modification of my original views which I, however, see no reason to adopt'. Snow's primary concern here was to distinguish himself from Budd.[2]

Simon's first independent reference to Thiersch's experiments shows both proximity to and distance from Snow's theories. Writing in 1857 of the preventability of certain kinds of diseases, he referred particularly to 'diseases of which it is no metaphor to say, they consist in the extension of the putrefactive process from matters outside to matters inside

---

[1] *Scientific Enquiries Report*, pp.59, 497 ff. 'A disease simulating cholera may be reproduced in guinea pigs and newborn rabbits by certain experimental procedures . . . The cholera vibrio when given by mouth, or injected *per rectum*, is harmless to mice, rabbits, guinea pigs and monkeys . . . Intraperitoneal injection of mice is fatal in 24 to 48 hours': G.S. Wilson and A.A. Miles (eds.), *Topley and Wilson's Principles of Bacteriology and Immunity*, 2 vols. (1964), i. 656. The 'animal models' most widely used at the present time are newborn rabbits; the ligated intestinal loop of young adult rabbits; and young adult dogs. Dogs, which meet the need for a larger 'model', have only been used since 1966. With modern techniques, *c.* 40 per cent develop choleraic disease; another 30 per cent develop diarrhoea: Barua and Burrows, *Cholera*, Ch. 9.

[2] *Snow on Cholera*, p.112; Snow, 'The Mode of Propagation of Cholera', *Ass. Med. J.* 4 (1856), 135.

the body: diseases of which the very essence is filth'. Cholera, diarrhoea, and dysentery constituted one such group. The mucous membrane or lining of the alimentary canal 'is the excreting surface to which nature directs all accidental putridities which enter us ... There as their universal result they tend to produce diarrhoea — simple diarrhoea, in the absence of specific infections; specific diarrhoea, when the ferments of cholera and typhoid are in operation.' In a note, Simon gave his summary of the 'peculiar [i.e. idiosyncratic] doctrine' of Snow, and applauded the practical results of its appearance before the public. In the same place he referred to the 'interesting and important' experiments of Professor Thiersch, and related these to the work of Acland and of Pettenkofer, both of whom had evolved notably mulitfactoral theories of cholera. He then concluded:

It is encouraging to sanitary reformers to observe that cases of apparent introduction of cholera contagion by human intercourse are essentially different from such cases of infection as are presented by measles or smallpox. The multiplication of poison in the latter diseases takes place exclusively within the human body; it has no immediate dependence on differences of medium; and wherever human beings can cross each other's path, the susceptible person may contract the infection ... for diffusing the contagium of cholera, if truly the disease be contagious, foulness of medium seems indispensable. Indeed it is no ordinary foulness which taints air or food or water with the leaven of decaying excrement. Therefore as regards cholera it seems highly probable that the immigration of infected persons might occur to any extent without exciting epidemic outbreaks, if it occurred only in places of irreproachable sanitary conditions, especially as regards the supply of water and continuous removal of house refuse.[1]

In many ways, Simon's views in 1866 were not different from these, because he never entirely accepted the exclusiveness of Snow's position. The repetition of communicability experiments other than Thiersch's led to similarly positive, but not 'exclusive', results.[2] The 'wandering ferment', however, was dispensed with, possibly under the added influence of Budd's

---

[1] Simon, Introduction to Greenhow, *Sanitary Papers*, PP, 1857–8, XXIII. 277, 281.

[2] This is deplored with respect to Villemin by Cummins, *Tuberculosis in History*, pp.139–40, but not placed in the context of contemporary interest in the phenomena of irritation, inflammation, and putrefaction, and in diseases as ultimately 'idiopathic'. This interest was clearly reflected in other work carried out under Simon by Sanderson.

views on typhoid. The communicability of cholera was accepted with less reserve, although it is still obvious that to accept this was not equivalent to accepting Snow's theory. In general, these changes may be seen as an approach towards Snow's view of cholera as analogous to smallpox, although, as we shall see, Snow's use of this analogy was less consistent than that of Budd.

7

THE SMALLPOX ANALOGY:
WILLIAM BUDD

I

Budd's use of the smallpox analogy is definitive of his theories of disease, and of the means he used to support them. This analogy, as he said, had for him as much force as a law; and he defined progress in the epidemiological field as the rate at which 'non-infectious diseases were transferred to the group typified by smallpox'.[1] In his argument, the smallpox analogy replaced reference to such exemplars as fermentation and muscardine and allowed him to limit severely his discussion both of the nature of the agent and of the disease process. This is not, of course, the sum of his views. Where convenient he used other analogies, and no difference in kind can be made out between his theories and those of Grove, Cowdell, Henle, or Snow.

Continued fever, the subject of Budd's major work, was one of his earliest interests. Clinical experience in France in the late 1820s and early 1830s convinced him that there was a disease characterized by an ulcerated condition of the alimentary canal, and that these ulcers corresponded to the crop of vesicles which appeared on the skin in smallpox. Thus, the alvine discharges of typhoid constituted the peculiar product of that disease, and it was some minute portion of this product which brought about the same disease in another person. The circumstances of epidemics which took place in confined localities, rather than the epidemiology of towns, persuaded Budd that typhoid was only less contagious than smallpox because of the manner in which the poison left the body and was affected by the contingencies of the environment.

---

[1] Budd, 'Government and the Prevention of Infectious Disease', *Trans. Nat. Ass. Soc. Sci.* 1869, p.387.

The picture which Budd built up of typhoid allowed him to apply the smallpox analogy wholeheartedly to cholera. Cholera did not obviously resemble smallpox, either in its pathology or its mode of distribution; typhoid, as Budd saw it, provided a rational link between them. In typhoid, the poison entered the bloodstream, and having increased was cast out of the body by exanthematous structures in the lining of the alimentary canal. Budd agreed with Snow that in cholera the blood was affected only by the loss of its constituents, and he placed no stress upon the equivocal 'desquamation' of the lining of the canal, which to some observers involved a shedding of epithelial cells. He might have claimed, as Spooner did, that this effect was analogous to the lesions in the gut in typhoid and thus to the pustules of smallpox.[1] On the other hand, the most characteristic product in cholera was, as in typhoid, the discharge from the bowels, and the behaviour of the two diseases in the field was much the same. They were regarded by Budd's contemporaries as related diseases, once typhoid had been defined as a condition in its own right.

In Budd's published work the smallpox analogy was deployed largely to prove an already developed case, and the arguments which he based upon it tend in sum to be self-supporting if not circular. However, something of the way in which he must have pursued the analogy in the first instance can be detected in his brief discussions of such diseases as yellow fever and diphtheria, which he progressively added to the smallpox family. Budd was convinced from a very early period that most if not all epidemic diseases would be found to belong to this group. The first consideration was if the disease appeared, *under ideal conditions*, to be contagious; and the second (which in part dictated the terms of those conditions), was if the disease resulted in the excretion of a specific product. If it did, it followed that the agent, whatever its nature, was contained in this discharge, and that the disease could be expected to show in the field a degree of ease of propagation deducible from the mode in which the

---

[1] Baly and Gull, *Reports on Epidemic Cholera*, p.118; E.O. Spooner, 'Contagion of Asiatic Cholera', *Prov. Med. Surg. J.* 13 (1849), 36–7.

discharge left the body. Collateral points were, whether there was a latent period between exposure to a source of infection and the appearance of the disease; whether immunity was conferred following one attack; and whether in a community there were persons exposed to the poison who did not take the disease. These points could be established independently, by the 'objective' statistical methods favoured by Budd's contemporaries; once established, they proved to Budd the 'position and natural affinities, as well as the true pathology' of the disease to which they belonged.[1] There was, of course, the largest possible basis (to Budd, an 'experimental' basis) for taking these factors to be characteristic of smallpox.

In an address on method delivered in 1863, Budd gave as one cause of the slow rate of progress in epidemiology an 'exaggerated estimate of the difficulties of the subject', and stated that 'the problem of the epidemiologist has in it at least one element of simplicity which is denied to the student of other disease; namely, that its chief concern is with the history of a single cause'.[2] This confident single-factor approach may be traced directly to the analogy with smallpox. On that basis, the existence of 'specific and definite' agents was assumed; all else was secondary. What had to be known was where and how the 'specific causative poisons' bred and multiplied. To this power of multiplication were attributable not only the diseased condition of the patient, but also the rise and spread of epidemics. It was clear that even a short sequence of victims would produce a vast quantity of infective matter; enough to induce the disease in whole populations.[3] The rise and fall of epidemics was for Budd regulated by the susceptibility of the population, and by contingent circumstances affecting the mode of propagation of the disease. The extension of the disease was facilitated, and often made to appear mysterious, by the ability of the poison to remain dormant in a dried state. Budd also argued from such incidents as the introduction of smallpox into the countries of

---

[1] Budd, 'On the Contagion of Yellow Fever', *Lancet*, 1861, i. 337–8; idem, 'Diphtheria', *Br. Med. J.* 1861, i. 575–9; idem, 'On Intestinal Fever' (1859), p.55; idem, *Typhoid Fever*, p.34.

[2] Budd, 'Variola Ovina, Sheep's Smallpox', p.141.

[3] For an actual 'calculation', see *Typhoid Fever*, pp.51–3.

the New World, stating that since all conditions other than the importation of smallpox poison had existed previously without their being able to produce the disease, then the relation between importation and outbreak must be that of cause and effect. It is, perhaps, important here to stress that modern bacteriology has returned to a multifactoral approach.[1]

According to Budd, things 'like each other and like nothing else' must be related, and the relation between diseases was at least analogous to that subsisting between groups and between individuals in natural-history classifications. What the investigator of an epidemic disease had to determine, therefore, was 'the biography of a single species'. The differences between diseases were truly specific, since diseases could not 'interbreed', nor could (for example) a case of smallpox give rise to one of measles. Generation of one thing by another was the 'highest proof of specific identity that can be had'.[2] Budd invoked various 'natural laws', but the most ubiquitous was the great 'law of continuous succession'. The 'analogy of living types' also told what were the 'invariable characteristics' attached to the dissemination of entities known to be propagated according to the law of succession. The geographical distribution and spread of diseases was similar to that of animals and plants.[3] As we shall see, Budd drew heavily on this 'analogy of living types' when dealing with the problem of spontaneous generation.

The types which were of most use to him were the animal parasites, especially the more highly developed forms.[4] Budd referred to this group as early as 1841, when he defined 'cancer cells' as parasitic growths on the grounds that they nourished themselves at the expense of the body, but were otherwise independent of it; and compared (in order to discount) the difficulties in the way of the supposition that

---

[1] See e.g. criticism of Budd by E.W. Goodall, 'Budd, A Forgotten Epidemiologist', *Proc. R. Soc. Med.* 25 (1931–2), 277–94: 289.

[2] Budd, 'Remarks on Cancer', *Lancet*, 1841–2, ii. 270.

[3] Here Budd cited Holland, and referred to Charles Darwin: 'Observations on Typhoid', p.605; p.626 n.

[4] See W.D. Foster, *A History of Parasitology* (Edinburgh and London, 1965); R.J.C. Hoeppli, *Parasites and Parasitic Infections in Early Medicine and Science* (Singapore, 1959).

the cancer germs came from without, with the difficulties in accounting for the origin of 'true [obligate] parasitic animals'. In 1849, he expressed his belief in the specificity of cholera in terms of the extreme specialization shown by some parasites, and though referring generally to the 'enormous chemical power' of plant life, ascribed the whole effect on the body in cholera to the fungal parasite's appropriation of the perfected juices of the blood. The animal parasites of the gut, in particular, resembled cholera in their mode of propagation, their fecundity, and the minuteness of their 'germs'. Some years later, in 1862, Budd recommended that the investigation of epidemic and epizootic diseases be associated with that of the diseases caused in man by living parasites, giving as his reasons firstly that 'at many points, the [parasites and the contagions] blend insensibly one into the other'; and secondly, 'that with the advance of knowledge, diseases are constantly being transferred from the group of common contagions, to the group of parasites'; and thirdly, that 'there already exists among the most advanced thinkers . . . a shrewd suspicion that the two groups will eventually coalesce, and be found to be in their essence, identical'. Elsewhere he speculated on the existence of 'whole tribes' of parasitic morbific principles, constituting an order to themselves, and being 'in their mode of growth and perpetuation, in their likenesses and differences . . . the exact reflex of the organic types that people the world without and on whose substance they prey'.[1] It is in such connections that Budd referred to Charles Darwin.

Because of its geology, and the polyglot population of its port, Bristol offered special advantages to those interested in questions of classification and descent. Two Bristolians known to Budd and prominent in the field were J.C. Prichard, and John Beddoe, a foundation member of the Ethnological Society (1857) and author of *The Races of Britain* (1887). J.A. Symonds, and David Davies (Medical Officer of Health for Bristol 1866–86, and a close friend of Budd and of Beddoe) both wrote (in 1869 and 1871 respectively) on the relation between evolutionary theory and epidemic disease,

---

[1] Budd, 'Remarks on Cancer', pp.269, 269; idem, *Malignant Cholera*, pp.9, 11; idem, 'Investigation of Epidemic and Epizootic Diseases', p.357; idem, 'Variola Ovina, Sheep's Smallpox', p.148.

presented by Davies as a 'somewhat bold idea'. Davies's son David Samuel Davies, who became Medical Officer of Health on his father's death, had similar interests. He thought that the evolutionary history of the parasites of man should illuminate the life histories of parasitic micro-organisms. Earlier, Symonds had referred to Darwinism as one of the current approaches towards 'that simplification of cause and unity of plan which has ever been the highest aim of philosophy'. At that time the merits of the 'great hypothesis' had yet to be decided upon.[1]

Budd was aware that Darwin's evolutionary theory at last promised (indirectly) an account of the origin and distribution of disease and of the phenomenon of obligate parasitism, but he was content to suggest this without committing himself to the theory or indeed placing much importance upon it.[2] This cautious interest may be contrasted with his attitude to the controversy over spontaneous generation. This is, of course, to speak only of Budd's opinion on each subject as he declared it in public. However, he had substantial reasons for being wary of Darwin's theory of evolution, since another of its tendencies was to give a new credibility to the doctrine of spontaneous generation. Medical men in general saw early the unifying power of Darwin's interpretation but, with obvious exceptions (for example Farr, W.B. Carpenter), left it to others to debate; later, when it was better established, they deployed it where this seemed appropriate.[3] Much of this interest naturally arose only with the conviction that disease was in some way caused by living matter; this led to a reaction

[1] Symonds, *Miscellanies* (1871), p.397; D. Davies, 'On the Origin of Species in Zymotic Diseases', *Bristol Naturalists' Society Procs*, 1871, p.4; D.S. Davies, 'Some Modern Aspects of Preventive Medicine', *Bristol Med.-Chir. J.* 18 (1900), 289; Symonds, *Ten Years* (1861).

[2] Budd, 'Observations on Typhoid', pp. 625 n., 626 n; reproduced in *Typhoid Fever*, though see in addition p.181. For a brief speculation on evolutionary lines, see Budd, 'Variola Ovina, Sheep's Smallpox', p.148. Darwin himself had not gone into the subject of parasitism: *On the Origin of Species* (1964), p.[500]. The evolution of parasites is still a matter for debate: see A.E.R. Taylor (ed.), *Evolution of Parasites* (Oxford, 1965).

[3] On some aspects of medicine and evolution see B. Towers, 'The Impact of Darwin's *Origin of Species* on Medicine and Biology', *Medicine and Science in the 1860s*, ed. F.N.L. Poynter (1968), pp.45–55. Ellegård's survey, *Darwin and the General Reader*, includes the *British Medical Journal* and *The Lancet*. T.H. Huxley gave some attention to the relation of Darwinism to the emergent germ theory;

in which the role of the environment was stressed as a factor in the evolution of organisms and in particular the determination of their pathogenic capabilities. Grounds were also found for an attack on the absolute specificity of disease, as well as for the origin of new diseases.[1]

Budd's views were not well adapted to demonstration by statistical or consensus methods, and Budd himself thought these methods very limited. It was part of his position that '*prima facie* evidence, which to the common eye seems irresistible, offers no guarantee that the conclusion on whose behalf it is cited may not be utterly false'. It was necessary, then, to experiment according to particular ideas. The analogy between smallpox and other diseases of man could furnish an argument, but it could not be put to experimental use. After 1860, Budd began to apply the smallpox analogy to diseases of the lower animals, using arguments similar to those already described: in particular, the contagiousness of these diseases and the specific appearances on the skin or gut. He saw sheep-pox, and pig typhoid and cattle plague, not as identical with smallpox and typhoid respectively, but as strictly analogous to these conditions. The differences were established by experiment, and confirmed his views on specificity. This form of the analogy was productive: through the diseases of the lower animals, 'all the questions that you wish to put to yourself may be decided experimentally'. In addition, animal populations provided ideal conditions for the study of disease in the field; in the case of an epidemic of sheep-pox, Budd demonstrated to his own satisfaction that all aspects of the phenomenon could ultimately be referred to a single infected sheep. It was also possible to demonstrate on the equivalent diseases of animals the means of prevention suggested by theory for human diseases.[2]

Darwin himself (though an admirer of Pasteur) appears to have left this to others: Darwin, *Life and Letters of Darwin* (1887), iii. 206, 234. In the context of his theory of pangenesis he adopted the contemporary habit of making use of the fixed nature of smallpox, and also used recent research by L.S. Beale and John Burdon Sanderson to support his own views: *The Variation of Animals and Plants Under Domestication* (1875), ii. 372–3.

[1] See e.g. J.T.C. Nash, *Evolution and Disease* (1915).

[2] Budd, 'Observations on Typhoid', p.457; idem, *Second Report of Royal Sanitary Commission*, PP, 1871, XXXV. 605; idem, 'Variola Ovina, Sheep's Smallpox', pp.143 ff., 147, 149.

Of the theorists dealt with in Chapter 5, Henle is most fittingly compared with Budd. As well as being interested in the subject, Budd was well read in German, and one cannot assume he never knew Henle's work in full. However, he did not refer to it, even in 1849, and mentioned its author only once, in connection with Schwann and some heat-experiments disproving spontaneous generation.[1] Both Budd and Henle made general theoretical statements, although it is important to notice that Henle was comprehensive in order to adjust and prove the fit of an explanation, whereas Budd covered a large area merely by asserting the universality of a small set of principles. In spite of the considerable differences in approach and in language, their theories were much alike. Both were conscious of the limits or limitations of direct evidence, although with Budd, as we saw in Chapter 5, this was in part a matter of learning by experience. Both saw disease not as 'intestine strivings between rival destructive and preservative tendencies supposed to be resident in the body itself', but as 'the reaction of living material against "abnormal external action"' or elements in the body's environment injurious to its welfare.[2] In this both differed from Liebig, although from the latter's account of contagions and miasms it might at first appear otherwise; and in their emphasis on specificity they differed from the Virchow school.[3] This specificity was clinically based, but none the less referable to the disease agent. 'Where the disease appears with such specific characteristics,' wrote Henle, 'we . . . have a right to consider its cause as something constant and unchangeable, as a distinct species.' Henle, like Budd, saw an analogy between diseases and living types. Both saw the relationship between diseases as referable to the relationship between their causes; and both took these causes to be 'endowed with individual life' and

---

[1] Budd, 'Observations on Typhoid', p.604 n.

[2] J.B.S., 'Henle', pp.vi-viii. The author was here referring specifically to the 'Romantic' school of pathology to which Henle opposed his 'rational' ideal: *Miasms and Contagions*, p.923.

[3] See G.A. Lindeboom, 'From the History of the Concept of Specificity', *Janus*, 46 (1957), 12-24:17-19; also E.H. Ackerknecht, *Rudolf Virchow* (Madison, 1953), p.107; W. Pagel, 'The Speculative Basis of Modern Pathology. Jahn, Virchow, and the Philosophy of Pathology', *Bull. Hist. Med.* 18 (1945), 1-43: 26 ff.

standing 'in the relation of a parasitic organism to the diseased body'.[1] Budd arrived at these views by considering the case of smallpox; Henle, ostensibly, by a process of elimination. In fact, he probably owed his convictions as much to the examples of fermentation and muscardine.

Henle, having surveyed all forms of propagation in disease, defined three disease types: the miasmatic, the miasmatico-contagious, and the fixed contagious. Budd took only one group, that typified by smallpox, and gradually increased its membership by including the doubtful diseases, typhoid and yellow fever, but also tuberculosis, cancer, and diphtheria. The characters of Budd's group most obviously resembled those of Henle's second type, but in some important respects those it shared with Henle's third type are more significant. The diseases of the third type (which Henle divided into two subtypes, typified by syphilis, a generalized disease, and cancer, a local) were 'not produced anew, but . . . rather always only transmitted from one body to another'. For Budd, this was true of all epidemic diseases, even if, as was *not* the case in the diseases of Henle's third group, the contagion was transmitted indirectly. Budd thought of his agents as independent, but as most closely resembling the obligate parasites. Henle also thought of his agents, at least in the case of the miasmatico-contagious diseases, as independent animals or plants, but he also thought that they must be capable of development and multiplication outside the body. This he assumed from there being not only single cases, but also single epidemics, of miasmatico-contagious diseases like influenza or cholera in which 'no contagious matter is formed, or in which contagious cases are at least exceptions'. Since some of these epidemics of 'low contagiosity' went on for some time, it could not be supposed that all cases arose merely as a result of the renewed activity of the infective material 'left over' from the last epidemic of the disease.[2]

There was also, for Henle, the fact that epidemic diseases often originated in the putrefaction of large quantities of

<hr>

[1] Henle, *Miasms and Contagions*, pp.962, 923.
[2] Ibid., pp.972, 957.

animal or vegetable matter.[1] Since he believed that all forms of putrefaction were brought about by infusoria or fungi, it was consistent with the rest of his argument to assume that some of these organisms could cause miasmatico-contagious disease. That Budd was entirely opposed to any such assumption is a point indicating not only the difference in first principles, but also, more particularly, Budd's comparative aloofness from the problems of contemporary mycology and protozoology. This point will be developed later, when Murchison's pythogenic theory is discussed. In relation to Henle, this difference can be referred to differences of opinion on the disease process. It should be noted that pathology was a part of the subject on which Budd had little to say. Apart from the few cardinal points, there are only isolated remarks: for example, Budd spoke of the inoculation of anthrax poison as setting up a 'series of malignant zymotic changes, which are propagated thence to the whole system'. Even this remark may only have referred to the process of putrefaction, since anthrax was a 'putrid' disease.[2] Henle, on the other hand, wrote as a pathologist and there is much in his theory of his particular views on fever and inflammation. For Budd, the agent's multiplication *was* the disease, and the typical rash or discharge, a kind of critical evacuation. Henle also saw the regular course of infectious disease as a reflection of the life history of the disease agent, but not exclusively as such. To him, local changes were of primary importance, and he criticized as 'entirely hypothetical' all the usual assumptions concerning the 'assimilation of the miasma and the contagion into the blood and its critical secretion from the blood by means of or into the exanthema'.[3] The depredations made on the blood or organic substance by the agent as it multiplied were important in producing symptoms and the changes which allowed exemption from further attack, but he gave an

---

[1] Ibid., p.958.

[2] Budd, 'Observations on Malignant Pustule', *Br. Med. J.* 1863, i. 87. Budd none the less continued to be interested in the physiology of the nervous and circulatory systems: see below. See also idem, 'On the Treatment of Croup', *Med. Times Gaz.* 1852, i. 611–15; note the chemical bias of this account.

[3] Budd, 'Observations on Typhoid', p.627; see also idem, 'Remarks on Cancer'. Henle, *Miasms and Contagions*, p.918.

equal part to local inflammatory processes and, as already noticed, he thought some diseases could occur without the agent's multiplying at all.

Having noted the differences in their arguments there is little point in also looking for differences between the views of Henle and Budd on the nature of the agent, though one may observe that Henle was prepared to consider that the agent in some fixed contagious diseases might be an elementary part of the body, and therefore only relatively animate. This gives him a closer relation than Budd to the developmental germ theorists.[1] Having arrived at his general conclusion, Henle relied on analogous cases such as muscardine to suggest particular properties. It seems probable that Budd adhered throughout life to the principle of his statement of 1849. After the events of that year, he publicly put the question aside as being of little practical importance; and used, as if algebraically, such expressions as 'virus', to stand in the place of the agent. Since, however, he was careful to point out how different was 'morbid poison' from 'poison' in the chemical sense; made constant use of the analogy with natural species; and showed an early interest in Pasteur, Casimir Davaine, and in such phenomena as Virchow's 'vibrio', it is unlikely that even his contemporaries were in doubt about his views.[2] Even in 1854, in his first communication on cholera since 1849, he found it possible to say that 'the probabilities are in favour of the supposition that the cause of cholera is a living organism'.[3] None the less, Budd had no part in the germ theory debate as it developed after 1865, and when he took note of its findings he did so in his own terms.

Correspondingly with his limited pathology, almost the only properties which Budd required of the agent were those of independent life and self-propagation. In his early paper on cancer it is these properties alone which are given to the

[1] Henle, *Miasms and Contagions*, p.971. Cf. Budd on the 'cancer cell', 'Remarks on Cancer', pp.268 ff.

[2] Budd, 'Variola Ovina, Sheep's Smallpox', p.147; idem, 'Observations on Typhoid', p.604 n.; idem, 'Bacteridia and Malignant Pustule', *Lancet*, 1865, i. 47.

[3] 'Common Sense' [Budd], 'Cholera: its Cause and Prevention', *Ass. Med. J.* 2 (1854), 1156. See also W. Michell Clarke, 'William Budd', *Br. Med. J.* 1880, i. 165.

'cancer cells'. These were, of course, not minor attributes, but properties expressed less in form than in function which gave great distinctiveness and power to the organism. One might add that the agent was required to be specifically adapted to a certain environment. A more realized property, of the agent of cholera at least, was its 'natural tendency except under special conditions, to rapid decay and extinction', which for Budd explained many otherwise mysterious circumstances. Budd described this state of the agent in terms which show him to have been as affected by Liebigian science as most of his contemporaries. In 1861 he stated that:

The powers of all the contagious poisons appear to be due to their being in an active state of metamorphosis, and to be proportioned to its intensity in each particular case. Where the conditions necessary to reproduction are present a rapid multiplication of the poison is the result. Where they are absent an equally rapid destruction of the original stock.

This spontaneous destruction occurred by a process of putrefaction or fermentation, and was more rapid where the poison was concentrated because 'the great characteristic of this process is to communicate itself with great rapidity to everything in contact with it, that is susceptible of taking on the same change'. In 1854 and in 1861, Budd used as an analogue the case of yeast. In 1854, he also described the 'powers which issue in rapid reproduction' as catalytic; and further speculated that the metamorphoses referred to which were set off by the exposure of the agent to oxygen, might be 'necessary for a renewal of that germinal force which gives to the poison its power over the body, as well as its own faculties of infinite reproduction'.[1] As we have seen, an apparently chemical view of process was not at all incompatible with biological explanations.

It is not surprising, given the similarity of his views to Budd's, that Henle was against the concept of *generatio aequivoca*, and tried to avoid invoking it even in the case of the entozoa.[2] Except for some of his references it does not at

---

[1] Budd, 'Memorandum on the Propagation and Prevention of Asiatic Cholera', *Memoranda on Asiatic Cholera* (1866), p.14; School of Hygiene Papers, Budd to G.M. Ogilvie of Lucknow, 16 Aug. 1856 [copy]; Budd, 'Cholera: its Cause and Prevention', p.1156.

[2] Henle, *Miasms and Contagions*, p.963, p.965 and note.

first appear to the modern reader that Henle was repudiating a concept any different from that opposed by Francesco Redi some two centuries before. This is primarily because Henle's agent, though hypothetical, was a free-living organism of fixed species; he would have been reluctant to resort to spontaneous generation to account for its origin not only because this would have jeopardized his concept of specificity, but also because, in such a case, the explanation would have been regarded by his contemporaries as unscientific. Writers who speak of the concept of spontaneous generation as lingering on well into the nineteenth century before being finally crushed by Pasteur, must necessarily be against the view that there were, according to context, different versions of the concept. One version arose at about the time Henle was writing, as a result of developments in organic chemistry and the first formulations of the cell theory. It was not so much a single concept as a series of approaches evolved in response to the newly defined problems of development and differentiation in living material. Carpenter, for example, in explaining the presence of fungi in the body, spoke of reproduction as a peculiar modification of nutrition: since its regular performance led to the evolution of germs, which when developed resembled the parent, it 'was not irrational to suppose that it may be so far perverted, as to give origin to beings of simpler organisation'. Somewhat later, Alfred Smee attempted to generate organisms in solutions by electricity, his aim being to determine how far a totally different organic being could spring from another made up of cells, as a result of the action on the cells of external forces.[1]

The 'old' and the 'new' versions were necessarily hard to distinguish, and some writers took advantage of this. One of these was Budd, who saw the concept as constituting a major threat to his theory as well as to the thorough application of his methods of prevention. He dealt with this threat (as with that of contingent contagionism) by imposing a kind of drastic oversimplification on contemporary opinion. Thus, in the case of spontaneous generation he ignored the 'new'

---

[1] Carpenter, *Principles of Physiology* (1839), p.63; *Lond. Med. Gaz.* 9 (1849), 591. For Smee (1818–77), M.R.C.S. 1840, F.R.S. 1841, see *DNB*. Smee also put forward an animalcular theory of the potato blight.

versions of the concept altogether. His account reads very much like those of many modern commentators, and was doubtless a source for some of them.[1] According to Budd, the concept had been gradually relinquished by naturalists from Aristotle onwards as they were forced to recognize the true complexity of lower and lower forms of life. The rejection of the notion that diseases arose *de novo* was simply the next stage in this enlightenment. In 1841, he wrote of the 'cancer cell' that 'it is . . . very difficult to conceive that a thing so specific in its nature, and endowed with such remarkable properties . . . can be actually engendered from the mere normal materials of the body under the influence of common agencies — This, to say the least, is treading very close upon the heels of spontaneous generation.' Here Budd was plainly referring only to the 'old' concept, and was taking advantage of the fact that his contemporaries, like himself, regarded the 'old' concept as no better than superstition. Elsewhere in the same paper he showed an awareness that the question was currently being reformulated, but again defined it in his own terms.[2]

His later arguments were of the same kind. The supposition that diseases arose *de novo*, he stated, 'discounted the whole analogy of nature'. Whether or not it was easier to conceive of a contagious fever originating anew, the fact remained that the evidence for spontaneous generation in animals and plants, as well as in diseases, was purely negative, and that if cholera had to generate spontaneously because one case could not be traced to another, then the same must be held not only of smallpox, but of known species of animals and plants. It should, perhaps, be emphasized that although Budd's contemporaries recognized that there was in pathology a question of the origin of contagion similar to that of the origin of species in physiology, there was little reason, apart from Budd's insistence, for them to equate the two. In 1863, Simon, after reporting on the work of Pasteur, contemplated the possibility that the two might be phases of one question;

---

[1] See e.g. Goodall, 'Budd, A Forgotten Epidemiologist', pp.279 ff.; idem, *William Budd*, pp.92 ff.; Dolman, art. 'Budd', *DSB*.

[2] Budd, 'Observations on Typhoid', p.605; idem, 'Remarks on Cancer', pp.296, 298.

but concluded that while there was little reason to suppose that contagion was frequently 'spontaneously generated', this was not to say that a contagious disease could not arise without contagion; and there were cases, such as the 'traumatic infections', in which 'spontaneous generation' of the disease was of very frequent occurrence.[1] Other authors have already been quoted to the same effect.

Because of his references to natural species, Budd's views might also be compared with those of John Grove, but there is probably more interest in a comparison with the obscure E.O. Spooner. This provincial surgeon was possibly a brother of William Charles Spooner, the veterinarian and agricultural chemist.[2] His only known appointment was that of Medical Officer to a Union Workhouse in Blandford, Dorset. His obscurity notwithstanding, he had had his medical education at St. Bartholomew's Hospital, University College, and in Paris. He was evidently active, at least in the middle of the century, in the Provincial Medical and Surgical Association, and was a lively critic of the views of both the General Board of Health and the Royal College of Physicians. In 1849, Spooner, having examined some of Joseph Griffiths Swayne's specimens, pronounced that the Bristol findings merited more careful investigation than that provided by the Royal College of Physicians, but that the fungoid theory had been 'too hastily put together' by Dr. Budd.[3] Spooner cannot be called a germ theorist, but he did believe that the 'doubtful' diseases were all, like smallpox, due to a single efficient cause, and that this agent was contained in the specific discharges or emanations from the sick.[4] In February 1849, well before Budd or Snow had published any statement on cholera, he wrote that 'the contamination of faecal evacuations . . . is the most fertile source of the disease'. He thought that morbid epithelial cells from the alimentary canal might generate the

---

[1] See e.g. Budd, 'Observations on Typhoid', p.604. Simon, *Public Health Reports*, ii. 151-2 nn.

[2] For Edward Oke Spooner (1808-87), L.S.A. 1829, M.R.C.S. 1830, F.R.C.S. 1852, see *Plarr*.

[3] Spooner, *Lond. Med. Gaz.* 9 (1849), 1078-9. Spooner also thought Snow's 'hydropathic theory' too narrow.

[4] But see Grove's use of Spooner's observation of 'cells' in smallpox matter: *Epidemics Examined*, pp.32-3.

specific poison involved. For the most part, he argued for the contagiousness of cholera on epidemiological grounds. Like Budd and Snow, he asserted that in this area a positive instance was worth more than a negative because, if not, smallpox itself would have to be regarded as non-contagious. He further remarked very succinctly that 'a disease cannot be contingently contagious, though it may spread or not according to certain contingencies...' Like Budd, he provided instances of diseases being imported into limited or susceptible populations. Most striking are his references to an epidemic of whooping cough in a nearby village, and his stress on the analogies provided by recent epidemics of sheep-pox.[1]

II

Budd is not an isolated figure like Snow; his interests were broader, and the influences upon him more numerous.[2] He was one of a large medical family brought up in the village of North Tawton in Devon, which, during 1839–40, was the scene of Budd's most definitive field work. Between 1828 and 1837 he studied in Paris, with several intervals which have been put down to cholera and political unrest in that city, and a severe attack of typhoid in Budd himself.[3] Among his teachers were Orfila, Broussais, Lisfranc, Andral, and Louis. Of these he probably had most contact with Broussais; but although he may have gained something from Broussais's emphasis on the condition of the alimentary canal in fever, his views as a whole on such subjects were entirely different from those of his teacher. A single letter written by Budd

[1] Spooner, 'The Contagion of Asiatic Cholera', pp.95, 37, 36, 93, 34, 91.

[2] William Budd (1811–80), M.D. Edinburgh 1838, F.R.S. 1871; educated Paris, London, Edinburgh. Taught himself French, German, Italian. Asst. physician to *Dreadnought* Hospital Ship, 1840. Asst. physician at St. Peter's Hospital, Bristol, 1842; physician to Bristol Royal Infirmary, 1847–62. Lecturer in medicine at Bristol Medical School, 1845–55. Member of first Board of Directors of Bristol Water Works Co. For critical biography and bibliography, see Goodall, *William Budd*; idem, 'William Budd, A Forgotten Epidemiologist'. Many of the letters now in the Wellcome Institute were not seen by Goodall. For personal impressions, see Prichard, *A Few Reminiscences*, p.87; the inaccurate Clarke, 'William Budd'. For Budd and Bristol, see R.C. Wofinden, 'Public Health in Bristol: Some Historical Aspects', *Public Health*, 69 (1956), 124–9. Most later accounts depend on Goodall; e.g. Dolman, art. 'Budd', *DSB*.

[3] Goodall, *William Budd*, pp.33–6.

from Paris praised Lisfranc, whose *clinique* he was then attending, and described Broussais as ageing, but 'very glad' to see him. Broussais later showed Budd 'the most remarkable phrenological specimen I ever saw'. Budd was his pupil for physiology, pathology, and clinical medicine in 1828-9, and clinical medicine in 1833-4.[1] Budd also studied clinical medicine under Louis, and admired him as a methodologist; later he depended upon him as 'the greatest of authorities, living or dead' on the natural history of enteric fever. He also admired Joseph Piedvache and Gendron de l'Eure for their grasp of the epidemiology of small localities or confined areas.[2] Budd's theory of typhoid, which led to his views on other diseases, coincides in many respects with that of Andral and of the 'school' of Pierre Fidèle Bretonneau (1778-1862). This does not mean that his theory was derivative; he alone was responsible for its unity and coherence. On his own account, Budd did not know of Bretonneau's similar views until 1857. He gave him credit for recognizing the eruptive nature of typhoid, but stated that neither in Bretonneau's papers nor those of his pupil de l'Eure was there 'the slightest hint of either the part the discharges play in the work of propagation or of the need of measures to disarm these discharges of their contagious power'. Bretonneau, although reaching a wider audience through his pupils, spent most of his life in Tours, and left the bulk of his work unpublished. Budd had a general, though not uncritical, respect for French writers; in later life, and on subjects other than typhoid, he referred to them continually, either for authority on particular points, for data, or in order to make points of his own.[3]

At Edinburgh, Budd was most impressed by Christison, the

---

[1] School of Hygiene Papers: Certificates; Budd Letters, William to Samuel, 6 Dec. 1833; Goodall, *William Budd*, p.26. For Budd on Broussais see also Budd, 'Contribution to the Pathology of the Spinal Cord', *Med. Chir. Trans.* 22 (1839), 176; idem, 'On Diseases Affecting the Body Symmetrically', ibid. 25 (1842), 111-12; idem, *The Times*, 26 Sept. 1849.

[2] Budd, *Typhoid Fever*, p.32. Piedvache was a hospital physician in Dinan (Côtes-du-Nord); both he and Gendron remain obscure. Piedvache's critical study, 'Recherches sur la contagion de la fièvre typhoide, et principalement sur les circonstances dans lesquelles elle a lieu', *Mémoires de L'Acad. Roy. de Méd.*, 15 (1849), 239-372, includes excerpts from Gendron's memoir.

[3] Budd, *Typhoid Fever*, p.50 n. In 1842-3 Budd was planning, as a part of his campaign to establish himself professionally, to submit his work on symmetry in

Regius professor of botany Robert Graham, and the physiologist John Reid.[1] Much local interest had been aroused by Reid's work on the reflex function in the nervous system and, as well as his thesis on rheumatic fever, Budd wrote another, on the spinal cord. He also worked on emphysema, carrying out experiments and making comparisons with the lower animals.[2] In 1841, after a trip to Dublin and a further period in North Tawton, he settled finally in Bristol.

The letters written by the Budds during this period make little mention of what are supposed to be William Budd's main interests. Later remarks indicate that he was keeping records of typhoid cases throughout the 1830s, as well as during the North Tawton epidemic of 1839–40; he wrote an essay on fever (the subject being given) in 1839, and was planning a book on the subject as early as 1842; none the less, the letters are, apart from points of practice, almost entirely concerned with the physiology and pathology of the blood and nervous system. In 1841, Budd wrote to the brother he loved most that he hoped to make the nervous system 'the work of my life. It is the finest subject in nature, and offers a richer harvest than any other field of enquiry, since nothing has yet been gathered from it.' At this period he was evidently hoping to make his name as a pathologist, and was exploring the consequences of a decision to take the research road to success: by which he meant reputation and then an increased practice. The most striking feature of the letters is Budd's constant calculation; research subjects, in particular, are chosen as much for their being topical or unexplored as from inclination. Budd subjected himself to constant criticism with

---

disease as an entry for the Monthyon prize: Budd Letters, William to Richard [1842. Tagged, 'On symmetry. 1st letter']; idem to idem, 'Monday' [1842]; idem to idem, November 1842 [Tagged, '1842']. Snow made a similar attempt at a lucrative French prize, in 1855: see G. Edwards, 'John Snow and the Institute of France', *Med. Hist.* 3 (1959), 249–50. For the Monthyon (or Montyon) prize in experimental physiology, see Olmsted, *Magendie*, pp.86–8 and *passim*.

[1] Budd Letters, William to Richard [November 1837]; William to George [20 Aug. 1838]. Budd wrote singling out Graham (1786–1845) among the staff of the Infirmary at Edinburgh, especially for his mode of investigation. Graham's only medical treatise was *Practical Observations on Continued Fever* (1818); Kay-Shuttleworth's *Autobiography* mentions Graham's work in an Edinburgh fever hospital, *c.* 1826: pp.5–6. Reid (d. 1849) also influenced W.B. Carpenter.

[2] Budd Letters, William to George [26 Feb. 1838].

respect to his level of application to research projects. In a characteristic outburst that followed the first reference in his letters to his interest in a law of symmetry in disease ('I see cases of it all the time and am already convinced that it is the most important law in diathesis ... Only the molecular actions of chemistry produce works of such delicacy'), Budd wrote to his brother Richard: 'It seems nothing short of culpable, to waste one's best years as I am doing, in specious idleness – Valuable and strong powers lying dormant and without use – Oh! for shame –. I must soon lay down some plan of action in the world. At present very jaded and weary.'[1]

Given Budd's early career, and those of other medical men of his period without family or similar connections, like James Paget or William Baly, one can no longer assume that the translation of a book or the publication of a paper indicates an interest in the subject itself, although the tendency to make the two kinds of interest coincide was of course strong. Budd's early exercises, like Snow's first and last, were intended to meet the necessity of establishing proprietary rights in a certain area. The Budd letters also contain interesting assessments of other courses open to a man not yet set up in practice, such as lecturing (in a provincial medical school), and editorship of a medical journal or similar publication.[2] In 1838, Budd thought that if he went to a large town (he suggested Norwich), he would give a course in physiology, if there was a school attached to the local hospital. He noted that there were many provincial schools already, and that 'the new London University' would probably multiply them. It is possible that Budd went to Bristol because of its school, although he twice turned down the offer of the 'chair' of forensic medicine, before becoming lecturer in medicine in 1845.[3]

---

[1] Ibid., William to Richard [1841]; idem to idem [November 1842]; idem to idem, 7 Nov. 1842; idem to idem, 22 Mar. 1841. William's breakdown in later life was mental as well as physical; other brothers (Samuel, George) suffered more consistently from depression.

[2] For similar material on a provincial physician of less calibre, see Foster, 'Dr. William Henry Cook'.

[3] Budd Letters, William to Richard [4 Jan. 1838. Tagged, 'Edinb. Visit to Wemyss']. Cf. Goodall, *William Budd*, p.56; on the advantages and disadvantages of the forensic (or any other) 'chair', see Budd Letters, William to Richard [Tagged, '1842']. However, 1845 was a year of financial crisis: idem to idem, 16 Nov. 1845 [Tagged, '1845. His gt. losses'].

Budd's choice of Bristol was probably also determined by the proximity of his family and brothers, who were dispersed around the West Country.

In discussing the nature of Budd's preoccupations and the influences which led to them, account must be taken of his sensitivity to suffering. A morbid form of this concern was a symptom of his breakdown in later years.[1] One of the reasons why Budd concentrated on the epidemic diseases was surely his conviction that they were entirely preventable. Typhoid in particular was constantly occurring and involved an unusually protracted period of suffering and anxiety.[2] Budd's insistence on the merits of his methods of prevention cannot be attributed entirely to a desire either to establish a name for himself or to provide a final proof of his theories.

Budd retained an interest in the action of substances through the blood and the means which determined them to different or corresponding areas of the body, and here he was influenced by Holland and by Liebig. As already mentioned he met Liebig in 1842. The coincidence of their interests is indicated in a review by W.B. Carpenter of Liebig's *Animal Chemistry*. Budd used cases of symmetry in disease to prove that many such local actions must be the effect of elective affinities operating after the agent had entered the blood. Carpenter, in commenting upon Liebig's explanation of the influence of medicinal agents on 'vital transformations', stated that 'the views of Liebig render more precise our ideas of this local action; and take from W. Budd's supposition the uncertain character of a hypothesis, conferring on it the definiteness of a theory'.[3] At about the same time Budd described as the 'three great books of the age' Marshall Hall's *Diseases and Derangements of the Nervous System* (1841), Marie-Jean-Pierre Flourens's *Recherches experimentales sur le système nerveux*

---

[1] Prichard, *A Few Reminiscences*, p.87. See also Budd's condemnation of the vivisectionism of some French physiologists: 'Retrospect of Anatomy and Physiology', *Trans. Prov. Med. Surg. Ass.* 13 (1845), 189–90. This aversion may have led Budd to favour the chemical, experimentless physiology of Liebig and Dumas.

[2] Budd, *Typhoid Fever*, pp.1–2. Budd himself had suffered twice from this disease; see Budd Letters, and Goodall, *William Budd*, pp.33–4, 37–8.

[3] On his own account, Budd had been interested in constitutional disease from 1836: 'On Diseases Affecting the Body Symmetrically', p.101 n. Carpenter, *Br. For. Med. Rev.* 14 (1842), 520.

(first edition, 1824; second edition, 1842), and Liebig's *Organic Chemistry*.[1] Like his contemporaries Budd was struck by the 'simplicity and sublimity' of the new organic chemistry as expounded by Liebig and Dumas, and was more tolerant than many of Liebig's physiological explanations.[2] Interestingly but consistently, he stated in 1845 that Liebig's observations on fermentation, putrefaction and decay were 'quite decisive in showing the purely chemical nature of the agency which the ferments and other bodies in a state of change play in these processes'.[3]

After the success of his first paper on symmetry, Budd planned a second and a third, one holding that the same type of effect took place in internal as in external structures, and the other, on the 'effects of morbid matters in blood, as affected by the rate and manner of their elimination'. He was interested in the action of 'blood medicines' such as potassium iodide, and thought that the occurrence of symmetrical appearances in disease provided an excellent natural opportunity for the controlled test of remedies.[4] As previous chapters have shown, this early work of Budd's may be seen as closely related to current estimates of the pathology of epidemic diseases. The phenomenon of elective affinity, which had recently been detected as characteristic of ordinary nutrition and of chemical action itself, was first observed as an effect of poisons. By a further use of analogy, and with the adoption of a humoral pathology, it could be freely asserted that elective affinity was also shown during the elimination of morbid poisons from the body. In 1848 Carpenter, after recognizing the claims of Robert Williams, gave credit to Budd for pointing out 'that the existence of a *materies morbi*

---

[1] Budd Letters, William to Richard, 'Monday' [1842]. Budd's titles are approximate.

[2] Ibid., William to Richard [Tagged, '1842']. See e.g. Budd, 'Retrospect of Anatomy and Physiology', pp.148 ff., 180 ff., 190 ff.

[3] Budd, 'Retrospect of Anatomy and Physiology', pp.190–1; see also p.174.

[4] Budd Letters, William to Richard [Tagged, '1842']; idem to idem [Tagged, '1841']; idem to idem, 30 Nov. 1843 [Tagged, 'Skin Diseases, 1843']. See Budd, ' "On the Employment of Potassium Iodide", by M. Melsens', *Br. For. Med. Chir. Rev.* 11 (1853), 201–24. 'Blood medicines' was Budd's own term: 'On Diseases Affecting the Body Symmetrically', p.126.

in the blood may often be predicted from the *symmetrical* nature of the disordered action induced by it'.[1]

On first going to Bristol, Budd had complained of the absence of congenial intellectual society to the kindly William Bowman of King's College. Bowman suggested that he see more of Carpenter, 'a clever fellow, but likely to be writing himself dry'.[2] Budd had already noted without much enthusiasm Carpenter's contributions to the debate over reflex function, but he evidently followed Bowman's advice, and in 1841 recorded with pleasure Carpenter's reaction to his paper on symmetry: 'Dr. Carpenter . . . thinks the whole quite new and highly original, and pays it the great compliment of likening it to Dr. Holland's production[s?].' Budd was pleased because Carpenter 'besides being a very clever fellow very generally underrates the productions of other men'. By 1842 the two men were evidently familiar, and it was through Carpenter's mentioning his work to Liebig, that Budd and the latter met. For a time Budd shared Carpenter's opinions as to the effect on the blood of the inspiration of putrid effluvia.[3]

Mention ought also to be made of Sir Thomas Watson, who gave Budd valuable support throughout his career.[4] Budd was first a pupil of Watson's at the Middlesex Hospital, and afterwards sent his teacher copies of his earliest productions. Watson publicly praised both the essay on symmetry and the paper on cancer, and commended the work of Budd and his brother George (who had also been a student at the Middlesex) in a letter to Budd: 'lucubrations such as these, which tend to elucidate great practical questions, are of great importance in our imperfect science'. Of Watson's public support Budd

---

[1] Ibid., pp.106, 110, 143 ff., 157; Carpenter, 'Taylor and Copland on Poisons', p. 197. See also Watson, *Principles and Practice of Physic*, ii. 692. For Budd on the mode of action of poisons and morbid poisons see also his 'The Frog as a Detector of Tetanic Poison', *Lancet*, i. 90–1.

[2] Budd Letters, W. Bowman to [William] Budd, November 1841.

[3] Budd Letters, William to Richard, January 1840; idem to idem [Tagged, '1841']. Budd, 'Observations on Typhoid', p.550.

[4] See *DNB* art., 'William Budd', quoting Tyndall. For Sir Thomas Watson (1792–1882), B.A. Cantab. 1815, M.A. 1818, L.R.C.P. 1822, M.D. Cantab. 1825, F.R.C.P. 1826, F.R.S. 1859, professor of medicine at University College, 1828–31, then of King's College, President of the Royal College of Physicians, 1862–5, see *Venn*; *Munk*.

wrote exultantly to his brother Richard, 'One would positively think he was in my pay ... I should think Watson would be worth [to] me a hundred a year at least.' In reply to Budd's avowal that he would if necessary get up a 'round robin' of Bristolians to persuade Watson to publish his own clinical lectures, Watson wrote (with great modesty, given their respective professional positions) that he would 'receive any criticisms of yours on them as a great favour'. Whether it need be supposed that either in any way influenced the other is not clear, but Budd had reason to think well of the *Principles and Practice of Physic*, since in many respects Watson's views on epidemic diseases were similar to his own. This was especially true of the former's idea of smallpox, including the circumstances of its propagation and prevalence, and the analogy of smallpox with other diseases, especially continued fever. The latter Watson regarded as a single, graduated entity, which originated in an 'animal poison', was contagious, and belonged like smallpox to the category of the exanthemata; this term being taken to signify not cutaneous but 'blood' diseases showing characteristic but not essential local appearances.[1]

The paper on cancer, which was read locally and attracted less notice from contemporaries, sufficiently indicates the early maturity of Budd's characteristic theories of epidemic disease.[2] It also represents his earliest published microscopical work. Although he saw cancer as analogous to the contagious diseases (especially syphilis), Budd evidently chose to publish on cancer rather than on some more typical representative because of its topicality.[3] His paper refers to the cell theory

---

[1] Budd Letters, William to Richard, 7 Nov. 1842 [Tagged, '1842']; Watson, *Principles and Practice of Physic*, ii. 658 ff., 669 ff., 696 ff., 661 ff.; Budd, 'Observations on Typhoid', pp.524, 576.

[2] Budd, 'Remarks on Cancer'. This paper was given in Bristol: Budd Letters, William to Richard [1842]. Budd wrote of this work to Richard Budd, who is found later asserting the contagiousness of cancer: William to Richard, 'Sunday' [1841, Tagged, 'On a monument to Father'] (for William on the microscopical technique to employ with cancer cells); idem to idem [Tagged, '1842']; idem to idem, 7 Nov. 1842 [Tagged, '1842']; R. Budd, 'Is Cancer Contagious?', *Lancet*, 1887, ii. 1091; Budd Letters, [draft of letter to journal?] by Richard, September 1894.

[3] On theories of cancer, see J. Ewing, *Neoplastic Diseases* (Philadelphia, 1928); H. Butlin, *Three Lectures on Unicellula Cancri* (1912); E.H. Ackerknecht, 'Histori-

of Schwann, and to Müller's major work on the microscopical anatomy of cancer (1838).[1] Budd went further than Müller in asserting the peculiarity of the cancer cell, which he thought must lie not in its 'minute anatomical elements' (since these appeared to be the same for all cells), but in its 'independent powers of life and nourishment'. The cancer cells or 'germs' were at first localized; then, like pus cells in 'general purulent infection', they were disseminated by the blood, and eventually lodged in other tissues, their distribution being determined, as in the case of pus and mercury globules, largely by 'mechanical conditions'. In considering the origin of the cancer germ Budd suggested two analogies, that of 'true parasitic animals', and that of the 'blood globules', according to whether the germs were to be considered as coming from without or within. Although clearly preferring the first alternative, Budd stated that he was prepared to wait for the solution to the current 'great question', 'whether or not, and under what limitations, things specific in their nature, and which multiply by propagating their own kind, may also be engendered in other ways'. It is possible that this discovery of an agent of disease which was capable of self-multiplication and 'an object of sight, of definite shape, and an organised form', and for which it was certain that 'increase is not the result of a chemical state, but the growth of a living thing', may have encouraged Budd in the adventure of 1849.[2]

The years between 1852 and 1864 were those in which Budd was most active, and will receive more attention here.[3] We shall be concerned mainly with a comparison of Budd's views

---

cal Notes on Cancer', *Med. Hist.* 2 (1958), 114–19. For the different views of Snow on cancer, see *Snow on Cholera*, p.xliv.

[1] See J. Müller, *On the Nature and Structural Characteristics of Cancer*, Pt. I, trans. C. West (1840). For Budd on cell theory see also 'Diseases Affecting the Body Symmetrically', p.152 n.

[2] Budd, 'Remarks on Cancer', pp.298, 269.

[3] It has not been possible to make a proper investigation of Budd's views in their public aspect, although their effect on John Simon must be a result as important as any. Budd did not of course have to enforce all his views in order to induce local and other authorities to adopt his system of prevention: see Budd, *Memoranda on Asiatic Cholera*; idem, *Cholera and Disinfection* (1883). Budd maintained a very successful collaboration with D. Davies, the city's Medical Officer from 1866. He also made representations to a range of health authorities, especially in the 1850s: see School of Hygiene Papers, and Goodall, *William Budd*, pp.65–6. See also Budd, 'Government and the Prevention of Infectious Disease'.

with Snow's, and with Budd's opposition to the prevailing
climate of contingent contagionism. Many of Budd's papers
were compiled in these years, well before they were actually
published. His views on tuberculosis, released in 1867, had
been held back for a decade;[1] while the book on fever, which
finally appeared in 1873, was composed largely of matter
published in the earlier period. The later years did bring public
recognition of Budd's particular expertise by, for example,
government and the British Medical Association. Budd
produced some valuable pieces for the Association, but
declined to join the Royal Commission on the cattle plague
(1865) because of the pressure of his professional commitments.[2] He was not elected a Fellow of the Royal Society
until 1871. Among those supporting his candidature from
'personal knowledge' were: Sir Thomas Watson (his proposer),
Sir Henry Holland, W.B. Carpenter, Professor E.A. Parkes,
and John Simon.[3] Towards the end of the 1860s his health
broke down and he barely finished the book on fever before
collapsing entirely in 1873. This means, among other things,
that criticisms contained in his book on fever cannot be
taken as a true reflection of the state of opinion at that later
date. For example, in the 1850s Budd with perfect justice
singled out the General Board of Health as a source of
anticontagionist opinion having 'unlimited printing power'
at its disposal, and expressed his doubt that the fall of one
Board and the rise of another had produced much change in
official doctrine.[4] The papers containing these and similar
criticisms were incorporated almost unchanged into the main
work published nearly twenty years later.

There is no evidence that Budd and John Snow ever met
to exchange views, although Budd described Snow as 'my
friend Dr Snow' and each very likely sent copies of his works
to the other. An isolated letter records George Budd's response to Snow's gift of the second edition of his work on

[1] Budd, 'Memorandum on the Nature and Mode of Propagation of Phthisis',
Lancet, 1867, ii. 451–2. For reactions, see ibid., pp.466, 550–1, 594–5.

[2] *Br. Med. J.* 1865, ii. 450.

[3] Bristol Medical Library, William Budd Box: W. Bulloch to E.W. Goodall,
January 1932; idem to idem, 30 Jan. 1932. This honour came very late and could
almost be regarded as consolatory.

[4] See e.g. Budd, 'On Intestinal Fever', *Lancet*, 1856, ii. 694; ibid. 1859, p.4.

cholera. George Budd was Snow's physician in the 1850s, and with Charles Murchison attended him in his last illness.[1]

The comparison of Snow and Budd is best begun by considering the six 'letters' on 'Cholera: its Cause & Prevention' which Budd published during 1854–5. Except for a paper on croup these constituted Budd's first communication on the subject of infectious disease since 1849; the first four letters were published under a pseudonym, 'Common Sense'. The author of these communications put aside the possibility of direct evidence, and provided instead the first development of the smallpox analogy and a series of 'instances in which cholera was imported into previously healthy districts, and there propagated by persons who had contracted it in distant places'. Such cases, Budd wrote, 'not only prove malignant cholera to be a catching disorder, but, so long as the specific agent which is the material cause of the disease eludes detection, *they contain the highest order of evidence of which the fact is susceptible*'.[2] Snow, who depended so much on epidemiological evidence, might also have written this, yet Budd was critical of the way in which Snow supported the theory which was so like his own. To explain this is to discover the differences between them.

Both Snow and Budd wanted to expand the definition of contagiousness to include different modes of propagation, but when Budd stated of typhoid, as he might have done of cholera, that 'contagion is the master fact in its history' he was not showing any particular interest in whether the disease was transmitted directly, or in air, or in water. Words such as 'contagious' or 'infectious' which commonly signified different modes of propagation could all be dropped in favour of the single word 'catching'. The 'catching' diseases were defined by their 'pathology'. This difference between Snow and Budd is best expressed by the fact that in extending his ideas to other diseases, Budd gave them the features of smallpox; Snow

---

[1] George Budd to Snow, 3 Jan. 1855. The essence of this letter has been published by K. Bryn Thomas, 'The Clover/Snow Collection: Papers of Joseph Clover and John Snow in the Woodward Biomedical Library, University of British Columbia, Vancouver', *Anaesthesia*, 27 (1972), 436–49: 447. I am grateful to Dr. Bryn Thomas for a xerox copy of the letter. *Snow on Chloroform*, p.xli.

[2] Budd, 'Cholera: its Cause and Prevention', p.951. Budd's italics.

merely asserted that other diseases might be waterborne.[1]

From the first Budd's wider view allowed him to be less exclusive than Snow. In 1849 he put forward all Snow's arguments and some of his own in support of the proposition that 'water . . . is the chief vehicle of the poison' but he thought it no less clear that cholera also diffused itself through the air; a single-factor explanation of cholera epidemics was otherwise impossible. In 1854, when he began to use epidemiological case histories, rather greater emphasis was placed on the air. In particular he used the case of a hospital in which the patients suffered from cholera according to whether they had access to a particular privy. It was plain that the patients who took cholera had it from the effluvia of specific discharges; and this, Budd stated, was the real explanation of 'the broad and now quite notorious connexion of malignant cholera with the effluvia arising from defective sewerage'. The poison was doubtless more concentrated in water than in air, but since foul privies and drains were universal, and their communication with water supplies comparatively rare, then the air had to be the more common vehicle of the poison. As in 1849, the presence of the poison in the air allowed Budd to refer all the phenomena of epidemics to the properties of the agent alone. Because of its rate of multiplication, 'the poison accumulates on so vast a scale that, exhaling into the air, *it broods like a great miasm* over large districts, and in a manner to admit of its being carried by currents of air to indefinite distances with its deadly powers intact'.[2]

Budd also thought that in typhoid, which was even more notoriously a filth disease, communication by infection of the air was 'by far the more common case'. In 1873 he found it necessary to contradict an assertion that it was 'impossible for typhoid fever to spread widely in any community provided with pure drinking water'. It should however be noted that except in making these points Budd did not normally in his case histories specify the means by which the poison travelled from the sick to the healthy. In 1855 Snow explicitly defined this difference between himself and Budd:

[1] *Snow on Cholera*, pp.125 ff.
[2] Budd, *Malignant Cholera*, pp.21–2; idem, 'Cholera: its Cause and Prevention', pp.976, 928. My italics.

Dr. Budd entirely agrees with me that the cholera poison is produced only in the alimentary canal and acts only on that canal, which it reaches by being swallowed . . . there is no difference between us respecting the essential mode of communication of the disease, but only as to the extent to which it is communicated through the air . . . In my opinion the cholera poison only produces its effects through the air when carried by insects or when the evacuations become dry, and are wafted as a fine dust.

It is true as Snow claimed that Budd's few arguments from clinical pathology were identical with his own and that he had published them first. In general however Budd's more deductive approach encouraged him to ignore pathological questions.[1] He did not, for instance, go into the consequences of his having suggested two possible modes of entry to the body in cholera.

We now turn to the epidemiological evidence used to support these similar views. Budd's epidemiology was, as already mentioned, that of the 'ideal situation'. Instead of rising to every challenge he looked for limited localities and isolated communities: country villages, ships, camps, and institutions. Only these cases were worth considering, because 'numberless cases . . . *necessarily* occur, in which it is no more possible to trace the individual case to the particular previous case in which it originated, than it is to trace the mildew which springs up in a pot of preserve to the particular mildew plant from which the sporules of the new crop came'. Budd believed that it was necessary to demonstrate a disease's contagiousness only once in order to fix its type; it was in order to make good these (as well as other) arguments that he took up an adamant position on spontaneous generation, and it was from this standpoint that he was critical of Snow. In 1857, at a time when cholera was not abroad in London, Snow sought to explain a localized outbreak in Abbey Row, West Ham, by tracing it to the ejecta of a seaman which had been thrown into the Thames. In order to make this connection, Snow had to embrace certain improbabilities. The *British Medical Journal*, which printed his paper, commented:

That cholera evacuations may be conveyed from one person to another by means of water and thus spread the disease, is most probably, under

---

[1] Budd, 'Observations on Typhoid', p.627; idem, *Typhoid Fever*, p.116; Snow, *Edinb. Med. J.* 1 (1855-6), 668.

certain circumstances, the case; but Dr. Snow should scarcely have floated his cholera germs with such unerring accuracy for two miles up a great tidal river and its tributary, into a sewer, and thence into a well, in order to account for the deaths of six people from cholera in Abbey Row.[1]

Budd, alarmed that Snow should so jeopardize their common interest, published a letter of his own. Snow, he said, was only weakening a case already made out by bringing forward an instance like that of West Ham, where 'the evidence is certainly neither clear or decisive, and is not at all likely to be accepted by the public generally'. As well as being of 'no scientific use' such evidence was unnecessary. As in the case of smallpox, 'having . . . learnt by direct observation where the poison breeds, and in what way it multiplies, we can afford to be very careless as to the manner in which, in any particular instances, its germs have become disseminated'.[2]

The advantages of 'village epidemiology' as practised by Budd have been dwelt upon by other writers, and it is not necessary to do so here.[3] As we have seen, and as Budd himself recognized, evidence based on operations in the field is always a matter of probabilities, and Budd's own case histories, although of a higher degree, rested on the same basis. Budd relied not on epidemiological evidence but on analogy to dispatch the claim that the poison was not bred in men's bodies, but merely mechanically carried about by them. P.E. Brown states that 'if it had not been for Budd's premature adoption of the fungus theory . . . his more careful epidemiological studies might well have supplanted those of Snow in the history of preventive medicine'.[4] There is no evidence that Budd's adventure of 1849 affected anyone more than himself, and as we have seen, he was not afterwards unduly inhibited by it. Considering the two kinds of epidemi-

---

[1] Budd, 'Cholera: its Cause and Prevention', p.928; Snow, 'Outbreak of Cholera at Abbey Row'; *Br. Med. J.* 1857, ii. 910.

[2] Budd, 'The Cholera at West Ham', *Br. Med. J.* 1857, ii. 955. See Richardson on Snow: 'had he put his labours before the world, and trusted in them and the world's justice, never replying a syllable, he would have avoided an extremity of argument which was often not merely unnecessary . . . but injurious to them, as reasonings overstrained': *Snow on Chloroform*, p.xxxviii.

[3] See e.g. W.N. Pickles, *Epidemiology in Country Practice* (Bristol, 1939), pp.1-2; Brown, 'Snow, the Autumn Loiterer', p.528.

[4] Budd, 'Cholera: its Cause and Prevention', p.951; Brown, 'Snow, the Autumn Loiterer', p.528.

ology purely on their merits as then perceived, one would imagine that Snow's work attracted more immediate attention not because he was being rewarded for 1849 and Budd punished, but because large-scale statistical investigations were more attractive to their contemporaries. In any case as we shall see Budd's case histories were not always ignored. Given also that different diseases were involved, that Budd seldom placed any stress on the exact mode of communication of infection, and that Budd's most detailed studies were not published until after Snow's death, there are definitely limits to how far contemporary reactions to each may usefully be compared.

It should be noted that Budd's own theory was made to depend on a 'popular experiment': that is, prevention by disinfection. It was for this feature of his theory that Budd claimed priority after allowing Snow's claims to other elements. The method was to bring to the theory 'its final and crowning proof'. Budd no doubt envisaged that disinfection would become precisely defined by the laboratory experiment, but this did not happen in time for it to be useful to him, and the 'final proof' of his theory continued to be dependent upon the results of trials conducted in the field.[1] P.E. Brown points to Snow's failure to recommend the chemical treatment of cholera evacuations 'although his own hypothesis seemed to demand it', and sees this as an ill-advised rejection of the sound parts of the cholera-fungus theory. Snow recommended disinfection not externally, but internally: 'Medicines should be chosen which have the effect of destroying low forms of organised beings.'[2]

Norman Longmate speaks of the 'unfortunate coincidence' of Budd and Snow's publications in 1849 as leading to 'endless confusion which irritated both parties'. This is unwarranted. There was no such confusion in 1849. After the next epidemic,

---

[1] Budd, 'Mode of Propagation of Cholera', p.259; *Typhoid Fever*, pp.128 ff. For contemporary theory and practice in disinfection see Condy, *Disinfection and the Prevention of Disease*. For later, experimental work on disinfection see E.B. Baxter, 'Report on an Experimental Study of certain Disinfectants', Appendix to *6th Rep. (NS) of Med. Officer of the Privy Council and Local Govt. Board*, PP, 1875, XL. 216–56.

[2] Brown, 'Snow, the Autumn Loiterer', p.521; Snow, 'Principles on which the Treatment of Cholera Should be Based', p.181.

W.P. Alison came out in (qualified) support of Budd, and Snow was piqued at not being mentioned.[1] Yet Alison's views were not of a kind which Snow wished to support.[2] Alison wanted only to establish that cholera was capable of being propagated from the sick to the healthy in a British climate, without committing himself to any other opinion as to its mode of communication or as to the existence of other modes. Furthermore he was inclined to believe that the poison of cholera, like other known animal poisons (such as that causing erysipelas or puerperal fever) was 'developed during the decomposition of the animal matter, the appearance of which is most characteristic of the disease'.[3] This Liebigian view was, as we have seen, not at all agreeable to Snow. Budd, however, was prepared to consider it, and was also less interested in modes of communication. It is hardly likely that Alison would have confused Snow's views with Budd's. Longmate bases his statement largely on a similar case in which Snow's concern for his own priority was again aroused; this case also illustrates the greater flexibility of Budd's views and his lesser estrangement from the contemporary context. In an address, Sir James Kay-Shuttleworth referred to the discovery of Ignaz Semmelweis with respect to puerperal fever, and to 'Dr. Budd's discovery of one mode of the dissemination of cholera by a poison evolved in the early stage of decomposition of the specific secretions'. This is again Liebigian; Sir James was referring (on the basis, it may be suspected, of a purely second-hand knowledge of the sources) not to epidemiology but to humoral pathology.[4]

Since Snow was criticized chiefly for his exclusiveness, and Budd was less exclusive, one would expect Budd's views to be the more popular. To some extent this was the case. Budd was perhaps less uncongenial to the sanitarians than Snow, and

---

[1] Longmate, *King Cholera*, pp.208–9; Alison, 'On the Communicability of Cholera by Dejections', *Edinb. Med. J.* 1 (1855–6), 481–92, 1112–25; Snow, ibid., p.668.

[2] As was indicated by the editor of the *Edinburgh Medical Journal*, who gave his preference to Alison: ibid., p.670.

[3] See also Alison, 'The Application of Statistics to Medical Science', *Edinb. Med. J.* 1 (1855–6), 388; 389.

[4] See Snow, 'Mode of Propagation of Cholera' (1856); Kay-Shuttleworth, *Ass. Med. J.* 4 (1856), 117.

his 'letters' of 1854-5, which contain the most temporizing account he ever gave of his views, were perhaps his most successful propaganda exercise.[1] They were referred to by B.W. Richardson who, noting Snow's opinion that choleraic and other poisons had to be swallowed to produce their effects, stated that 'although . . . we are prepared to go great lengths with Dr. Snow in support of his peculiar views, we are obliged to stop whenever we meet with this absolute conclusion . . . we are glad to see supported by Dr. William Budd . . . the view that the specific cause of cholera may be carried by the air into the lungs'.[2] There is also Alison's support, although Alison was himself more compatible with the profession in general, than with the London sanitarians. In spite of these and other indications, however, Budd did not fare so much better than Snow. He had his own form of exclusiveness; his theories were directly opposed to the climate of contingent contagionism.

This is best illustrated in the context of Budd's views on typhoid, which was his main interest for many years after 1855. His activity at this later period was to a large extent provoked by that of others. For twenty years at least after the distinction between typhus and typhoid was first established in France, ulceration of the intestines in fever was recognized by the majority as a distinct condition or variety, but not as the mark of a specific disease. Hence the importance of William Jenner's work in the London Fever Hospital from 1847 to 1851. The classification of the 'continued fevers' was still a matter for controversy in the 1860s. Budd, like his brother Richard, took his interest in Louis's 'fièvre typhoide' with him to Edinburgh, and in 1839 produced his essay asserting it to be a specific contagious disease; but although he was among the earliest to make such a claim he took no real part in promoting its acceptance, except to teach his views to his students at the Bristol medical school.[3]

---

[1] See e.g. School of Hygiene Papers, G.M. Ogilvie of Lucknow to William Budd, 16 Aug. 1856; E. Harris of New York to William Budd, 31 Aug. 1866.

[2] Richardson, *J. Publ. Hlth Sanit. Rev.* 1 (1855), 134-5.

[3] Budd, 'On Intestinal Fever' (1859), p.5. See Goodall, *William Budd*, pp.41 ff. This essay was Budd's entry for the Provincial Medical and Surgical Association's 'Thackeray Prize'. The Association's choice of topic ('Causes and Mode of Propagation of the Common Continued Fevers in Great Britain and Ireland') was highly

'Fever', it will be remembered, was the sanitarians' chief concern. It was indigenous, took a constant toll and was unmistakably associated with deprivation and filth. As both typhoid and typhus became better defined, the former disease emerged as the more important from a sanitary point of view. It was more common than typhus by the second quarter of the century, and its incidence seemed to depend not on contagion but almost entirely on local conditions. Sir James Clark was representative in seeing typhoid as one of the retributive diseases which came as a punishment for the violation of natural law. Budd sent to Clark in 1862 a 'pamphlet, *The Propagation of Typhoid Fever*'.[1] In reply Clark contended for the spontaneous origin of typhoid in isolated districts, and rejected both the analogy between the pathologies of smallpox and typhoid, and the equivalence asserted by Budd to subsist between the spontaneous origin of diseases and that of organisms. Clark found it not surprising but rather in accordance with 'the moral and physical government of the world' that the whole body should enter a morbid state when all the physiological laws were broken that were known to regulate health. He ended his letter: 'The subject is a most important one and it is of vital consequence that the truth should be elicited. — I fear if the public should adopt your views the necessity of careful drainage would . . . be less considered. It would be unfortunate if such should be the result.'[2] As we shall see, Clark's letter epitomizes the general response to Budd's attempts to establish his views.

typical of current interests. The prize went (in 1840) to Dr. W. Davidson of Glasgow. Budd Letters, William to Richard, 4 Jan. 1841 [Tagged, '1841. In love'], includes a rather cryptic reference to Davidson's essay as being 'well overloaded'. William added that his own essay could be greatly expanded, and that he was then revising it. See also Goodall, *William Budd*, p.42. In 1859 he still possessed a manuscript copy, which seems now to be lost. However Budd evidently published most of its contents in the 1850s and again in 1873. See Budd, 'On Intestinal Fever' (1859), p.5 n. where he also recorded that he had read an abstract to the 'Bristol Medical Library Society' in 1843.

[1] No such pamphlet is known. It was evidently not made up of the papers published in and after 1859: see next note. It may even have been the 'lost' essay.

[2] School of Hygiene Papers, James Clark to William Budd, 29 Sept. 1862. Snow's views were criticized on similar grounds: *Snow on Chloroform*, p.xxv. Budd replied to Clark at length, enclosing the papers published as 'On Intestinal Fever' in 1859 and 1860. See Budd's endorsement of the letter just cited, and School of Hygiene Papers, Budd to [Clark], 2 Oct. 1862 [draft or copy].

Another reason for typhoid's emerging as a subject for particular concern was that it was found to attack the rich as well as the poor. This, as *The Lancet* and others hastened to point out, was because the houses of the rich were very often badly drained or otherwise defective; a fact which had gone unnoticed in the earlier, heroic period of sanitary improvement.[1] The concern over typhoid reached a peak with the death of the Prince Consort in 1861. Cholera was of course not epidemic in England from 1855 until 1865.

For many medical writers typhus ceased to be of interest as it appeared to decrease in incidence and was joined to the well-known (if inscrutable) group of specific eruptive fevers. The nature of typhoid, on the other hand, was a question which raised all the current issues. More than any other such disease it appeared to be caused by some change akin to putrefaction in the organic substances which were or had been part of the body. Jenner's distinction was based partly on a difference in causation; typhoid became associated with one kind of filth, that is the faecal pollution of air and water. This of course coincides with the situation in respect of cholera. Thiersch's results, and Liebig's interpretation of them, were naturally held to be as relevant to typhoid as to cholera. The same variety of contingent-contagionist positions was taken up. Those who held these positions often had little more in common than the view that typhoid, like cholera, was sometimes contagious and sometimes not. Many formed the view purely on the grounds of typhoid's behaviour in the field, and were seemingly regardless of other considerations and of the nature of the disease process in particular. Others like Acland and Alison who were more aware, were content simply to establish a basis for prevention.[2] The most common opinion was that the poison increased or was developed outside the body but some held that this could happen inside the body as well. Pettenkofer's theory, devised first for cholera

---

[1] *Lancet*, 1862, i. 75.

[2] Murchison, *Treatise on Continued Fevers*, p.6. H.W. Acland, *Fever in Agricultural Districts* (1858). For the multifactoral theory constructed by Acland to meet his conclusion, based on epidemiological grounds, that cholera was contingently contagious, see his *Memoir on the Cholera at Oxford*, especially pp.73 ff. Note references to Budd and to Alison, p.73.

and then extended to typhoid, was perhaps the most highly developed compromise solution. For Pettenkofer, cholera and typhoid were transmissible but not contagious in that they could be transmitted from one locality to another but not from one individual to another. The body of the patient produced a specific germ or ferment, but this could not of itself produce disease in another person. There had in addition to be a faecalized material or soil, which received the first factor and gave rise to a fermentation; this generated a miasma, which excited disease if it was inhaled at a certain level of concentration by susceptible subjects.[1]

Some writers like Armand Trousseau who shared Budd's views as to the specificity of typhoid and the entirely ancillary role played by local conditions in the production of the disease, were counted by him as contingent contagionists, because they assumed, purely on logical grounds, that if typhoid had arisen spontaneously in the first instance, then it was possible for it to do so again.[2] This as we have seen was a typical assumption, and allowed even by Snow to hold for 'septic diseases'; it was however denied by Southwood Smith.

Budd's theories were quite in opposition to this climate. With one or two exceptions he did not deal with its components in detail, but rather, as in the related case of spontaneous generation, imposed his own views upon it. His theory admitted only the existence of two poles; if a disease were not 'essentially contagious' then it could not be contagious at all. Budd misrepresented his opposition to correspond with this. In 1873 he stated that 'the great majority not of the laity only but of the profession also, still remain anticontagionists'. In 1865, Simon had commented: 'When phenomena of pestilence are under popular discussion, and most of all when quarantine is being spoken of, frequently language is used which seems to imply a belief that the medical profession is divided as it were into two camps, respectively of "contagionists" and

---

[1] See E.E. Hume, 'Pettenkofer's Theory of the Aetiology of Cholera, Typhoid Fever, and Other Intestinal Diseases — A Review of His Arguments and Evidence', *Ann. Med. Hist.* 7 (1925), 319–53; N. Howard-Jones, 'Gelsenkirchen Typhoid Epidemic of 1901, Robert Koch, and the Dead Hand of Max von Pettenkofer', *Br. Med. J.* 1973, i. 103–5. *Med. Times Gaz.* 1854, ii. 550.

[2] Budd, 'Observations on Typhoid', p.625.

"anticontagionists".' Simon's own view was that, 'speaking of course of the medical profession as represented by its acknowledged teachers', no such duality of opinion existed. No one denied the fact of contagion itself, nor that contagion was modified by different circumstances in different diseases. Opinion was not dictated by any *a priori* belief, but had been arrived at pragmatically in each different case.[1] This view is a just one, and it is a demerit of Budd's work that it has encouraged the oversimplified view.

None the less it may have been his only possible approach, given the diversity and even inconsistency of the views which differed from his own. Budd could rarely be sure, for instance, when the word 'contagious' was used, that it held any meaning which he himself would recognise. Other writers found it possible to say that a contagious disease under certain circumstances became epidemic, or even that a disease when strongly epidemic became contagious. For Budd this language could only mean that the morbific agent was supposed to come into being in some condition and in some mode of development other than that which occurred when it was propagated directly from one individual to another. To say of typhoid that it was by nature non-contagious, but that it could become contagious under certain circumstances was, unless it were meant only that its *propagation* required certain conditions, a 'flagrant inconsistency'.[2]

As early as 1849 Budd used the argument that many human diseases could not be induced in the lower animals most closely resembling man, and that if the poison could not reproduce itself in this similar environment it was extremely unlikely that it could do so in mere filth.[3] Here Budd had a problem which Henle, who allowed his agents an active life outside the body, would not have had. The more Budd's contemporaries agreed with him that morbid poisons were in some way peculiar to the body, the less likely they were to think of them as independent organisms of fixed species. One trend was part of the germ theory as it was then developing;

---

[1] Budd, *Typhoid Fever*, p.5; Simon, *Public Health Reports*, ii. 236–7.

[2] Budd, 'Variola Ovina, Sheep's Smallpox', pp.146–7; idem, *Typhoid Fever*, p.37. For a similar statement by Snow, see *Snow on Cholera*, pp.171–2.

[3] Budd, *Malignant Cholera*, pp.14–15.

the other was not. Budd's only resource, the analogy of obligate parasitism, was an insufficient one.

Budd's first reaction to Liebig's account of Thiersch's experiments was enthusiastic, but the chief if not the only reason for this was Liebig's inference that cholera was to be prevented by the use of 'the well known preventives of fermentation and putrefaction', that is by disinfection; Budd was delighted to have such support. Even so he was careful to add (respectfully) that his own interpretation of the experiments differed 'in many essential points' from that of the Munich chemists. It was, in short, more specific. This latter principle he retained; but some years later he stated that he had 'long ago observed that the discharges of typhoid fever and of Asiatic cholera do not develop their full infectious power at first'. The reason for this was, he thought, that in these diseases as well as in phthisis the excreta were cast off in pellets, and some kind of fermentation was required before the germs could be freed of this 'organic husk' and released into the air as impalpable atoms. In 1873, he emphasized that this fermentation conferred no new powers but merely brought those already existing into play. In a note on Thiersch's experiments he criticized them on the grounds first that mice were probably not susceptible to cholera, and second that it had not been shown that mice thus poisoned had the power to communicate cholera to other mice, in the same way as (in his view) cholera-stricken men communicated cholera to other men.[1] Budd's explicitness at this later time was probably due to the increasing influence in Germany if not in England of Pettenkofer's theory, which Thiersch's experiments were said to support. This theory was difficult to combat because of its complexity, and because Pettenkofer himself concentrated on finding instances of the local and seasonal conditions he had previously defined. While apparently agreeing with Budd and later with Koch as to the nature of the agent, he made

---

[1] Liebig, 'Etiology of Cholera'; School of Hygiene Papers, William Budd to [Dr. A. Smith], 23 Dec. 1854 [copy?]; Budd, 'Cholera: its Cause and Prevention', pp.1156–7. Idem, *Second Report of Royal Sanitary Commission*, p.45 [603]; idem, *Typhoid Fever*, pp.75, 91–2 n. Budd did not mention Sanderson's experiments, in which material from 'mice thus poisoned' was used to induce the same condition in other mice. For Budd's appreciation of 'Koch's postulates', see 'On the Occurrence of Malignant Pustule in England', *Lancet*, 1862, ii. 164.

all its powers depend on events outside the body. Budd complained that Pettenkofer's theory was 'couched . . . in terms so vague and mysterious that I never myself feel quite sure of exactly understanding what it involves'.[1] He combated it not by trying to find counter-instances but by stressing, in the terms already described, that the agent was sufficient in itself to cause disease.

The rival conception to which Budd paid most attention was the pythogenic theory. This term was the creation of Charles Murchison, author of the standard compendium on continued fevers. Murchison, a close relative of the geologist Sir Roderick Murchison and the intimate friend and editor of the botanist and palaeontologist Hugh Falconer, took up the profession of his father and graduated in medicine with high honours at Edinburgh in 1851. After gaining further education and experience in Turin, Edinburgh, Dublin, and Paris, he entered the service of the East India Company and made observations on the climate and diseases of India and of Burma. He settled in London, and began taking up medical appointments, in 1855; most importantly in the present context, he was assistant physician and then physician to the London Fever Hospital from 1856. Of considerable reputation as a clinical teacher, he was also a prolific and fluent author and achieved European recognition for his works on fever and diseases of the liver. Murchison further exercised his characteristic talents as a botanist and chemist. He was said to possess 'the genius of thoroughness' and to be 'essentially British . . . in his solidity, in his honesty, in his plainness'.[2] A follower of Louis, Murchison showed every sign of commitment to the prevailing 'inclusive' methodology.

On his own account Murchison was taught (about 1850) to regard typhus and typhoid as mere varieties of the one disease, and altered this view when he joined the London Fever Hospital and read the works of A.P. Stewart and of

---

[1] Budd, *Typhoid Fever*, p.91. For a tabulated comparison between Pettenkofer's and Koch's theories, see Hume, 'Pettenkofer's Theory', pp.343 ff.

[2] Obituary, *Br. Med. J.* 1879, i. 648. For Charles Murchison (1830–79), M.R.C.S. Edinburgh 1850, M.D. Edinburgh 1851, M.R.C.P. 1855, F.R.C.P. 1859, F.R.S. 1866, see *DNB*.

William Jenner.[1] He subsequently classified the continued fevers into four types. Of the three which were specific (the fourth being 'simple' fever), typhus and relapsing fever were 'epidemic'; enteric, typhoid, or 'pythogenic' fever was 'endemic'. Pythogenic fever provided a link between the contagious continued fevers (like typhus), and the remittent fevers, and its analogies were with these latter rather than with the eruptive diseases like smallpox. Like the remittents, pythogenic fever was not contagious. The remittents were caused by the emanations from decaying vegetable matter; pythogenic fever, similarly, by the poison arising from certain forms of (animal) organic matter in a peculiar state of decomposition. Fever caused by air and water polluted by putrefying sewage was always pythogenic fever. Although contact with the sick was neither sufficient nor necessary to bring it about, the disease was communicable. 'As in dysentery and cholera, the alvine discharges appear to constitute the chief, if not the sole, medium of communication.' However, no specific poison was given off by the bowels; the fresh evacuations were harmless. As in cholera, the poison was developed during their putrefaction. Thiersch's experiments had been done solely with the specific discharges; Murchison therefore went so far as to say it was probable that 'the stools of enteric fever are more prone than ordinary sewage to the specific fermentation by which the poison was produced'.[2] This form of communication was, however, rare; more often the disease originated spontaneously.

Murchison's work was a faithful reflection of the contemporary context, and this is only a little less true of the edition of 1873, in which he made certain adjustments to his theory. One must therefore be critical of the large class of writers of which Adam Patrick is an example: 'Charles Murchison, the best known fever physician of his time, believed that typhoid might originate spontaneously from dirt. This old fashioned

---

[1] Murchison, *Treatise on Continued Fevers* (1862), Preface. Murchison's history with respect to his ideas on typhoid fever was not unusual; for the views of older medical men in the late 1850s see Acland, *Fever in Agricultural Districts*. Acland was fifteen years older than Murchison; Simon, notably, was only a year younger than Acland.

[2] Murchison, *Treatise on Continued Fevers*, pp.3, 466, 487.

view of his was rather surprising, for he was only 32 when his great treatise . . . was published.'[1] Murchison's work 'pythogenic', which he introduced in 1858, did not mean 'born of filth' but 'born of putrescence' and therefore signified as much the *process* taking place in the substance, as the substance itself. Sufficient has been said of the contemporary interest in and importance of this concept of process. An indication of its part in the germ theory is given by Murchison himself.

The recent researches of Beale, Sanderson, and Chauveau [he stated] . . . have gone far to prove that the virulence of contagious liquids is due to the presence of minute solid particles of organic matter derived from the human organism, and these particles are probably the degraded offspring of some kind of normal living matter incapable of returning to its previous healthy state but capable of being *developed de novo* in plants and animals living under conditions adverse to health.

There was no proof, he concluded, that these particles were endowed with the power of self-multiplication. Probably, like tubercle or pus corpuscles, they excited '*by contact*' a fresh formation of similar particles in the human body.[2]

In addition, of course, it is wrong to say that Murchison thought typhoid arose spontaneously in dirt. Like the majority of his contemporaries, Murchison thought that typhoid might arise in organic matter which had been part of an animal body, by a variety of molecular action.

The *Treatise* became a standard work because it was comprehensive and informative. Its method was avowedly that of Louis; matters of symptomology, pathology, and aetiology were if possible reduced to a numerical expression. Murchison's membership of the London Medical Society of Observation was evidently better than nominal. The backbone of his work was the extensive case-histories and other records kept by the London Fever Hospital. His most striking evidence for the non-contagiousness of typhoid was statistical: between 1848 and 1870, he stated, the hospital admitted 5,988 cases of enteric fever but in that time only seventeen of its residents contracted the disease.[3] Matters of policy in hospitals, such

[1] A. Patrick, *The Enteric Fevers, 1800–1920* (Edinburgh, 1955), p.22. Dolman, art. 'Budd', *DSB*, is a more recent example.

[2] Murchison, *Treatise on Continued Fevers*, p.12. Murchison's italics.

[3] Ibid. (1862), Preface. Ibid. (1884), p.462; for an earlier version covering ten years, see idem, 'Contributions to the Etiology of Continued Fever', *Med. Chir. Trans.* 41 (1858), 219–306.

as whether enteric cases should be distributed among patients labouring under other, non-infectious diseases, were decided on the basis of these figures. This evidence is the same in kind as that offered by Snow in his comparison of London water supplies. Murchison's use of case-histories of epidemics also resembled Snow's rather than Budd's; that is, instead of being selective, on the basis of theoretical or methodological premisses, he thought that there was the same requirement of explanation in each case. His theory therefore represents the sum total of these requirements. Of Budd's mode of reasoning he said, significantly, 'If, because a disease can be proved to be in a few instances communicated by the sick, it can never arise in any other way, there is an end of all discussion of the matter; but this does not seem to me to be a scientific decision of the question at issue.'[1]

To some extent the danger for Budd of Murchison's theory lay in its resemblance to his own. Like Budd, Murchison thought that the diseases he dealt with were specific, and among the grounds he adduced were firstly that one kind or species never gave rise to another, and secondly that a given attack conferred immunity from that and no other disease. It was also his belief that 'no new species of continued fever had appeared among us, and the type of each has changed little, if at all'. Opinions to the contrary were to be ascribed to imperfect diagnosis; the reason why diagnosis was imperfect and why many thought the continued fevers were all phases of the one disease, was that too much reliance had been placed on symptomology and pathology, and not enough on causation. As in cases of poisoning, 'the most philosophic classification [of diseases] must be one which is based on their aetiology'. Simon praised Murchison for this 'effort to trace different fevers to different aetiological relations'. Murchison adopted a multifactoral structure, but one that was specific; he was able to say that 'if certain conditions are present, we can, with almost certainty [*sic*] predict the result'.[2] A

---

[1] *Br. Med. J.* 1879, i. 649; Murchison, *Treatise on Continued Fevers*, pp.462, 485.

[2] Murchison, *Treatise on Continued Fevers*, p.7. Idem, 'On the Nomenclature and Classification of Continued Fevers', *Edinb. Med. J.* 4 (1858–9), 320, 325; Simon, *Sanitary Institutions*, p.287 n.

cardinal difference between Budd and Murchison was that Murchison thought he could account for the actual origin of the disease.

Budd's later papers on typhoid were written specifically to refute the pythogenic theory, and the later edition of Murchison's *Treatise* in turn dealt explicitly with Budd's work. The arguments used were based on the differences already described. Probably the only difference which might be thought of as crucial (although it was not, during Budd's active lifetime) was that which subsisted between them on the question of spontaneous generation. Neither could 'disprove' the other's theory by resorting to epidemiological evidence. Instances in which a typhoid case could not be traced to a previous one were regarded by Budd as negative evidence; to Murchison they were positive. Both accepted the principle that positive was not to be outweighed by negative evidence. In the event, Budd's theory was 'contained' in Murchison's, in the same way that Snow's was contained in the conclusions of the Committee for Scientific Enquiries. The best illustration of this is provided by a well-known epidemic of typhoid fever in Windsor in 1858. The circumstances of this epidemic were made the subject of a special investigation by Simon as Medical Officer of the Privy Council, and were used in evidence by both Murchison and Budd. Simon's surveyor discovered that one specific fault had pervaded the sewerage (much of it new) of the town. Systematically, it was without adequate exterior ventilation, and systematically, it was inferred, it must have ventilated itself into the houses which communicated with it. Furthermore, in a part of the Castle which had a drain of its own, separate from the town system, there were no cases; in a part of the Royal Mews which connected with the town drains, there were several. The implication of these findings was accepted by all parties. 'That the fever was due to the emanations from the sewers', stated Murchison, 'was the un-disputed opinion of all who investigated the circumstances.' Budd, however, made the apparently gratuitous assumption that these emanations arose only from the excreta of typhoid patients. He was not, of course, able to enforce this assump-tion, and it was concluded on all sides that Simon and Murchison had between them 'very satisfactorily' disposed of the notion that the disease was imported into the town, or was of a contagious nature.[1]

Simon had not been forward in recognizing the distinction between typhus and typhoid, and during his first few years as Medical Officer Budd found nothing to distinguish his views from those of the old General Board of Health. His earliest statement on typhoid came in 1858, when he accepted the definitions of Murchison and Jenner. On the question of contagion, Simon was cautious. He ended by explaining that he could still speak of the continued fevers only as they were registered, as a single form; and that, while the profession might be divided on questions of theory, it was united on the practical point that 'Fever is fostered and spread through those impurities which sanitary measures are intended to banish.'[2] By 1861 his views had undergone a change which Simon himself attributed to the influence of the papers published by Budd in 1859-60.[3] After giving a very fair account of Budd's theory Simon stated that 'the facts which Dr. Budd adduces from his own experience and from that of other observers are, in my opinion, sufficient to prove that the contagion of typhoid fever is importable by persons who have the disease'. On this point Simon found Budd's account of the North Tawton epidemic 'more conclusive than anything previously known to me', but he was not only impressed by the epidemiological evidence. Budd's arguments were also 'cogent to this general effect, — that specially the bowel discharges are means (*yet not therefore necessarily the sole means*) by which a patient, whether migrating or stationary, can be instrumental in spreading the infection of typhoid fever'. As Simon's reports are at this time the sole source of information as to his state of mind one can only conclude that he was impressed by Budd's arguments and by his 'village

---

[1] Murchison, 'On the Causes of Continued Fevers', *Med. Times Gaz.* 1859, i, 253-4; Budd, 'On Intestinal Fever' (1860), pp.187-90, 239-40; idem, *Typhoid Fever*, pp.56 ff.; *1st Rep. of Med. Officer of Privy Council*, PP, 1859, XII. 274; Murchison, *Treatise on Continued Fevers*, p.481; *Med. Times Gaz.* 1858, ii. 634.

[2] Simon, Lecture XII, *Lancet*, 1850, ii. 227; Budd, 'On Intestinal Fever' (1856), p.694; Simon, *Public Health Reports*, i. 444-7. Rather appropriately Simon was quoting this unifying practical dictum from Thomas Watson.

[3] For Budd himself on Simon's change of opinion see 'Mr. Simon on Typhoid Fever at Bedford', *Lancet*, 1861, i. 630; ibid. 1861, ii. 17, and idem, 'Observations on Typhoid', p.457.

epidemiology' to the extent of perceiving a close analogy to exist between typhoid, and cholera as he then saw it. 'Typhoid fever seems to be in its causes as in its nature, very intimately related to other diarrhoeal infections.' It was of practical importance to learn 'whether it is in all states and in all circumstances, *or only in certain states and under certain circumstances*, that the bowel discharges of typhoid fever can effect what is here imputed to them'. Simon then quoted the passage he had written in 1858 referring to the experiments of Thiersch and the theory of Pettenkofer.[1] He singled out a passage of Budd's stating that typhoid was 'one of the great group of diseases which infect the ground'. This may indicate that Simon was responsive to Budd because of his affinity to Pettenkofer, although it must have been clear that Budd merely thought the specific discharges were cast on the ground and could from there infect both air and water.

Simon agreed with Budd to the extent of stating that 'where any disease is possessed of infectious powers, the discharges which characterise the disease are likely to be its chief means of spreading infection', but it is plain that he thought of typhoid not as akin to smallpox but as forming a special class with cholera. After 1861, the two alvine diseases, cholera and typhoid, were dealt with together.[2] In this connection Simon may be described as a contingent contagionist, some little distance from Budd but about the same distance from Murchison.

Budd could achieve no more than this with indirect evidence, a fact of which he was himself well aware. Given the circumstances, especially the peculiar status of typhoid fever, it was not an inconsiderable achievement. Budd's contention that experimental evidence was the basis of further progress was also borne out by the event, and possibly prompted some of the research carried out by Simon's department during its period under the Local Government Board.[3] Budd's own

[1] *3rd Rep. of Med. Officer of Privy Council,* PP, 1861, XVI. 344 n., 345 n. My italics.

[2] See e.g. in 1863: Simon, *Public Health Reports,* ii, 153.

[3] See e.g. E. Klein, 'Report on the Pathology of Sheeppox', Appendix to *3rd Rep. (N.S.) of Med. Officer of Privy Council and Local Govt. Board,* PP, 1874, XXXI. 403–14; idem, 'Report on the So-called Enteric or Typhoid Fever of the Pig', Appendix to *8th Rep. (N.S.) of Med. Officer of Privy Council and Local Govt. Board,* PP, 1876, XXXVIII, pp.569–79. On Klein, see Lambert, *John Simon,* p.569.

willingness to go beyond a single proposition, combined with the integrity of his approach, and his concern for the relief of unnecessary suffering, were respected by his contemporaries, if not often understood.

8

CONCLUSIONS

The years after 1865, dominated as they were by the successes of Pasteur, Lister, and Koch, have been the subject of so much adulatory and other attention that little further comment need, perhaps, be attempted. In any case, the 'dawn of the germ theory' cannot be described here, although it should be emphasized that, as there is a continuity of interest detectable through the first part of the century, so there is no discontinuity between later developments and those which have been of most concern in this book.[1] The experimental work done under the Cattle Plague Commissioners in 1865–6, and the 'Scientific Researches' instituted by Simon in 1865, may be said factitiously to have marked a kind of transition. 1866 was also the last year in which cholera prevailed in England as an epidemic. A feature of interest connected with this outbreak was the revival of the fungus theory of cholera. Ernst Hallier announced in Germany that the cause of the disease was proved experimentally to be a form of a fungal parasite of rice. This theory at first caused some sensation, and was then rapidly abandoned.[2] Its failure indicates how little the emergent germ theories were concerned with free-living organisms of recognizable species as the agents in disease.

The practical instructions issued by Simon at the time of the last cholera epidemic are indicative both of the influence upon him of original theories like Budd's and Pettenkofer's, and of the limits of that influence. In Simon the medical profession and 'official doctrine' became reconciled, but the dichotomy between medical theory and sanitary practice emphasized in the first chapters remained. This dichotomy,

---

[1] This is made clear by J.K. Crellin in 'The Dawn of the Germ Theory — Particles, Infection, and Biology', *Medicine and Science in the 1860s*, ed. F.N.L. Poynter (1969), pp.57–76.

[2] That cholera might in some way be related to an affection of rice was proposed at the time of the first epidemic.

or discrepancy, is perhaps bound to persist where practical issues are able to take precedence; but Simon's position is made clearer when it is realized how much scope there still was for simple sanitary improvement. The sanitary generalizations of the early period were carried well into the 1870s, but this was not a measure so much of conservatism as of their continued relevance to existing conditions.[1] The most difficult institutional and political problems remained; health had been shown to depend upon the public ownership of water companies, legal powers of compulsion and prosecution, and a uniform control of local administration. These changes were resisted under the usual rubrics by a variety of forces and interests, which were able to bring about a situation regarded by some reformers as retrogressive.

How much sanitarianism had been able to achieve in real terms remains difficult to assess, but it cannot be assumed that any form of interference necessarily produced a situation better than (as opposed to different from) that which had existed before. Cholera stayed away after 1866, but a formidable outbreak of smallpox, a disease which had been preventable since the eighteenth century, caused 42,000 deaths in England and Wales during 1871 and 1872, and scarlatina destroyed 82,000 persons between 1868 and 1870.[2] Water (and milk) supply had not reached that state of perfection necessary for the prevention of typhoid; cholera, as already mentioned, was probably held at bay chiefly by a combination of natural factors and improved measures of quarantine. This is, of course, to speak in terms merely of epidemics, which, as previously stressed, were not responsible for the major proportion even of preventable deaths. The historian's concentration on epidemics is in part a result of the sanitarian's attempts to establish a category of preventable diseases, together with the natural tendency of the public mind to fasten briefly upon noticeable excesses of disease. Attention tends to be given to the centralized phase of sanitarianism more or less automatically, but occasionally on the ground that no earlier phase can be regarded as effec-

---

[1] See **A.P. Stewart** and **E. Jenkins**, *Medical and Legal Aspects of Sanitary Reform* (1867; 1969).

[2] Creighton, *Epidemics*, ii. 614–15, 627.

tive. Clearly the criterion of effectiveness must be carefully defined if it is not, when strictly applied, to exclude later as well as earlier periods.

There have been few attempts to do justice to the theoretical developments of the first half of the nineteenth century. This applies especially to theories of fever, which were fundamentally related to issues in epidemiology. It is generally assumed that the years before 1850 were, in England, distinguished by their human and political rather than their scientific qualities. The second half of the century then provides a direct contrast, in seeing the growth of experimentalism and scientific medicine in general, as well as the beginnings of modern bacteriology. The period of public-health reform is made an immediate precursor of the bacteriological period, even though health reform, being integrally related to other aspects of reform, had begun on the local level very much earlier. It may also be noted that such a chronology does not allow for the coincidence, in the latter half of the century of strenuous and probably more effective sanitarianism with the early successes of bacteriology. That the sanitary period immediately preceded the bacteriological is one of the assumptions made by those who see nineteenth-century epidemiology in terms of a struggle between opposites, with the health of the population at stake — the historical irony allegedly being that, although one theory was wrong and the other right, the health of the population (at least potentially) did almost as well out of one as the other. The competing theories involved in this particular historical approach were, of course, the miasmatic theory of the sanitarians, and the *contagium vivum* theories of such pioneers as Snow and Budd. A later refinement of this interpretation is that nineteenth-century medicine was in some state of crisis or revolution, corresponding to a similar state in society as a whole, and that crisis naturally breeds 'new things' and opposite opinions.

This is the traditional view, which persists in such studies as Underwood's introductory essay to Creighton's *History of Epidemics*, a work now widely used by historians in general, as well as by specialists. It is also the view adopted in the only major attempt to estimate the merits and wider significance of the epidemiology of the first half of the century.[1] Although written as long ago as 1948, Ackerknecht's paper has not been superseded, and is still regularly if not exclusively used to cover this aspect of nineteenth-century history. It is only fair to its author to concede that his work has enjoyed this long supremacy partly because it refers to an extremely wide range of sources, French, German, and American as well as English, and pays particular attention to active and previously neglected writers including Charles Maclean. Ackerknecht's main conclusion is that an attitude of thought appropriately called anticontagionism attracted liberal-minded activists early in the century, and increased in influence until a peak was reached in the middle of the century, just before its final downfall:

> It was, curiously enough, in the first half of the 19th century, that is shortly before their final and overwhelming victory, that the theories of contagion and the contagium vivum experienced the deepest depression and devaluation in their long and stormy career, and it was shortly before its disappearance that 'anticontagionism' reached its highest peak of elaboration, acceptance, and scientific respectability.[2]

Ackerknecht gives as evidence for this mid-century peak, a number of recommendations issued with respect to the second cholera epidemic, and the conclusion that anticontagionist views had received government sanction for the first time, in the reports of Chadwick's General Board of Health. His argument is based partly on the attitudes taken towards quarantine, an issue which is treated as inextricably related to the question of contagion.[3]

As well as asserting the reality of these radical shifts of opinion, however, Ackerknecht also states that the rival explanations were so finely balanced, and both so inadequate to explain the phenomena, that each man's decision was determined not by scientific but by social, economic, and political factors:

> I am afraid that, forced to decide ourselves a hundred years ago on the

---

[1] viz. Ackerknecht, 'Anticontagionism 1821–1867'.

[2] Ibid., p.565.

[3] Historically, this was in a sense true, but the relation was as complex as all other contemporary relations between theory and practice. See e.g. Chadwick in the more conciliatory *Second Report on Quarantine*, where a belated attempt was made to dissociate the two questions: pp.2 ff.

basis of the existing materials, we would have had a very hard time. Intellectually and rationally the two theories balanced each other too evenly. Under such conditions the accident of personal experience and temperament, and especially economic outlook and political loyalties will determine the decision. These, being liberal and bourgeois in the majority of the physicians of the time brought about the victory of anticontagionism. It is typical that the ascendancy of anticontagionism coincides with the rise of liberalism, its decline with the victory of the reaction.[1]

Anticontagionism therefore presents what the author himself sees as a paradox, that of an eminently progressive movement based on a wrong (and therefore retrogressive) scientific theory.

The present book has dealt only with the English scene, and it seems certain that a different series of situations prevailed in France at least. This is certainly what was believed by English writers of the time. However, Ackerknecht's whole approach is open to strong objections. Although one welcomes the incorporation into the argument of factors other than what are regarded as the purely scientific, the result in this case is a very uneasy alliance between a recognition of the importance of these factors, and a conviction of the superiority of *contagium vivum* theories of any description, and of the inferior claims of what is set up as their opposite, the miasmatic theory. All theories of contagion are treated as having some essential relation to *contagium vivum* theories, and all theories of contagion and *contagium vivum*, as if they entailed eventual adherence to nineteenth-century germ theory. The latter in its turn is regarded as an early form of twentieth-century bacteriology. Similarly, all theories involving miasma, and all 'filth theories', are identified as anticontagionist. Thus Liebig, because he opposed biological explanations in disease as well as in other areas, becomes an anticontagionist.[2] Again because Ackerknecht deals in opposites, he has to find that the convinced anticontagionist majority of the 1850s reverted to contagionism in the 1860s. This shift, as might be expected, presents him with no diffi-

---

[1] Ackerknecht, 'Anticontagionism 1821–1867', p.589. This duality of intention is evident throughout the article, and corresponds to the author's inclusion of statements apparently modifying his main conclusions: see e.g. ibid., pp.568–9.

[2] Ibid., p.580.

culties of explanation, since it merely represents the gradual but inexorable and inevitable effect of theories such as those of Snow and Budd, which brought about the 'final and over-whelming victory'. The reader will remember that it was the period around 1860 which saw the notably contingent approaches to typhoid fever of John Simon and Charles Murchison.

Very little indication is given of the content or implication of the decision for or against contagion. The reader is merely obliged to assume that this was regularly correlated with other factors, and in sum as considerable as decisions taken to determine social, religious, or political allegiances. Yet, it is also claimed that the medical man's commitment was decided not by anything in contagionism or anticontagionism itself, but by other factors entirely.

The over-simplification of the more medical aspects is necessarily matched by an equal over-simplification both of the structure of the medical profession during the period in question, and of political change and opinion either at any one time in the first half of the century, or over the period as a whole. This tendency includes an important misrepresentation of the peculiarly complex relation in the nineteenth century between theories and practical decisions. Ackerknecht treats this relation as invariably direct or even as one of identity: practical decisions are no more than the 'supreme test of one's convictions'.[1] Thus the relation between sanitary theory and practice is misrepresented by the historian, as it was by Chadwick and Southwood Smith as a matter of policy a century before.

With respect to the specific areas of interest of this book, the chief objection to Ackerknecht's account must be his dependence on the 'official status' of the miasmatic theory as evidence of its dominance in mid-nineteenth-century epidemiological thought. Apart from the more theoretical aspects, it is obvious that Chadwick's General Board was not comparable as an institution with the Royal College of Physicians; its adoption of theoretical principles was not the last stage in the adoption of these principles by the medical

---

[1] Ibid., p.589.

profession at large. Instead, the Board operated independently of, and latterly in opposition to, the profession. The anti-contagionism which existed in the 1850s was, as we have seen, not a reflection of the will of the profession, but a repetition of earlier polemic, produced in haste as an attempt to dominate executive opinion and pre-empt anticipated opposition. This being the case, it is hardly necessary to suggest that however 'bourgeois' the 1840s and 1850s, these decades could hardly be called triumphantly liberal, and the 1860s by contrast a period of reaction. Nor can Chadwick and Southwood Smith, the most steadfast adherents of a position legitimately called anticontagionism, be defined except as advocates of State interference, a position which was then compatible with a belief in the freedom of capital.[1]

Another point which may be stressed is the number of current factors tending towards an independent assessment of each disease or disease state, even where 'varieties' rather than 'species' were thought to be in question, and where a range of conditions was regarded as attributable to a single cause. Under such conditions a bilateral division of opinion is not to be expected. Moreover, aetiology was itself not a single concept, or by any means a constant or dominant pre-occupation. English medical men were, as already pointed out, resistant to continental developments aimed at undermining the 'natural history' concept of disease, and this commitment to specificity was further reinforced by the clinically and epidemiologically oriented English equivalent of the French pathologico-anatomical school. The English therefore reacted more or less flexibly to the increased prevalence of the not-very-infectious diseases like typhoid and cholera.

The most adaptable were conditioned by their consideration of intermittent, remittent, and continued fevers as a set of related conditions dependent for their variety upon a range of factors (especially the environmental), and for their causation on the putrefaction of organic matter. However, it should be stressed that most of the profession saw the relevant developments of the early and mid-nineteenth century as contributing to a modification of the definition of con-

---

[1] But see Finer, *Life of Chadwick*, pp.475 ff.

tagion; although the activity of the period cannot be assessed in such narrow terms without misrepresentation. It will be remembered that the reviews of Southwood Smith's work of 1830 were as concerned about his mode of treatment, his denial of the existence of simple or essential fever, and the likelihood that his book would mislead the young practitioner, as they were about his 'anticontagionism'. This reflects the normal balance of interests, which became distorted, as it very often did in the nineteenth century, by the necessity of deciding on a public position. However, it is interesting that when the reviewers dealt with Smith's definitions of 'contagion' and 'epidemic', he was attacked as much for the first as for the second, in terms very similar to those used against the Board of Health's reports in the medical journals of the late 1840s. It is clear from this that professional opinion in general was at a very early stage thinking in terms of the influence of environmental factors in combination even with the contagion of archetypally contagious, indigenous diseases.

The implication of these objections seems to be that Ackerknecht's account, for all its apparent concessions to science and medicine as integrally related or even similar to other contemporary activity, is really only a sophistication of the unhistorical accounts found in such sources as Frazer's *History of English Public Health*. It is particularly indicative that Ackerknecht gives very little attention to the complexities of 'continued fever' which, at least with respect to England, is a far more accurate and comprehensive index to current concerns than cholera or yellow fever.[1] The terms 'contagionist' and 'anticontagionist' are an entirely inadequate and misleading summary of these concerns. As far as possible in this book they have been used only in respect of a limited period, or a few specific individuals. Here again the situation for present-day historians has tended to become as confused and as unproductive as it was for some nineteenth-century

---

[1] Ackerknecht considers 'Typhus and Anticontagionism' for little over a page (op. cit., pp.586–7), pointing to the difficulty of analysis because of the late differentiation of typhoid and typhus. Typhoid itself is mentioned only in passing. The 'later representatives' of anticontagionism, 'the English sanitarians (Chadwick, Southwood Smith, John Simon, etc.) or Pettenkofer and his followers' are treated in a 'very summary way', because of the existence of recent discussions elsewhere: ibid., pp.569–70.

theorists. Unless it is seriously misleading, this terminology lacks the content which would entitle it to any level of significance or general application. When it is used, or described as having been used, it cannot stand alone, without explicit definition.

The complexity and sense of compromise more characteristic of the whole period in question, were most obviously expressed in the widespread use of analogy. A dependence on analogy, whether admitted or not, was, as has been shown, common not only to Budd, Snow, and other 'germ theorists', but also to the majority of those interested in the subject of epidemic disease. It is noticeable that, in times of emergency, medical men were at once more likely to use analogies, and less likely to tolerate this form of reasoning in others. Obviously one would not wish to claim that the profession was at all times as dependent upon analogy as it was in relation to the problems imposed by the doubtful diseases. None the less, it is clear that in considering the growth of any branch of medicine in the nineteenth century, attention must be given to a wide range of other developments occurring at the same time. The influence of Liebigian chemistry on mid-nineteenth-century theories of disease is the plainest proof of this.

Stress has been placed on Liebig's provision, by analogy with his account of fermentation and putrefaction, of a notion of process in epidemic disease. The immediate and generalized use of his ideas means that interest in this aspect of the disease phenomenon was current rather earlier than some writers have imagined. It is claimed that 'the history of biology gives evidence of the growing reliance of the biologist on mechanical and physical analogy', and in this the use by sanitarians and medical men of Liebig's version of 'contagious molecular action', as well as their adoption of the details of the fermentation analogy, could perhaps be included.[1] However, it should be stressed that this usage was to a large extent self-conscious, the aim being to acquire the status and benefits of the methodology of natural philosophy. Other ideas and attitudes existed, especially in medicine, which tended to limit the scope of reductionism, or to make it controversial. Again,

---

[1] E. Mendelsohn, *Heat and Life* (Camb., Mass., 1964), p.3.

as in the case of the 'contagionism versus anticontagionism' dichotomy, the reader must place contemporary usage in its context, and estimate its weight.

As some later nineteenth-century writers were aware, bacteriology, like the cholera fungus, provided no substitute for the explanations of the disease process offered by biochemical theories.[1] Bacteriology was, as Shryock has remarked, inherently dramatic; but while it may have revitalised the practical side of medicine, it is permissible to emphasize that, in spite of its successes, it offered no satisfactory explanation of disease.[2] One school of thought defines progress in epidemiology as progress towards the doctrine of *contagium vivum*; at the other extreme, nineteenth-century bacteriology is seen as a deviation from the norm of substituting physico-chemical for special biological explanations. It is perhaps more reasonable to regard bacteriology and biochemistry as parallel developments, historically rather different from the separate disciplines of today, which were complementary, but which sometimes clashed. Liebig and Pasteur were brought into confrontation but, whatever the nature of Liebig's personal defeats, he was by that time not responsible for the further development of 'extracellular' biochemistry, and it cannot be maintained that this development was made discontinuous by his disputes with Pasteur. More importantly, Liebig and Pasteur cannot be categorized as representing reductionism and vitalism respectively.

It has been claimed that, as the prevailing climate of opinion was anticontagionist, so contagionist theories were uniquely at a disadvantage in the mid-century period. The extent and depth of the cholera-fungus controversy of 1849, should perhaps be sufficient to cast doubt on this assumption. However, it has occurred to few later writers to doubt the justice of Baly and Gull's conclusions, and the modern reader, even if unimpressed by the College's report itself, might be tempted to think the 'cholera-fungus' irrelevant to the history of disease theory except as an unfortunate aberration on the

---

[1] See e.g. Thudichum, 'On the Discoveries of Liebig', p.128.

[2] R.H. Shryock, 'Nineteenth-Century Medicine – Scientific Aspects', *J. World Hist.* 3 (1956–7), 881–908: 900.

part of William Budd.[1] Several arguments may be advanced against this narrow view, some of them historiographical, and all of them having ultimate reference to the theoretical context in which the investigation took place. One historian, Shryock, is prepared to state that 'most of the basic ideas and even some of the procedures shortly to be utilised in the rapid development of bacteriology, parasitology and immunology between 1865 and 1880, had already been marked out by the middle of the century'. Frazer, typically of a certain historical approach, asserts of the middle period that there was 'available' to sanitarians and miasmatists an 'alternative and more cogent' theory, that is, the 'theory of specific contagia'. Shryock's statement rightly emphasizes the continuity between the 'pre-bacteriological' and 'bacteriological' periods; both writers, in rather different ways, invite the question of why, if what they say is true, the cholera-fungus theory should have been so easily dismissed. Paradoxically, however, writers of Frazer's persuasion would be among the first to describe the same theory as aberrant, even though they would extend credit to other investigations made at this time, and would now be obliged to admit that, even on their own terms, the agent in cholera was 'discovered' perhaps four times before Koch isolated it in 1882. These posthumously creditable claims were dismissed or overlooked by contemporaries more or less (according to their different contexts) as easily as were those made by the Bristolians. That Budd's contemporaries had not any anachronistic intuition of the inferior claims of the Bristol investigations, corresponding to the conviction of present-day scientists and some historians, is indicated by the claims occasionally made for them at a later date. In 1885, Francis Fowke was inspired by Koch's recent work to claim for the Bristolians priority in the discovery of the bacillus. This is of interest in that, in the case of cholera, the direct evidence which Koch had for the causal relationship was little different from that offered by the Bristol investigators. In 1884, Arthur Hassall had contested a claim similar to Fowke's in order to establish the priority of

---

[1] See e.g. Simon, *Public Health Reports*, ii. 332; Goodall, *William Budd*, p.91; Brown, 'Snow, the Autumn Loiterer', p.521.

his own observations made in 1854.[1] These claims are significant not for their validity, which is doubtful, but for the effective changes in context which they reflect. It may be noted that in the mid-century, others besides Budd, who are now also regarded with some reverence, were inclined to think along similar lines.[2]

The interests of the present-day scientist and the historian are therefore somewhat divorced. Historically, the cholera-fungus controversy must be regarded as a series of events at least as valid and interesting as others similarly based. Several of the answers to the main question, that is, why the claims of the Bristolians were so easily discounted, have already been given. As we have seen, the Bristol theory did not fail because of fallacies in the original investigation, or through a lack of publicity. It was not opposed by better or more thorough research. Instead, research of a lower standard won greater respect. Institutional factors were important, as much in the origin of the theory as in its trial and defeat. Shared methodological or philosophical preconceptions were also operative. Most importantly, as we have seen in earlier chapters, a broadly based theoretical commitment to which biological explanations appeared irrelevant, was already in existence. The chemical and instrumental resources which also prompted the cholera-fungus theory and decided the terms in which it was discussed, were regularly and consistently an integral part of this commitment, which included an emphasis on physiology and humoral pathology. The demand made of *contagium vivum* theorists in the early 1840s, that they produce 'ocular proof' of their hypotheses, was highly characteristic, chiefly as a reflection of current epistemology, but also as evidence of the reliance upon clinical and post-mortem observation and micropathology. The reception of the cholera-fungus theory, which might have been supposed to have pro-

---

[1] Shryock, *Development of Modern Medicine*, p.267. See also A.P. Usher, 'The Development of the Microscope and its Application to Medicine and Public Health', *Am. J. Pharm. Educ.* 15 (1951), 319–38: 332. W.M. Frazer, *The History of English Public Health 1834–1939* (1950), p.39; De, *Cholera: Its Pathology and Pathogenesis*, p.15; Fowke, 'The First Discovery of the Comma Bacillus', *Br. Med. J.* 1885, i. 589–92; Clayton, *Memoir of Hassall*, pp.7 ff.

[2] See e.g. Lister, *Third Huxley Lecture*, p.9.

vided the 'ocular proof', shows the difference in complexity between comment and actual response.

Writers adopting Frazer's approach are obliged to find incredible both the acceptance of the one theory (the miasmatic) and the repudiation of its opposite, 'more cogent' extreme, specific contagia. No such difficulty arises with respect to the theories of disease process and propagation based on the principle of contagious molecular action. The cholera-fungus theory, therefore, was predictably dismissed, although as much a reflection of its context, institutionally and philosophically, as the 'successful' theories just mentioned. Similar points may be made about Snow and Budd. Both were in many respects at odds with their contemporaries; their theories were regarded as unsafe, and unscientific. Generalized sanitary propaganda, rather than the dogmatic position occupied by Southwood Smith, was a success; this, being compatible with other important trends and in particular with the strenuous efforts made to inculcate the elements of normal physiology and the 'laws of health', prepared a doubting, and even condemnatory, response to single-factor theories. Yet even Snow and Budd were in certain respects typical; Snow used statistical methods, and Budd another contemporary resource, the smallpox analogy. Ironically enough, the content of Snow's speculations as to the nature of the disease agent were highly typical of his period.

The cholera-fungus controversy is a useful example because it resembles, and yet differs from, incidents on which emphasis is usually placed. This might have been an insufficient ground for selection, had not the controversy also been of interest as one of the chief incidents of a cholera year, involving a wide range of preconceptions, persons, and institutions. Less for its own sake than as a means to an end, it serves as a useful test of prevailing assumptions.

The nature of controversy is of interest as well as its subject matter, and one relevant concept identified by modern commentators is that of the priority dispute. A scientist's interest in recognition has been described as the 'motivational counterpart on the psychological plane to the emphasis on originality on the institutional plane'.[1] This description seems laborious, but its terminology is at least preferable to that of what can only be called sensationalist accounts of disputes between investigators. That recognition by his colleagues of his claim to a discovery is the scientist's only 'property right' is a fact of which struggling nineteenth-century doctors were perhaps more aware than are members of the highly developed research professions with which modern analysts are primarily concerned. Brittan and Swayne were, for example, the most newly qualified members of the Microscopical Subcommittee, and consequently had both leisure and motive for persevering with their discovery. Various claims were put in during the first week of the cholera-fungus controversy; most were claims to the 'first sighting' of what promised to be, if not the actual agent of disease, at least a new species of organism. One reason which might be given for this and similar exhibitions of the 'collector's spirit' is the want of a developed 'rewards system' in nineteenth-century English medicine and science. Again, with respect to medicine at least, this must refer to the inequities of professional competition within an established structure, rather than the entire absence of system or rewards.

It has also been pointed out that, since few can actually achieve the goal of originality on which such stress is laid, value is also placed on disinterestedness in the discoverer himself. Ideally, of course, there are no priority disputes, and a man is not obliged to defend his own claim. The values thus referred to are illustrated by Brittan's fortune in the cholera-fungus controversy, which was that of acquiring a credit in the profession which survived the rejection of the discovery itself. Brittan first won approval by submitting his facts to his professional peers before publishing them. Later, in his reply to Swayne's claim, he brought himself even further into line with avowed professional standards by taking the bold step of dispensing with the question of priority altogether.[2] The only claim he made was to the virtues of industry,

---

[1] R.K. Merton, 'Priorities in Scientific Discovery: A Chapter in the Sociology of Science', *The Sociology of Science*, ed. B. Barber and W. Hirsch (New York, 1962), pp.447–85: 455.

[2] Brittan, *Morning Chronicle*, 25 Sept. 1849.

method, and caution. His refusal to express an opinion on the implications of his discovery, and his deference to future investigation, made even Swayne's brief conclusions look like a major speculative excursion. Budd, of course, was almost universally disapproved of, though it should be stressed that there were forms of originality in medical thought and practice more likely to be tolerated than aetiological speculation.

This recognition of Brittan's merits was very general. In spite of the complaints that the medical men appointed to government posts were not those whom the profession would itself have chosen, it can be assumed that in appointing Brittan an Inspector, the General Board of Health was demonstrating that it shared some of the same values. It is important to notice that these values did not include that placed on originality of the most significant kind, since the Board was unlikely to appoint anyone of eccentric theoretical convictions, its own eccentricity notwithstanding. There is no doubt of the scientist's, or even of the general, recognition of originality in principle, but some analyses seem to ignore the immediate real effects of radical innovation. Many 'priority claims' are ratified or even made retrospectively, for to be deeply original in any field is to be estranged from a greater or lesser number of contemporaries for a greater or lesser length of time. Here the reception given Brittan may be compared with that experienced by both Budd and Snow. This contrast shows that the immediate approval of the group is reserved for conformity to certain behavioural and then methodological standards — commitments probably of longer term than any other. In the course of this book, many resemblances have been traced between the positions held by Snow and Budd and that taken up by Southwood Smith; the reactions of their different contemporaries were especially similar. In addition, Alexander Tweedie, in the context of the 1830s, serves as a contrast to Smith, and in that way, as a counterpart to Brittan.

In retrospect, it is found that innovation is readily distinguished from aberration, and the onus of self-justification is usually placed on those who resist: that is, in this case, the contemporaries of Snow and Budd, since Smith's reviewers would not be blamed for their attitude to his work. Much of this book has been concerned with defining the commitments which caused the 'delay' in acceptance of Snow's and Budd's theories. There is, in addition, the point that among the criteria for what constitutes a reasonable belief in a given context must be included the role of authority and of consensus. The assumption that evidence plus weight of authority balances apparently more substantial evidence from a less dignified source, must always be resented and usually justifiably, but it is tolerated in most communities. The critics of the Royal College of Physicians, for instance, all envisaged its having a legitimately authoritative role, which was later embodied in the *Reports on Epidemic Cholera* of 1854. The demands made at the time from outside this institution were that it should both advance science and 'preserve the truth'. Naturally, it was rarely seen that these demands might be conflicting. The only realistic demand made of the College at this time was that it should, like a constitutional monarch, give credit where the profession thought it was due.

If medicine can be said to have had a crisis of its own, I would prefer to describe this as one of professionalism, which led, among other things, to the airing in public of what had previously been private dilemmas. The overriding crises of the nineteenth century were social and political, to which medical men, not as a single class, but as members of a range of classes in society, responded according to their different convictions and interests. The intellectual response to crisis is not necessarily, or even generally, dogmatic. In nineteenth-century epidemiology the social and the scientific very plainly meet, and I would argue that the main product of mid-nineteenth-century epidemiology was a kind of compromise; not essentially an area occupied by moderates and the non-committal, but an intelligent position consistent with interest, experience, and methodology alike.

SELECT BIBLIOGRAPHY

No secondary works are entered in this bibliography. Only selected works of the authors of most concern are included, and only key contributions to journals. Most reviews, editorials, and obituaries are not listed. Official reports or submissions by individuals do not appear under the names of their authors but are entered under 'Parliamentary Papers'. Anonymous articles are listed under the name of the periodical in which they were published. Both here and in the footnotes, the place of publication was London unless otherwise stated.

MANUSCRIPT SOURCES AND COLLECTIONS

Dr. Richard Harper of Barnstaple:

> Family Papers

Bristol Central Library:

> Estlin Collection, Boxes 1–3. Unbound, uncatalogued papers of John Bishop Estlin and Mary Estlin.
> Volume of Public Notices, etc., Concerning Miscellaneous Bristol Institutions and Societies.

Bristol Medical Library:

> William Budd Box. Unbound, uncatalogued, miscellaneous.

See also Abbreviations, p. x.

PARLIAMENTARY PAPERS

1804, IV, Pt.2 [no. 28] Report from the Committee to whom the Petition of Members of the Society for Bettering the Condition of the Poor, Respecting the Fever Institution, was referred.

1818, VII. 1. Report from the Select Committee appointed to examine into the State of Contagious Fever in the Metropolis, and the Condition of the Institution for the Cure and Prevention of the Same.

1819, II. 537. Report from the Select Committee appointed to consider the Validity of the Doctrine of Contagion in the Plague.

1824, VI. 165. (Second) Report from the Select Committee appointed to consider of the Means of Improving and Maintaining the Foreign Trade of the Country; Quarantine.

1831-2, I. 323. A Bill for the Prevention . . . of the Disease called the Cholera, or Spasmodic or Indian Cholera, in England.

> 329. [——, Scotland].
> 335. [Bill amending the above].

1833, XXXIV. 99. [Apothecaries, Surgeons, etc. — Certificates, Byelaws, Statistics, and Accounts.]

312   SELECT BIBLIOGRAPHY

1834, XIII. 1. Report from the Select Committee on Medical Education with Minutes of Evidence and Appendix. Pt. I: Royal College of Physicians. Pt. II: Royal College of Surgeons.
1835, XXXVII. 597. [Apothecaries' Company. Copies of Regulations.]
1837–9, XXVIII. Fourth Annual Report of the Poor Law Commissioners. App. A, Suppl. No. I: 'Report on the prevalence of certain physical causes of fever in the metropolis, which might be removed by proper sanatory measures', by *N. Arnott* and *J.P. Kay* (pp.67–83 [215–31]; App. A, No. 2: 'Report on some of the physical causes of sickness and mortality to which the poor are particularly exposed; and which are capable of removal by sanatory regulations', by *T. Southwood Smith* (pp.83–94 [231–42]).
1839, XX. 1. Fifth Annual Report of the Poor Law Commissioners. App. C, No. 2: 'On the prevalence of fever in 20 Metropolitan Parishes or Unions during the year ending 20 March 1838', by *T. Southwood Smith* (pp.100-6 [112–18]).
1842, XXVI (Lords), 1. Report from the Poor Law Commissioners, on an Inquiry into the Sanitary Condition of the Labouring Population of Great Britain. 'Report on the Sanitary Condition of the Labouring Population of Great Britain', by *E. Chadwick* (pp.xxi-xxxii; 1–457).
   XXVII (Lords). Local Reports on the Sanatory Condition of the Labouring Population of Great Britain.
   XXVIII (Lords). Reports on the Sanatory Condition of the Labouring Population of Scotland. 'Report on the fevers which have prevailed in Edinburgh and Glasgow', by *N. Arnott* (pp.1–13); 'Observations on the Generation of Fever', by *W.P. Alison* (pp.13–33); 'Remarks on Dr. W.P. Alison's "Observations on the Generation of Fever"', by *N. Arnott* (pp.34–9).
1845, XVIII. 1. Second Report of Commissioners for Enquiring into the State of Large Towns and Populous Districts. 'Report on the sanatory state of Bristol', by *H. de la Beche* and *L. Playfair* (pp.61–75 [195–211]).
1846, X. 535. Report of the Select Committee on Metropolitan Sewage Manure.
1847, LVII. 9. Reports on Disinfecting Fluid. [Copies of Reports of *Southwood Smith, Grainger, Toynbee*, various physicians and surgeons at Dublin, etc.].
1847–8, IV. 511. Nuisances Removal and Diseases Prevention Act (Amended).
   XXXII. 1. First Report of the Commissioners appointed to inquire whether any and what Special Means may be requisite for the Improvement of the Health of the Metropolis.
   253. Second Report of the Same.
   LI. 535. Disinfecting Fluids and Metropolitan Sewers.
1849, XXIV. 1. Report by the General Board of Health on the Measures

adopted for the Execution of the Nuisances Removal and Diseases Prevention Act, up to July 1849.

137. Report of the General Board of Health on Quarantine. 'On the principles of ship ventilation', by *N. Arnott* (pp.144–51 [280–7]).

1850, XXI. 3. Report of the General Board of Health on the Epidemic Cholera of 1848 and 1849. App. A: Report by *J. Sutherland* (pp.1–149 [187–347], and Appendix); App. B: 'Sanitary report on epidemic cholera as it prevailed in London in 1848–49', by *R.D. Grainger* (pp.1–180 [367–546], and Appendix).

XXII. 1. Report of the General Board of Health on the Supply of Water to the Metropolis. App. III: 'Reports and Evidence (Medical, Chemical, Geological and Miscellaneous)' including 'On the air and water of towns', by *R.A. Smith* (pp.83–99 [751–67]).

1851, XV. 1. Minutes of Evidence taken before the Select Committee on the Metropolis Water Bill.

XXIII. Report by the Government Commission on the Chemical Quality of the Supply of Water to the Metropolis.

XLIII. 321. General Board of Health: Accounts and Statements.

1852, XX. 117. Second Report of the General Board of Health on Quarantine: Yellow Fever. Appendices.

1852–3, LXXXV. 1. Population (Great Britain). England and Wales: Pt. I.

1854–5, XIII. 413. Report of Select Committee on the Public Health Bill and Nuisances Removal Amendment Bill.

XXI. 1. Report of the Committee for Scientific Enquiries in Relation to the Cholera Epidemic of 1854. Appendices by *R.D. Thomson, G. Rainey, N. Arnott, A.H. Hassall, M. Faraday, G.W. Callender*, etc.

XLV. 1. Report of the Medical Council to the President of the General Board of Health.

69. Letter of the President of the General Board of Health to Viscount Palmerston, with Report of *Dr. Sutherland* on Cholera in the Metropolis in 1854.

227. Report by Mr. Thomas E. Blackwell to the President of the General Board of Health, on the Drainage and Water Supply of Sandgate, in connexion with the late Outbreak of Cholera in that town. Appendices by *W. Herapath, F. Brittan, R. Etheridge*, etc.

1856, LII. 357. Report on the Last Two Cholera Epidemics of London, as affected by the Consumption of Impure Water ... by the Medical Officer of the Board [*John Simon*].

1857–8, XXIII. 267. Papers relating to the Sanitary State of the People of England ... communicated to the General Board of Health by *E.H. Greenhow*, with an Introductory Report by the Medical Officer of the Board, on the Preventability of Certain Kinds of Premature Death.

1859, XII. 257. First Report of the Medical Officer of the Privy Council. Appendices.

1861, XVI. 339. Third Report of the Same. Appendices.

1864, XXVIII. 1. Sixth Report of the Same. Apps. 13 and 14: 'Report by *Dr. George Whitley* as to the quantity of ague and other malarious diseases now prevailing in the principal marsh districts of England' (pp.430–54 [434–58]); App. 15: 'Reports on the Hospitals of the United Kingdom', by *J.S. Bristowe* and *T. Holmes* (pp.463–743 [467–753]).

1866, XXII. 321. Third Report of Commissioners appointed to inquire into the Origin and Nature, etc., of the Cattle Plague. Appendices.

1867, XXXVII. 1. Ninth Report of the Medical Officer of the Privy Council. Appendix IX: 'Report by *Dr. Burdon Sanderson* on the experimental proofs of the communicability of cholera', with a note by the Medical Officer, pp.[434–58].

1868–9, XXXII. 301. First Report of Royal Sanitary Commission. Minutes of Evidence.

1871, XXXV. 1. Second Report of the Same. Minutes of Evidence.

1874, XXXI. 355. Third Report (N.S.) of the Medical Officer of the Privy Council and Local Government Board. App. 2: 'Report on the pathology of sheep-pox', by *E. Klein* (pp.49–60 [403–14]).

1875, XL. 1. Sixth Report (N.S.) of the Same. App. 6: 'Report on an experimental study of certain disinfectants', by *E.B. Baxter* (pp.216–56 [652–92]).

1876, XXXVIII. 455. Eighth Report (N.S.) of the Same. App. 4: 'Report on the so-called enteric or typhoid fever of the pig', by *E. Klein* (pp.91–101 [569–79]).

XLI. 227. Report of Royal Commission on the Practice of Subjecting Live Animals to Experiments for Scientific Purposes.

(For John Simon's official writings see also Simon, *Public Health Reports*.)

Annual Reports of the Registrar-General with
Appendices by William Farr

1839, XVI . . . .First Report   1844, XIX . . .Sixth Report
1840, XVII. . . .Second   1846, XIX . . .Seventh
                                                      [no Appendix by Farr]

1841, Sess. 2,
        VI. . . .Third   1868–9, XVI. .Thirtieth Report
1842, XIX . . . .Fourth   1877, XXV. . .Thirty-eighth Report
1843, XXI . . . .Fifth

Miscellaneous

Registrar-General [Farr, W.],   *Report on the Mortality of Cholera in England, 1848–9* (1852).

Sixteenth Annual Report of the Registrar-General of Births, Deaths and Marriages in England (1856).

(For William Farr's official writings see also Farr, *Vital Statistics*.)

PUBLISHED WORKS

Acland, H.W., *Memoir on the Cholera in Oxford in the Year 1854* (1856).
——, *Fever in Agricultural Districts* (Oxford and London, 1858).
Adams, J., *Observations on Morbid Poisons, Chronic and Acute* (2nd edn. 1807).
——, *Memoirs of the Life and Doctrines of the Late John Hunter* (1817).
Alison, W.P., 'Observations on the epidemic fever now prevalent among the lower orders in Edinburgh', *Edinb. Med. Surg. J.* 28 (1827), 233-63.
[——], 'Report on the registration of deaths. By the Edinburgh Sub-Committee', *Rep. of 5th Meeting of British Association* (1836), pp.251-5.
——, 'Notes on the application of statistics, to questions in medical science, particularly as to the external causes of diseases', *Edinb. Med. J.* 1 (1855-6), 385-99.
——, 'On the communicability of cholera by dejections', *Edinb. Med. J.* 1 (1855-6), 481-92, 1112-25.
Ancell, H., 'Liebig, his chemistry and reviewers', *Lancet*, 1842-3, i.
——, *A Treatise on Tuberculosis* (1852).
Anon., *Bristol Microscopical Society* (Bristol, 1878).
——, *Correspondence and Editorial Comments on the Points at Issue Between Dr. Tweedie and Dr. Murchison Concerning Identical Passages in their Respective Works on Fever* (n.pl., 1863).
——, *Curiosities of Animal Life: With the Recent Discoveries of the Microscope*, Religious Tract Society [1848].
——, *Memoir of the Bristol Institution* (Bristol, n.d.).
——, *The Penny Cyclopaedia*, 27 vols. (1839-43).
Baas, J.H., *Outlines of the History of Medicine and the Medical Profession*, trans. by H.E. Handerson (1889; reprinted in 2 vols. New York, 1971).
Baly, W., 'Note on the presence of peculiar microscopic bodies in the discharges of epidemic dysentery', *Lond. Med. Gaz.* 9 (1849), 580-3.
Baly, W., and Gull, W.W., *Report on the Nature and Import of Certain Microscopic Bodies Found in the Intestinal Discharges of Cholera* (1849).
——, *Reports on Epidemic Cholera* (1854).
Bell, C.W. 'The address in medicine, being an essay on the principal causes which unite in producing and diffusing disease', *Trans. Prov. Med. Surg. Ass.* 5 (1850), 1-47. Also as *An Essay on the Principal Causes . . .* (Worcester, 1849).
Bentham, J., *Works*, ed J. Bowring, 11 vols (Edinburgh, 1843).
Bernard, T., (ed.), *Reports of the Society for Bettering the Condition and Increasing the Comforts of the Poor*, Nos. 1-40, 7 vols. (1798-1817).
Blane, G., *Elements of Medical Logick* (1819).

Blyth, A.W., *Poisons: Their Effects and Detection* (2nd revised edn. 1884).

Boott, F., *Memoir of the Life and Medical Opinions of John Armstrong, M.D.*, 2 vols. (1833-4).

Bowring, J., *Observations on the Oriental Plague and on Quarantines, as a Means of Arresting its Progress* (Edinburgh, 1838).

——, 'Free Trade Recollections. No. VIII: Quarantines', *Howitt's J. of Literature and Popular Progress*, 2 (1847), 362-5; 'Free Trade . . . No. IX . . .', ibid., p.376.

——, *Autobiographical Recollections*, with a memoir by L.B. Bowring (1877).

Branson, F., 'New Hypothesis to account for the presence of fungoid growths in cholera', *Prov. Med. Surg. J.* 13 (1849), 614-15.

Bristol Med.-Chir. J. 50-1 (1933-4), 165-82: 'Bristol's contributions to medical progress'.

Brit. For. Med. Rev. 1 (1836), 34-70: 'Life and works of Dr. Armstrong'.

——, 19 (1857), 60-86: 'On the local causes of cholera'.

Brittan, F., 'Report of a series of microscopical investigations on the pathology of cholera', *Lond. Med. Gaz.* 9 (1849), 530-42.

——, *Blood Diseases and Blood Germs* (London and Bristol, 1874).

[Brodie, B.] , 'Mr. Chadwick's Report on the Sanatory Condition of the Labouring Population of Great Britain', *Brit. For. Med. Rev.* 15 (1843), 328-46.

[Brown, J.] , 'Locke and Sydenham', *N. Br. Rev.* 12 (1849), 53-85.

Budd, G., 'Statistical account of cholera, in the Seamen's Hospital, in 1832', *Med. Chir. Trans.* 22 (1839), 110-23.

Budd, G., and Busk, G., 'Report of twenty cases of malignant cholera that occurred in the Seamen's Hospital, Dreadnought, between the 8th and 28th of October, 1837', *Med. Chir. Trans.* 21 (1838), 152-86.

Budd, R., 'Is cancer contagious?', *Lancet*, 1887, ii. 1091.

Budd, W., 'Contributions to the pathology of the spinal cord', *Med. Chir. Trans.* 22 (1839), 153-90.

——, 'Remarks on the pathology and causes of cancer', *Lancet*, 1841-2, ii. 226-70, 295-8.

——, 'On diseases which affect corresponding parts of the body in a symmetrical manner', *Med. Chir. Trans.* 25 (1842), 100-66.

——, 'Retrospect of anatomy and physiology for the year 1843-44', *Trans. Prov. Med. Surg. Ass.* 13 (1845), 143-240.

——, *Malignant Cholera: Its Cause, Mode of Propagation, and Prevention* (1849).

——, 'On the treatment of croup by warm vapour and emetics', *Med. Times Gaz.* 1852, i. 611-15.

——, ' "On the employment of potassium iodide as a remedy for the affections caused by lead and mercury", by M. Melsens. Translated from *Annales de chimie et de physique*, June 1849', *Brit. For. Med. Chir. Rev.* 11 (1853), 201-24.

Common Sense' [pseud. Budd] 'Cholera: its cause and prevention', *Ass. Med. J.* 2 (1854), 928-9, 950-1, 974-8, 1152-7; 3 (1855), 207-8, 283.

——, 'Mode of propagation of cholera', *Ass. Med. J.* 4 (1856), 259.

——, 'The frog as a detector of tetanic poison', *Lancet*, 1856, i. 90-1.

——, 'On the fever at the Clergy Orphan Asylum', *Lancet*, 1856, ii. 617-19.

——, 'On intestinal fever: its mode of propagation', *Lancet*, 1856, ii. 694-5.

——, 'The cholera at West Ham', *Brit. Med. J.* 1857, ii. 955-6.

——, 'On intestinal fever' [running title] , *Lancet*, 1859, ii. 4-5, 28-30, 55-6, 80-2, 131-3, 207-10, 432-3, 458-9; 1860, i. 187-90, 239-40.

——, 'On the contagion of yellow fever', *Lancet*, 1861, i. 337-8.

——, 'Diphtheria', *Brit. Med. J.* 1861, i. 575-9.

——, 'Mr. Simon on typhoid fever at Bedford. Change in the doctrines of the General Board of Health', *Lancet*, 1861, i. 630; 1861, ii 17.

——, 'Observations on typhoid or intestinal fever: the pythogenic theory', *Brit. Med. J.* 1861, ii. 457-9, 485-7, 523-5, 549-51, 575-7, 604-5, 625-7.

——, 'On the occurrence (hitherto unnoticed) of malignant pustule in England', *Lancet*, 1862, ii. 164-5.

——, 'Observations on the occurrence of malignant pustule in England: illustrated by numerous fatal cases', *Brit. Med. J.* 1863, i, 85-7, 110-13, 159-61, 237-41, 316-18.

——, 'Variola ovina, sheep's smallpox; or the laws of contagious epidemics illustrated by an experimental type', *Brit. Med. J.* 1863, ii. 142-50.

——, 'Investigation of epidemic and epizootic diseases', *Brit. Med. J.* 1864, ii. 354-7.

——, *The Siberian Cattle-Plague; or, the Typhoid Fever of the Ox* (Bristol, 1865).

——, 'Bacteridia and malignant pustule', *Lancet*, 1865, i. 47-8.

——, 'On the cattle-plague', *Brit. Med. J.* 1865, ii. 205-6.

——, *Memoranda on Asiatic Cholera: Its Mode of Spreading and its Prevention* (2nd edn. Bristol, 1866).

——, 'Memorandum on the nature and the mode of propagation of phthisis', *Lancet*, 1867, ii. 451-2.

——, *Scarlet Fever and its Prevention* (2nd edn. London and Bristol, 1869). Reprinted from *Brit. Med. J.* 1869, ii. 23-4.

——, 'Can government, further, beneficially interfere in the prevention of infectious disease?', *Trans. Natn. Ass. Soc. Sci.* 1869, pp.386-402.

——, *Typhoid Fever: Its Nature, Mode of Spreading and Prevention* (1873).

——, *Cholera and Disinfection. Asiatic Cholera in Bristol in 1866* (2nd edn. Bristol, 1883).

Busk, G., 'Observations on parasitical growths on living animals', *Microscopic Journal*, 1841, pp.145-52.

——, 'On the occurrence of sarcina ventriculi in the human stomach', *Microscopic Journal*, 1842, pp.321-3.
See also Budd, G., 1838.

Butlin, H., *Three Lectures on Unicellula Cancri — the Parasite of Cancer* (1912).

Cabanis, P.J.G., *Sketch of the Revolutions of Medical Science*, trans. A. Henderson (1806).

Carpenter, W.B., *Principles of General and Comparative Physiology* (1st edn. 1839; 2nd edn. 1841). 2nd edn. unless otherwise specified.

——, 'Report on the results obtained by the use of the microscope in the study of anatomy and physiology. Pt. II: On the origin and function of cells', *Brit. For. Med. Rev.* 15 (1843), 259-81. See also Paget, J., 1842.

——, 'Taylor and Copland on Poisons', *Brit. For. Med. Chir. Rev.* 2 (1848), 172-201.

——, [Review of M. Marchal on epidemics], *Brit. For. Med. Chir. Rev.* 11 (1853), 159-77.

——, *Nature and Man*, with a memoir by J.E. Carpenter (1888; reprinted Farnborough, 1970).

Carrick, A., and Symonds, J.A. 'Medical topography of Bristol', *Trans. Prov. Med. Surg. Ass.* 2 (1834), 148-80.

Chadwick, E. 'Life assurances — diminution of sickness and mortality', *Westminster Review*, 9 (1828), 384-421. Also as enlarged edn. 1836.

——, 'Preventive police', *Lond. Rev.* 1 (1829), 252-308.

——, 'Centralization' [French medical charities], *Lond. Rev.* 2 (1829), 536-65.

——, 'On the best mode of representing by statistics the duration of life', *J. Stats. Soc.* 7 (1844), 1-40.

——, *The Comparative Results of the Chief Principles of the Poor-Law Administration in England and Ireland, as Compared with that of Scotland* (1864).

——, 'Administration of medical relief to the destitute sick of the metropolis', *Fraser's Magazine*, 74 (1866), 353-65.

[——], *University of London Election. Address to the Members of Convocation by E.C.* (1867).

——, *On Local Medical Appointments* (1872).

——, 'The plague', *J. Soc. Arts*, 27 (1879), 329-30.

——, 'Progress of sanitation: in preventive as compared with that in curative science', *Trans. Natn. Ass. Soc. Sci.* 1881, pp.625-49.

——, *On the Prevention of Epidemics* (1882).

——, *Report on the Sanitary Condition of the Labouring Population of Great Britain*, ed. M.W. Flinn (1842; Edinburgh, 1965).

——, *The Health of Nations*, ed. B.W. Richardson, 2 vols. (1887; 1973).

Christison, R., *A Treatise on Poisons* (Edinburgh, 1829).

——, 'Fevers', in *Library of Medicine*, Vol. I: *Practical Medicine*, ed. A. Tweedie (1840), pp.113-25; 'Continued fever', ibid., pp.125-88.

——, *The Life of Sir Robert Christison, Bart.*, ed. by his sons (Edinburgh, 1885-6).

Clark, J. *The Influence of Climate in the Prevention and Cure of Chronic Diseases* (1st edn. 1829; 2nd edn. 1830; 3rd edn. 1841). 2nd edn. unless otherwise specified.

——, *A Treatise on Pulmonary Consumption* (1835).

Clarke, W.M., 'William Budd, M.D., F.R.S. In memoriam', *Br. Med. J.* 1880, i. 163-6.

Condy, H.B., *Disinfection and the Prevention of Disease* (1862).

Conolly, J., 'A proposal to establish County Natural History Societies, for ascertaining the circumstances, in all localities, which are productive of disease, or conducive to health', *Trans. Prov. Med. Surg. Ass.* 1 (1832-3), 180-218.

Cowdell, C., *A Disquisition on Pestilential Cholera* (1848).

Creighton, C., *A History of Epidemics in Great Britain*, with additional material by D.E.C. Eversley, E.A. Underwood, and L. Ovenall, 2 vols. (1894; 2nd edn. 1965).

Cullen, W., *First Lines of the Practice of Physic*, supervised by J. Gregory, 2 vols. (Edinburgh, 1808). This edn. unless otherwise specified.

——, *Nosology, or a Systematic Arrangement of Diseases*, transl. by C.S. (Edinburgh, 1810). This edn. unless otherwise specified.

——, *Works*, ed. J. Thomson, 2 vols. (Edinburgh, 1827).

Daremberg, C. *Histoire des sciences médicales*, 2 vols. (Paris, 1870).

Darwin, C., *The Variation of Animals and Plants under Domestication*, 2 vols. (2nd edn. 1875).

——, *The Life and Letters of Charles Darwin*, ed. F. Darwin, 3 vols. (1887).

——, *On the Origin of Species*, with introduction by E. Mayr (1859; Camb., Mass., 1964).

Daubeny, C., 'On the influence of the lower vegetable organisms in the production of epidemic diseases', *Edinb. Phil. J.* 2 (1855), 88-113.

Davies, D., 'On the origin of species in zymotic diseases', *Bristol Naturalists' Society Procs*, 1871, pp.4-9.

Davies, D.S., 'Some modern aspects of preventive medicine', *Bristol Med.-Chir. J.* 18 (1900), 289-305.

Davies, W., 'Fever in its relations to sanitary reform, being the address in medicine', *Trans. Prov. Med. Surg. Ass.* 4 (1849), 67-95.

Dixey, F.A., *Epidemic Influenza* (Oxford, 1892).

Dublin Review, 25 (1848), 179-204: 'Liebig's philosophy'.

Edinb. Med. Surg. J. 73 (1850), 81-118: 'Documents on the hypothesis which ascribes cholera to the presence of fungi'.

Edmonds, T.R., 'Statistics of the London Hospital, with remarks on the law of sickness', *Lancet*, 1835-6, ii. 778-83.

Faraday, M., *The Letters of Faraday and Schoenbein 1836-1862*, ed. G.W.A. Kahlbaum and F.V. Darbishire (Basle and London, 1899).

Farr, W., 'Lecture introductory to a course on hygeine [*sic*], or the preservation of the public health', *Lancet*, 1835-6, i. 240-5; 'Lecture on the history of hygeine', ibid., pp.773-80.

——, 'On a method of determining the danger and the duration of diseases at every period of their progress. Art. I', *Br. Ann. Med.* 1 (1837), 72-9.

——, 'On the law of recovery and dying in smallpox. Art. II', *Br. Ann. Med.* 1 (1837), 134-43.

——, 'On prognosis', *Br. Med. Almanack*, 1838, pp.199-216.

——, 'On Mr. Farr's law of recovery and mortality in cholera', *Rep. of 8th Meeting of British Association*, Trans. of Sections (1838), pp.126-7.

——, 'On the law of recovery and mortality in cholera spasmodica', *Lancet*, 1838-9, i. 26-9.

——, 'History of the medical profession, and its influence on public health, in England', *Med. Ann., or Br. Med. Almanack*, suppl., 1839, pp.113-78.

——, 'Medical reform: an oration delivered at the last anniversary meeting of the British Medical Association', *Lancet*, 1839-40, i. 105-11.

——, *Report on the Nomenclature and Statistical Classification of Diseases for Statistical Returns* [1856].

——, *Vital Statistics*, ed. N.A. Humphreys, Sanitary Institute of Great Britain (1885).

——, 'Vital statistics; or, the statistics of health, sickness, diseases and death' in Farr, W., and Ratcliffe, H., *Mortality in Mid-19th Century Britain*, ed. R. Wall (1974). Originally in J.R. McCulloch (ed.), *A Statistical Account of the British Empire*, 2 vols. (1837), ii. 567-601.

Fleming, G., *Animal Plagues: Their History, Nature and Prevention*, 2 vols. (1871-82).

——, *A Manual of Veterinary Sanitary Science and Police*, 2 vols. (1875).

Fowke, F. 'On the first discovery of the comma bacillus of cholera', *Br. Med. J.* 1885, i. 589-92.

Fox, C.B., *Ozone and Antozone. Their History and Nature* (1873).

Fox, E.L., *Surmises Respecting the Cause and Nature of Cholera* (Bristol, 1831).

Fraser's Magazine, 74 (1866), 718-40: 'Was Lord Bacon an impostor?'.

Gairdner, W.T., *Public Health in Relation to Air and Water* (Edinburgh, 1882).

——, *The Physician as Naturalist* (Glasgow, 1889).

[Gooch, R.], 'Plague, a contagious disease', *Quarterly Review*, 33 (1826), 218-57.

Graham, T., *Elements of Chemistry* (1842).

Greenhow, E.H., *Papers Relating to the Sanitary State of the People of England*, with an introduction by C.F. Brockington (1858; 1973).

Griffith, J.W., and Henfrey, A., *The Micrographic Dictionary*, 2 vols. (3rd edn. 1874).

Grove, J., *On Sulphur as a Remedy in Cholera* (1848).
——, 'The vitality of the choleraic fungi demonstrated', *Lancet*, 1849, ii. 427–8, 451–3, 556–8.
——, *Epidemics Examined and Explained* (1850).
Gull, W.W., *A Collection of the Published Writings of William Withey Gull*, ed. T.D. Acland, New Sydenham Society, 2 vols. (1894–6). See also Baly, W., 1849 and 1854.
Guy, W.A., *Public Health: A Popular Introduction to Sanitary Science*, 2 vols. (1870–4).
——, *Miscellanea: Sanitary, Social and Political. IV: Statistics and Social Science* (1884).
Hassall, A.H., 'Memoir on the organic analysis or microscopic examination of water supplied to the inhabitants of London and the suburban districts', *Lancet*, 1850, i. 230–5.
Haygarth, J., *A Letter to Dr. Percival, on the Prevention of Infectious Fevers* (1801).
Henry, W., 'Experiments on the disinfecting powers of increased temperatures, with a view to the suggestion of a substitute for quarantine', *Phil. Mag.* 10 (1831), 363–9.
——, 'Further experiments on the disinfecting powers of increased temperatures', *Phil. Mag.* 11 (1832), 22–31; 'Letter . . . on a modified disinfecting apparatus', ibid., pp.205–7.
——, 'Report on the state of our knowledge of the laws of contagion', *Rep. of 4th Meeting of British Association* (1835), pp.67–94.
Herapath, T.J., 'An account of certain chemical and microscopical researches on the blood, excretions and breath in cholera', *Lond. Med. Gaz.* 9 (1849), 838–45.
Highmore, A., *Pietas Londinensis*, 2 vols. (1810).
Hirsch, A., *Handbook of Geographical and Historical Pathology*, transl. by C. Creighton, New Sydenham Society, 3 vols. (1883–6).
Hofmann, A., *The Life-Work of Liebig . . . Faraday Lecture for 1875* (1876).
Holland, H., *Medical Notes and Reflections* (1st edn. 1839; 2nd edn. 1840; 3rd edn. 1855). 3rd edn. unless otherwise specified.
——, *Recollections of Past Life* (1872).
Hunt, R. 'The probable causes in operation to cause pestilential cholera', *Lond. Med. Gaz.* 9 (1849), 473–5.
Hunter, J., *The Works of John Hunter*, ed. with a life by J.F. Palmer, 5 vols. (1835–7).
Jenner, E., *An Inquiry into the Causes and Effects of the Variolae Vaccinae* (1798).
Kay-Shuttleworth, J.P., *Autobiography*, ed. B.C. Bloomfield, University of London Institute of Education, *Educ. Libr. Bull.*, suppl. 7 (1964).
Knight, C., *Passages of a Working Life*, 3 vols. (1864–5).
Lancet, 1835–6, i. 1–13: 'List of the schools of medicine in London'.

Liebig, J., *Chemistry in its Applications to Agriculture and Physiology*, ed. L. Playfair (1st edn. 1840; 2nd edn. 1842). 2nd edn. unless otherwise specified.

——, *Animal Chemistry, or Chemistry in its Applications to Physiology and Pathology*, ed. W. Gregory (1st edn. 1842; 3rd edn. 1846). 3rd edn. unless otherwise specified.

——, *Familiar Letters on Chemistry, and its Relation to Commerce, Physiology and Agriculture*, ed. J. Gardner (1843).

——, *Familiar Letters on Chemistry. The Philosophical Principles and General Laws of the Science*, 2nd Ser., ed. J. Gardner (1844).

——, *Familiar Letters on Chemistry: in its Relations to Physiology, Dietetics, Agriculture, Commerce and Political Economy* (3rd edn., much revised and enlarged, 1851).

——, 'Etiology of Cholera, by Professor Liebig', *Med. Times Gaz.* 1854, ii. 515.

——, 'Lord Bacon as natural philosopher', *Macmillan's Magazine*, 8 (1863), 237–49, 257–67.

——, 'Was Lord Bacon an impostor?', *Fraser's Magazine*, 75 (1867), 482–95.

——, *Aus J. Liebigs und F. Wöhlers Briefwechsel in den Jahren 1829–73, unter Mitwirkung von E. Wöhler*, ed. A.W. Hofmann, 2 vols. (Braunschweig, 1888).

——, 'Justus von Liebig — an autobiographical sketch', *Pop. Sci. Mthly*, 40 (1891–2), 655–66.

——, *Animal Chemistry, or Organic Chemistry in its Application to Physiology and Pathology*, ed. W. Gregory, with additions (Cambridge, Mass., 1842; reprinted with a new introduction by F.L. Holmes, New York, 1964).

Lindsay, W.L., 'Clinical notes on cholera', *Ass. Med. J.* 2 (1854), 216–22, 330–5, 347–53, 410–14, 527–31, 670–6, 834–41, 896–900, 967–71, 1110–20.

Lond. Med. Gaz. 1 (1839–40), 333–6: 'Böhm on the morbid changes in cholera'.

——, 9 (1849), 507–11, 556–9, 600–2: 'History of the origin, progress and mortality of the cholera morbus'. Reprinted from *The Times*.

Macdonald, J.D. *A Guide to the Microscopical Examination of Drinking Water. With an Appendix on the Microscopical Examination of Air* (2nd edn. 1883).

M[aclean], C., *To the British Inhabitants of India* [1798].

Maclean, C., *Results of an Investigation, Respecting Epidemic and Pestilential Diseases*, 2 vols. (1817–18).

——, 'Summary of facts and inferences respecting the causes, proper and adventitious, of plague, and other pestilential diseases . . . intended for the use of the Select Committee of the House of Commons', *Pamphleteer*, 16 (1820).

——, *Evils of Quarantine Laws and Non-Existence of Pestilential Contagion* (1824).

Marshall, J., 'The communicability of cholera to animals', *Brit. For. Med. Chir. Rev.* 11 (1853), 390–409.

[—— *et al.*], *Report on the Cholera Outbreak in the Parish of St. James, Westminster* (1855).

[Masson, D.], 'Edwin Chadwick, C.B.', *N. Br. Rev.* 13 (1850), 40–84.

Mayhew, H., *The Unknown Mayhew*, ed. with introductions by E.P. Thompson and E. Yeo (Penguin edn. 1973).

Mayo, T., *Sequel to Outlines of Medical Proof* (1849).

Med. Times Gaz. 1854, ii. 550–1: 'Munich. Discussion on cholera'.

Mill, J.S., *A System of Logic*, 2 vols. (1st edn. 1843; 3rd edn. 1851).

——, *Autobiography*, ed. J. Stillinger (Oxford, 1971).

Müller, J., *Elements of Physiology*, transl. by W. Baly, 2 vols. (1st edn. 1837; 2nd edn. 1840).

——, *On the Nature and Structural Characteristics of Cancer*, Pt. I, transl. by C. West (1840).

Murchison, C., 'Typhus and typhoid fever', *Med. Times Gaz.* 1857, ii. 642–3.

——, 'Contributions to the etiology of continued fever: or an investigation of various causes which influence the prevalence and mortality of its different forms', *Med. Chir. Trans.* 41 (1858), 219–306.

——, 'On the nomenclature and classification of continued fevers', *Edinb. Med. J.* 4 (1858-9), 320–30.

——, 'On the causes of continued fevers, with special reference to the recent "Windsor epidemic"', *Med. Times Gaz.* 1859, i. 253–4.

——, *A Treatise on the Continued Fevers of Great Britain* (1st edn. 1862; 2nd edn. 1873; 3rd edn. ed. W. Cayley, 1884). 3rd edn. unless otherwise specified.

Murray, T.A., *Remarks on the Situation of the Poor in the Metropolis as Contributing to the Progress of Contagious Disease* (1801).

Nash, J.T.C., *Evolution and Disease* (Bristol, 1915).

Nicholls, G., *A History of the Scotch Poor Law* (1856).

Owen, R., *On Parthenogenesis* (1949).

Paget, J., *Report on the Chief Results Obtained by the Use of the Microscope in the Study of Human Anatomy and Physiology* (1842). Reprinted from *Brit. For. Med. Rev.*, 14 (1842), 259–96.

Parker, N., 'On the microscopical pathology of cholera'. *Lond. Med. Gaz.* 9 (1849), 668–71.

Parkes, E.A., *Researches into the Pathology and Treatment of Asiatic or Algide Cholera* (1847).

——, 'On the intestinal discharges in cholera', *Lond. J. Med.* 1 (1849), 134–52.

——, 'An inquiry into the bearing of the earliest cases of cholera, which occurred in London during the present epidemic, on the strict theory of contagion', *Brit. For. Med. Chir. Rev.* 4 (1849), 251–76.

——, 'Dr. Snow on the communication of cholera', *Brit. For. Med. Chir. Rev.* 15 (1855), 449–63.

——, *A Manual of Practical Hygiene* (1864).

Pettenkofer, M. von, 'Liebig's scientific achievements', *Contemporary Review*, 29 (1877), 865–87.

P[richard], A., 'William Budd, F.R.S.', *Bristol Roy. Inf. Reports*, 1 (1878–9), 361.

Prichard, A., 'The early history of the Bristol Medical School', *Bristol Med.-Chir. J.* 10 (1892), 264–91.

——, *A Few Medical and Surgical Reminiscences* (Bristol, 1896).

Prichard, J.C., *Researches into the Physical History of Man*, ed. G.W. Stocking (1813; Chicago and London, 1973).

Pringle, J., *Observations on the Diseases of the Army* (5th edn. 1765).

——, 'A discourse upon some late improvements of the means for preserving the health of mariners' (1775), in *Six Discourses*, with a life by A. Kippis (1783), pp.143–200.

Prov. Med. Surg. J. 13 (1849), 600–3: 'Report of the Microscopical Subcommittee of the Bristol Medico-Chirurgical Society'.

Richards, HC., and Payne, W.H.C. *London Water Supply*, ed. J.P.H. Soper (2nd edn. 1899).

Richardson, B.W., 'Water supply in relation to health and disease', *J. Publ. Hlth. Sanit. Rev.* 1 (1855), 130–40.

——, 'On the theory of zymosis', *Trans. Epidem. Soc.* 1, Pt. I (1859–60), 20–30.

——, 'On the theory and mode of propagation of cholera', *Trans. Epidem. Soc.* 2 (1862–6), 424–34.

——, *On the Poisons of Spreading Diseases* (1867).

——, 'The glandular origin of contagious diseases', *Nature*, 16 (1877), 480–6.

——, *Vita Medica: Chapters of Medical Life and Work* (1897).

——, *Disciples of Aesculapius*, with a life by Mrs. G. Martin, 2 vols. (1900).

Roscoe, H.E., 'Justus Liebig', *Nature*, 8 (1873), 27–8.

Ross J., *The Graft Theory of Disease* (1872).

Rumsey, N., Rumsey, H.W., and Ceely, R., 'Observations on the present condition of medical relief for the sick paupers, with recommendations for an altered and improved system', *Trans. Prov. Med. Surg. Ass.* 5 (1837), 441–55.

Ryan, M., *A Manual of Medical Jurisprudence and State Medicine* (2nd edn. 1836).

J.B.S., 'F.G.J. Henle', *Proc. R. Soc. Lond.* 39 (1885), pp.iii–viii.

Sanderson, J.B., 'Sir John Simon. 1816–1904', *Proc. R. Soc. Lond.* 75 (1905), 336–46.

Schwann, T., *Microscopical Researches*, trans. by H. Smith, Sydenham Society (1847).

Shadwell, A., *The London Water Supply* (1899).

Simon, J., *On the Aims and Philosophic Method of Pathological Research* (1847–8).

——, 'A course of lectures in general pathology', *Lancet*, 1850, i, and 1850, ii, also as *General Pathology* (1850).

——, *Report to the Local Board of Health of Croydon* (Croydon, 1853).

——, 'Results of inoculation with tubercular matter', *Trans. Path. Soc.* 18 (1867), 290–3.

——, *Experiments on Life* (1882).

——, *Public Health Reports*, ed. E. Seaton, Sanitary Institute of Great Britain, 2 vols. (1887).

——, *English Sanitary Institutions*, 2nd edn. (1897).

Smith, F., *The Early History of Veterinary Literature and its British Development*, 4 vols. (1919–33). Reprinted from *J. Comp. Path. and Therapeutics*, 1912–18.

Smith, R.A., 'Some remarks on the air and water of towns', *Phil. Mag.* 30 (1847), 478–82.

——, 'Science in our courts of law', *J. Soc. Arts*, 8 (1860), 133–42.

Smith, T.S., *Illustrations of the Divine Government* (3rd edn. 1822).

——, 'Use of the dead to the living', *Westminster Review*, 2 (1824), 59–97.

——, 'Contagion and sanitary laws', *Westminster Review*, 3 (1825), 134–67; contd. as 'Plague – typhus fever – quarantine', ibid., pp.499–530.

——, 'Anatomy', *Westminster Review*, 10 (1829), 116–48.

——, *A Treatise on Fever* (1830).

——, *The Philosophy of Health; or, an Exposition of the Physical and Mental Constitution of Man, with a View to the Promotion of Human Longevity and Happiness*, 2 vols. (1835–8).

——, *The Philosophy of Health; or, an Exposition of the Physiological and Sanitary Conditions Conducive to Human Longevity and Happiness* (11th edn., revised and enlarged, 1865). This edn. unless otherwise specified.

——, 'Lectures on forensic medicine', *Lond. Med. Gaz.* 1837–8, i, and 1837–8, ii.

——, *An Address to the Working Classes of the United Kingdom on their Duty in the Present State of the Sanitary Question* (1847). Extracted from *Howitt's J.* Reprinted in Lewes, *Southwood Smith – A Retrospect*, pp.111–22.

——, *Results of Sanitary Improvement* (1854).

——, *Epidemics Considered in Relation to their Common Nature, and to Climate and Civilisation* (Edinburgh, 1856).

——, *The Common Nature of Epidemics and Their Relation to Climate and Civilisation*, ed. T. Baker (2nd edn. 1866).

Snow, J. 'On the circulation in the capillary blood vessels, and on some of its connections with pathology and therapeutics', *Lond. Med. Gaz.* 1843, i. 810–16.

——, 'On narcotism by the inhalation of vapours', *Lond. Med. Gaz.* A series of 16 papers from 19 May 1848 to 11 Apr. 1851. Reprinted (Pts. 1–7), 1848; (Pts. 8–16), 1851.

——, *On the Mode of Communication of Cholera* (1st edn. 1849; 2nd enlarged edn. 1855; repr. of 2nd edn. 1936 and 1965).

——, 'On the pathology and mode of communication of cholera', *Lond. Med. Gaz.* 9 (1849), 745–52, 923–9.

——, *On Continuous Molecular Changes* (1853; reprinted 1936 and 1965).

——, 'The principles on which the treatment of cholera should be based', *Med. Times Gaz.* 1854, i. 180–2.

——, 'Cholera in the Baltic Fleet', *Med. Times Gaz.* 1854, ii. 170.

——, 'On the comparative mortality of large towns and rural districts, and the causes by which it is influenced', *Trans. Epidem. Soc.* 1 (1855), 16–24.

——, 'On the chief cause of the recent sickness and mortality in the Crimea', *Med. Times Gaz.* 1855, i. 157 8.

——, 'The mode of propagation of cholera', *Ass. Med. J.* 4 (1856), 135.

——, 'Cholera and the water supply in the south districts of London in 1854', *Publ. Hlth. Sanit. Rev.*, 2 (1856), 239–51.

——, 'On the outbreak of cholera at Abbey Row, West Ham', *Med. Times Gaz.* 1857, ii. 417–19.

——, 'Cholera, and the water supply in the south districts of London', *Br. Med. J.* 1857, ii. 864–5.

——, *On Chloroform and Other Anaesthetics*, ed. with a memoir by B.W. Richardson (1858).

——, *Snow on Cholera . . . with a biographical memoir by B.W. Richardson and introduction by W.H. Frost* (1st edn. 1936; reprinted New York, 1965).

Spooner, E.O., 'The contagion of Asiatic cholera', *Prov. Med. Surg. J.* 13 (1849), 34–7, 62–6, 91–7. Also enlarged as *The Contagion of Asiatic Cholera Deduced* (1849).

Stewart, A.P., and Jenkins, E., *The Medical and Legal Aspects of Sanitary Reform*, with an introduction by M.W. Flinn (1867; New York, 1969).

Swayne, J.G., 'An account of certain organic cells peculiar to the evacuations of cholera', *Lancet*, 1849, ii. 368–71, 398–9.

——, 'Observations on the Report of the College of Physicians relative to the organic bodies discovered in the evacuations of cholera patients', *Lancet*, 1849, ii. 530–2.

——, *Medical Diagnosis, Past and Present* (Bristol, 1880).

[——*et al.*] 'In memoriam Augustin Prichard', *Bristol. Med.-Chir. J.*, 16 (1898), 1–15.

Symonds, J.A., 'Remarks on the progress and causes of cholera, as it occurred in Bristol in 1832', *Trans. Prov. Med. Surg. Ass.* 3 (1835), 170–93.

——, *Our Institution and its Studies* (London and Bristol, 1850).

——, *Ten Years: an inaugural lecture delivered at the Bristol Institution* (London and Bristol, 1861).

——, *Miscellanies*, ed. J.A. Symonds the younger (1871). See also Carrick, A., 1834.

Thompson, T., (ed.), *Annals of Influenza or Epidemic Catarrhal Fever*, Sydenham Society (1852).

Thomson, J., *An Account of the Life, Lectures and Writings of William Cullen*, with W. Thomson and D. Craigie, 2 vols. (2nd enlarged edn. Edinburgh, 1859).

Thomson, R.D., 'Clinical researches on the nature and cause of cholera', *Lancet*, 1850, i. 154–5.

——, 'On the chemical conditions of cholera atmospheres', *Lancet*, 1856, i. 63–4.

Thudichum, J.L.W., 'On the discoveries and philosophy of Liebig, with especial reference to their influence on the advancement of arts, manufactures, and commerce', *J. Soc. Arts*, 24 (1875–6), 16, 80–6, 95–100, 111–16, 125–8, 141–5.

Tunstall, J., 'Petroleum in Asiatic cholera', *Prov. Med. Surg. J.* 12 (1848), 390–1, 471–2.

Tweedie, A., *Clinical Illustrations of Fever* (1830).

——, *Lectures on the Distinctive Characters, Pathology and Treatment of Continued Fevers* (1862).

——, (ed.) *Library of Medicine. I–V: Practical Medicine*, 8 vols. (1840).

Watson, T., 'Lectures on the principles and practice of physic', *Lond. Med. Gaz.*, 1840–1, i and ii; 1841–2, i and ii. Also as *On the Principles and Practice of Physic*, 2 vols. (1843).

Westminster Review, 15 (1831), 457–90: 'Spasmodic cholera'.

Wilkinson, J.S., 'Some remarks upon the development of epiphytes', *Lancet*, 1849, ii. 448–51.

Williams, R., *Elements of Medicine. I and II: Morbid Poisons* (1836–41).

——, 'On the decrement of weight in phthisis', *Lancet*, 1842–3, i. 629–30.

Yelloly, J., 'Observations on the arrangement connected with the relief of the sick poor, addressed to . . . Lord John Russell', *Trans. Prov. Med. Surg. Ass.* 5 (1837), 456–88. (This is a 2nd, enlarged edn.)

See also Abbreviations, p.x.

INDEX

Aberdeen, 128

Acland, Henry, 155-6, 175n., 246, 248, 283, 288n.

Adams, Joseph, 115

adulteration, 151

agriculture, 32, 34, 126-7, 129, 140n.

agues. *See* fever

airs, analyses of, 38, 105, 107, 141, 143, 165, 175, 176, 180, 182, 184, 187, 221n., 223

Albert, Prince, 128n., 283

alcohol, 118, 122

alcoholism, temperance, 5, 44, 91, 205, 214-15

Alderson, James, 222

Alexandria, 3

algae, 170n., 186n., 221n.

Alison, Archibald, 40, 41

Alison, William Pulteney, 26, 35, 41-6, 95n., 96-7, 101, 210, 280, 281, 283

America, 38n., 85, 184n., 189, 195, 298

ammonia, 107, 141

anaesthesia, 203n., 214n., 215

analogy, use of, 84, 95, 100, 102, 104, 109, 112-15, 117-20, 130, 138, 141, 151, 182, 189-91, 193, 197-201, 205, 206, 229, 232ff., 239, 247, 249, 250-3, 256, 257, 260, 261, 263, 265, 270, 272, 273, 275, 278, 282, 286, 303, 307

Ancell, Henry, 130, 133

Andral, Gabriel, 85, 96, 265, 266

animalculae, 88, 148, 149, 165, 190, 192, 193, 198ff., 201n., 208, 220-1, 262n.

anthrax, 137, 239, 259

anthropology, 85, 104, 109, 160n., 254

anticontagionism, 7, 24, 27, 30, 35, 44, 57-8, 63-7, 69-70, 73, 77ff., 139, 274, 284-5, 298-302, 304

Armstrong, John, 9, 19, 26, 28, 43, 54

Arnott, Neil, 6, 12, 31, 35, 36, 38, 39, 42, 44-5, 65, 66, 72, 73, 78, 87, 222

Ashmolean Society, 175

Athenaeum, The, 150

atomic theory, 62, 104, 124, 211, 214

Audouin, Jean Victor, 191

Aylesbury, 238

Babington, Benjamin Guy, 178n., 179, 222

Bacon, Francis, 29n., 53, 129, 133n.

Bacot, John, 222

Bacteriological Nomenclature, Committee on, 3

bacteriology, 1, 3, 253, 297, 299, 304, 305

Baly, William, 119n., 166, 178ff., 181-2, 183ff., 218, 222, 226-8, 240, 268, 304

Bassi, Agostino, 191

Bateman, Thomas, 9n., 43

Bavaria, 127, 244

Bayle, Gaspard Laurent, 95n.

Beale, Lionel, 256n., 289

Beddoe, John, 158, 254

Bell, Charles, 138n.

Bell, Charles William, 138, 139-40

Bennett, John Hughes, 142, 143, 155, 186n.

Bentham, Jeremy, 7, 29n., 31, 32, 82

Benthamism, 6n., 7, 10, 11, 28, 29, 42, 82, 230

Berg, Fredrik Theodor, 191n.

Berkeley, Miles, 177n., 185, 186n., 188, 200n.

Berlin, 160n., 181n., 236n.

Berlin Cholera Commission, 3n.

Bernard, Claude, 124

Bernard, James Fogo, 159, 161, 162, 165

Bernard, Ralph Montague, 159n.

Berthollet, Claude Louis, 121, 208

Berzelius, Jöns Jacob, 120

Bilston, 51n.

biochemistry, 1, 126, 304

biological theories of causation, 1, 73, 88, 104, 113, 121-2, 125, 134-6, 140, 141, 148, 149, 170-1, 175n., 181-2, 188-202, 207, 208, 220,

biological (*cont.*)
  233, 234, 253-64, 273, 282, 285,
  295, 297ff., 304-7
Bird, Golding, 132
Birmingham, 2, 70, 150, 158
Blacklock, A., 148-9
Blandford, 175, 209, 264
Blane, Gilbert, 27, 137
Boards of Health, 32, 50, 56, 86, 162.
  Central (1831), 51n., 238; Central
  (1854), 144, 220, 221-2, 231, 234,
  245, 274 (*see also* Committee for
  Scientific Enquiries); General (1848)
  7, 10n., 29, 34, 46, 51-2, 55, 57,
  63-80, 81, 114, 139, 142-4, 146,
  175n., 178, 179, 218n., 222, 232,
  264, 274, 292, 298, 300-1, 302, 309
Boehm, Ludwig, 194, 209
Boerhaave, Hermann, 136
Bowerbank, James, 153
Bowie, Robert, 59
Bowman, William, 271
Bowring, John, 81
Bretonneau, Pierre Fidèle, 16, 94n., 266
Bridgewater, 175n., 185n.
Bright, Richard, 178
Bristol, 156-61, 162ff., 167, 186,
  189, 192, 254, 267, 268-9, 271,
  273n.
Bristol Baptist College, 8n.
Bristol College, 159, 160n.
Bristol Gazette, 184
Bristol Literary and Philosophical
  Institution, 156, 157, 163
Bristol Medical Library Society, 158n.,
  282n.
Bristol Medico-Chirurgical Society, 157-
  8, 159, 164, 185. Microscopical
  Subcommittee of, 159-60, 161,
  163-4, 175, 308; other commit-
  tees, 160-1
Bristol Microscopical Society, 156-7,
  162, 177n., 186n.
Bristol Naturalists' Society, 156n.
Bristol School of Pharmacy, 156n.
British Annals of Medicine, 105
British Association for the Advance-
  ment of Science, 87, 93, 96, 97,
  126, 128, 150, 163
*British and Foreign (Medico-Chirurgical)
  Review*, 61-2, 72, 76-7, 87, 104,
  111, 129, 132ff., 141, 194
British Medical Association (1), 111

British Medical Association (2), 160n.,
  214n., 274. *See also* Provincial
  Medical and Surgical Association
British Medical Journal, 167, 172,
  185, 277
Brittan, Frederick, 72, 159, 160, 162,
  163, 164-7, 168ff., 172-3, 174,
  175, 180, 185, 187ff., 308-9
Broad Street (Soho), 218, 224-5, 241,
  246
Brodie, Benjamin Collins (snr.), 40-1,
  231
Broussais, François Joseph Victor, 15,
  16, 265-6
Brown, John, 53, 156
Brown, Robert, 152
Brown, Thomas, 20
Brussels, 99
Budd, George, 95n., 157, 174n., 178,
  179, 195, 268n., 271, 274-5
Budd, Richard, 267, 268, 272, 281
Budd, William, 1, 46, 161, 162, 170-3,
  201, 209, 250-94, 297, 300, 305.
  Biog. details of, 162n., 174n., 265-
  7, 274. On aerial transmission,
  141n., 166, 171, 275, 276, 281,
  286; on cancer, 174n., 253-4, 258,
  260-1, 263, 271, 272-3; on cholera,
  147, 161n., 162n., 163, 166, 167,
  170-3, 179n., 226, 251, 254, 260,
  261, 263, 264, 275-7, 280, 281,
  286; on contagion, 18, 23, 65n.,
  250-2, 254, 258, 260ff., 272-3,
  275, 276, 277-8, 284-6, 287ff.;
  on epidemic disease, 161, 171,
  179n., 250, 251-2, 257-8, 269,
  272, 275; epidemiological arguments
  of, 250, 256, 265ff., 275, 276-9,
  290, 291-3; and evolution, 255;
  and experimental investigation,
  239n., 252, 256, 267, 286; fungoid
  theory of, 148, 164, 170-3, 174,
  175, 182, 187, 191, 217, 278-9,
  304-5, 306; and Henle, 250, 257-
  60, 285; and Holland, 193, 253n.,
  269, 271, 274; and Liebig, 128-9,
  257, 261, 269-70, 271, 280, 286;
  measures urged by, 119, 171, 191,
  256, 262, 266, 269, 273n., 279,
  286; methodology of, 170, 174,
  251-3, 256, 257, 265, 275, 303;
  microscopical work of, 155n., 157,
  160, 163, 166, 174n., 191, 272; and

Budd, William (*cont.*)
  Murchison, 287, 290-2; on pathology, 170-1, 251, 252, 254, 256, 259, 267, 270, 271, 275ff., 281, 282; on physiology, 259n., 267, 269-70; reactions to, 171-2, 182, 200, 264, 270, 271, 273n., 274, 278-82, 291ff., 307, 309-10; and Simon, 248, 273n., 274, 291-3, 295; on smallpox, 213, 250-3, 256, 258, 265, 272, 275, 278, 282; and Snow, 171, 207, 213, 215ff., 247, 249ff., 265, 268, 272n., 274-81; on spontaneous generation, 253, 255, 262-4, 273, 277, 282, 291; on symmetry in disease, 193n., 266n., 268, 269, 270, 271; on typhoid, 248-9, 250-1, 256, 265, 267, 269, 274ff., 281-6, 291-2; on water transmission, 166, 171, 172, 182, 275, 276
Burma, 287
burn, 93, 163
Burnett, William, 58, 141n., 178
Burrows, George, 178, 179, 181n.
Busk, George, 157, 174, 175-7, 178, 181n., 182ff., 188, 208

Cagniard de la Tour, Charles, 122, 134, 135, 193
Callender, George William, 223
Cambridge, 5n., 161n.
camphor, 192
Canada, 61
cancer, 93, 174n., 236n., 253-4, 258, 260-1, 263, 271, 272-3
carbon, 148-9
Carlisle, 92
Carpenter, Lant, 159
Carpenter, William Benjamin, 119-20, 138-40, 143, 152, 155n., 156, 157, 170, 175, 196, 200, 255, 262, 267n., 269, 270-1, 274
Carswell, Robert, 95n.
catalysis, 120ff., 190, 196, 233, 261
cattle-plague, 110, 237, 239, 256, 274, 295
Ceely, Robert, 238
cell theory, 130, 134n., 135, 136, 153, 165, 174, 175, 204, 208-9, 211, 213, 262, 272-3
Chadwick, Edwin, 6-7, 8, 10-13, 31ff., 39-42, 46-53, 54ff., 82, 104, 140n., 220, 300, 301, 302n.. Biog. details of, 7, 10-11, 49, 70. On cholera, 31-2, 40, 46-58, 66, 78-9, 147; and disinfection, 60-1; and Farr, 40, 83-4, 85, 87, 110-11; and the medical profession, 12-13, 31, 40, 41, 52, 62, 72, 111; and poor law, 11, 42, 82; on public health and disease, 11-12, 31-3, 34, 39-41, 45, 56, 57, 67, 111, 245; and Southwood Smith, 7, 10, 12, 13, 31, 45; and statistics, 82, 86. *See also* Board of Health, General; Metropolitan Sanitary Commission.
chalky bodies, 183
Chalmers, Thomas, 44
Chauveau, Jean Baptiste Auguste, 289
chemistry, 37, 48, 73, 85ff., 94, 103, 105, 108, 110, 111, 118, 119, 121, 125-7, 128ff., 132, 135, 143, 145ff., 151, 155, 156, 160, 161n., 163, 175, 183-4, 187, 190, 207, 209ff., 219ff., 227, 228, 232-3, 237, 241, 243, 254, 259n., 261, 264, 268, 269n., 273, 287, 303, 306. Organic or animal, 16, 78, 118, 120-1, 125, 126, 131, 133-4, 141, 151, 208, 219, 232, 262, 270. *See also* Liebig.
childbirth, 98, 214n.
children, infants, 4, 42, 124, 191n.
cholera, Asiatic, 1-7, 18, 46-79, 108-10, 144, 146-51, 159, 162-97, 198ff., 203-9, 215-18, 222-9, 233-7, 239-49, 254, 260, 261, 265, 275-6, 283-4, 286, 295, 296, 298, 301, 302, 304ff. Cholerine, 102, 110; consecutive fever of, 49, 54; contagiousness or otherwise of, 7, 23, 28, 29, 46, 47, 49-50, 55, 57-8, 61, 66, 69, 71, 73, 139, 147, 195-6, 218, 227-8, 233-4, 236, 240-2, 246, 248-9, 251, 258, 263, 264-5, 275-8, 280, 283n., 284, 286; El Tor vibrio, 3n.; epidemiology of, 2, 29, 47, 67, 70-1, 100, 109, 114-15, 139, 180, 190-1, 193, 195, 203-4, 215, 218-19, 224-6, 227, 235-6, 265, 275, 276-8, 281, 283n., 290; and fever, 6, 31-2, 40, 46-9, 54-5, 57, 62, 64, 71, 78n., 79, 248-9, 251, 283, 288, 293; General Board of Health on, 7,

cholera (*cont.*)

10n., 46, 51-2, 55, 64, 66-72, 73ff., 78-9; literature on, 4-5, 147-8, 227; in lower animals, 3, 239, 240-3, 246-7, 286; mathematical laws in, 88, 89, 109, 223, 228; Metropolitan Sanitary Commission on, 46-51, 55-8, 61-2, 66; mortality from, 2-3, 52, 108-9; pandemics, 1-3; pathology, 71, 74, 78, 114, 147, 148, 159, 162, 166, 170-1, 175, 176, 179, 180, 181, 193, 194n., 196, 204, 205-7, 208, 209, 216, 217, 223, 226, 242, 244, 251, 254, 277, 281; and sanitarianism, 6, 7, 30, 40, 46-7, 56, 58, 65, 68, 74, 78-9, 100-1, 144, 248, 276, 295; subjects of, 2, 48, 64-5, 79, 146, 239; symptomology, 5, 51, 71, 74, 146, 148, 195, 200-1, 242, 243; *Vibrio cholerae*, 3, 247n., 305-6. *See also* diarrhoea; experimentation; *and other headings*

Christison, Robert, 43, 44n., 46, 65, 95n., 116-17, 266

Clark, James, 31n., 86-7, 95n., 128n., 222, 245, 282

climate, 2, 19, 21, 30, 37, 38, 43, 75, 86, 119, 287

Cobbett, William, 13n.

cod-liver-oil, 163

Coleridge, Samuel Taylor, 230

College of Chemistry, 128n.

Combe, Andrew, 86, 111

Combe, George, 86

Committee for Scientific Enquiries, 144, 183n., 222-6, 227, 236, 237, 244-5, 246, 247, 291. *See also* Board of Health, Central (1854)

Condy, Henry, 61

Conolly, John, 54, 86

consensus-enquiries, 162-3, 177, 180, 218, 223, 227, 256

contagion, 36, 44, 47, 64ff., 68, 70, 75, 76-8, 79, 90, 99ff., 103, 106, 107, 115, 123ff., 136, 138n., 141, 147, 192, 194, 196, 198, 201, 206ff., 218, 232-4, 238, 244, 248, 250-2, 254, 258, 260-1, 263-4, 275ff., 283-5, 289, 298-303. Common, 15, 22, 254; modified, 73; specific, 15, 22, 24; strict, 58, 61-2, 69, 73, 77

contagionism, 23-4, 27, 29, 46, 50, 196n., 284, 299-300, 304. *See also* anticontagionism

contagious or continuous molecular action, law of, 121ff., 125, 133-4, 135, 144-5, 208, 210, 212, 289, 303, 307

contingent contagionism, 18, 22, 44, 57, 61, 67, 73, 76-8, 105-6, 111, 118, 138-9, 162, 172, 206, 248, 258, 262, 264, 265, 274, 281, 283-5, 293

Cooper, Bransby, 142

Copland, James, 195

Cowdell, George, 169, 189, 190, 191n., 194-6, 198ff., 250

cowpox, 17, 238. Vaccinine, 238. *See also* vaccination

croup, 96, 101, 275

Cullen, William, 14-15, 18, 20, 21, 26, 53, 92, 94, 95

Currie, James, 65

Cuvier, Georges, 85, 95

Dalton, John, 95n., 104n.

Darwin, Charles, 229, 253n., 254-6

Daubeny, Charles, 175, 189, 190, 193, 201n.

Davaine, Casimir, 260

Davidson, W., 282n.

Davies, David, 254-5, 273n.

Davies, David Samuel, 255

Davy, Humphry, 192

Davy, John, 148

Day, G. E., 196

deficiency theories, 148-9

deodorants, 58, 61

diarrhoea, 18, 43, 48, 55, 56, 109n., 110, 165, 242, 247n., 248, 293. Premonitory, 51-2, 56, 147, 168

diphtheria, 98, 251, 258

disinfection, 48, 58, 60-1, 124, 150, 178, 191-2, 238, 279, 286

dispensaries, 9, 13, 51, 105, 130. Bristol, for Diseases of the Skin, 159n; Bristol Eye, 160n.; Eastern, 9; Edinburgh New Town, 43; Finsbury, 183n.; Public, 9n.

Dorchester, 169, 194n.

'doubtful diseases', the, 9, 18, 22, 23, 47, 67, 73, 79n., 139, 140ff., 258, 264, 303

dropsy, 53

Dublin, 96, 159n., 160n., 161n., 267, 287
Dumas, Jean Baptiste, 126, 269n., 270
Dupuytren, Guillaume, 84
dysentery, 18, 70, 101, 181, 182, 248, 288
dyspepsia, 95n.

East India Company, 27, 45n., 287
Edinburgh, 8, 9, 14n., 41ff., 45, 93, 96-7, 116, 155, 159n., 161n., 175, 186n., 192, 240, 241n., 242, 265n., 266-7, 281, 287
Edinburgh Medical and Surgical Journal, 26, 186
Edmonds, T. R., 95n.
education, 7, 12-13, 44, 45, 84, 111, 127, 210, 211
Egypt, 24, 37
electricity, 67, 79, 120, 148ff., 196, 262
Elliotson, John, 65n.
emphysema, 267
epidemic atmosphere, 22, 55, 113. Constitution, 16, 55, 73; influence, 62, 66-8, 75, 76, 78, 113, 139, 143, 144
Epidemiological Society of London, 99, 197, 214n., 222, 231, 239
epithelium, 165, 176, 194n., 208-9, 251, 264
epizootics, 55, 238, 239, 242, 254, 256. *See also* cattle-plague, *etc.*
erysipelas, 100, 101, 102, 137, 213, 280
d'Espiné, Jacob-Marc, 97, 99
Estlin, John Bishop, 157
Estlin, John Prior, 192
Ethnological Society, 254
de l'Eure, Gendron, 266
Examiner, The, 7, 10, 11, 31-2, 48, 49, 53ff., 70n.
exanthemata, 20, 43, 76, 209, 251, 272. *See also* smallpox, *etc.*
Exeter, 175
experimentation, research, 3, 16, 37-8, 53, 58, 62, 63, 65, 70, 103, 107, 116n., 118, 124, 136, 137, 141, 143, 144, 149, 165, 177-8, 191, 204n., 206, 220, 222-3, 227, 232, 235-44, 252, 256, 257, 267, 269n., 285, 289, 293, 295, 297, 306. In cholera, 3, 50, 110, 148, 163ff., 174, 181ff., 224-5, 235-6, 239-44,

245, 246-7, 248, 279, 286; 'crucial', 29, 50, 224-5; 'popular', 236, 237, 279; vivisection, 269n. *See also* airs; water

Falconer, Hugh, 287
Faraday, Michael, 58n., 127, 129, 192, 238
Farr, William, 36, 81-112, 113, 255. Biog. details of, 82, 84-7, 105, 231. And Chadwick, 40, 83-4, 85, 87, 110-11; on cholera, 86, 88, 89, 100ff., 108-10, 144, 222, 226, 229; on contagion, 90, 99ff., 103, 105-6, 107, 111, 199, 229; disease classification of, 40, 46, 83-4, 90, 92-101, 105, 108; on epidemic diseases, 88, 89-91, 92, 93, 96, 100-1, 105, 106, 141-2; on fever, 92, 94, 95n., 98, 99; and Henle, 87-8, 194, 199; humoral pathology of, 94, 102ff.; influence of, 82, 83, 89, 91, 92, 97, 98, 108, 112; and Liebig, 84, 87, 94, 95n., 96 101ff., 104-5, 141-3, 229; mathematical laws of disease of, 88-91, 104, 107-8, 109, 112, 223; and the medical profession, 83, 93, 95-6, 103ff., 110-12, 132; methodology of, 84, 91, 103, 110, 112, 193, 229; on poisons, 102-3, 105-6, 108, 141; sanitarianism of, 31, 83, 91, 93, 106-8, 111ff.; on smallpox, 88, 90-1, 93, 99ff., 141, 238; and Snow, 109, 110, 203, 218, 228-9; statistical work of, 39, 83, 85ff., 112; and Sydenham, 87ff., 95, 103, 104, 111, 142; on zymosis, 90, 99, 101-8, 109-10, 143
Farr, William (of Nice), 86n.
fermentation, 53, 95, 101-2, 103-4, 108, 113, 120, 121-3, 124, 125, 133, 134-6, 138, 140, 143-4, 189ff., 196, 199-200, 201, 208, 210, 211, 213, 233, 234n., 244, 246, 247, 251, 258, 261, 270, 284, 286
fever, 5, 14-26, 31-2, 34-8, 41-8, 89, 132, 207, 233, 259, 267, 281-93, 297. Agues, 17, 38, 99, 115, 117; Alison on, 41-5; Armstrong on, 28, 55n.; Arnott on, 6, 42, 44; Chadwick on, 30-1, 40, 41-2; changes in nature of, 54-5, 94, 290; and cholera, 6, 32, 40, 46, 47-

334 INDEX

fever (*cont.*)
9, 54-5, 57, 62, 64, 71, 78n., 79, 251, 283, 288, 293; Christison on, 43, 44n., 46, 95n., 116-17; consecutive (of cholera), 49, 54; contaminative, 24, 65; continued, 4, 6, 15, 16n., 18, 19, 26, 30, 32, 38, 43-4, 68, 76, 80, 250, 272, 281, 287, 288, 290, 292, 301, 302; Cullen on, 15, 21, 26; and destitution, 41-2, 43, 45, 48; and diarrhoea, 56; 'dothinenteric', 94; economic importance of, 32, 39, 41ff.; 'endemic', 288; enteric, 98, 266, 288, 289-90; 'epidemic', 288; epidemic continued, 101n.; eruptive, 142n., 283, 288 (*see also* exanthemata; smallpox); Farr on, 92, 94, 95n., 98, 99; 'fever nests', 31-2, 37, 49, 64, 71; in France, 15-16, 43, 250, 266, 281; idiopathic, essential, or simple, 15-16, 21, 288, 302; infectious, 24, 65; inflammatory, 15, 136; intermittent, marsh ague, 17ff., 38, 80, 102, 105, 140, 233, 301; low nervous, 136; Murchison on, 287-91, 300; pestilential, 136; Poor Law reports on, 6, 31, 35-9, 40, 45-6, 222n.; puerperal, 98, 102, 138, 280; putrid, 66, 136, 137, 139, 140; pythogenic theory of, 10, 259, 287-91; relapsing, 4, 18, 43-4, 288; remittent, 18, 38, 80, 288, 301; rheumatic, 267; simple continued, 98; Southwood Smith on, 6-7, 9, 10, 13, 18-25, 31, 41-44, 54, 66, 68, 95n., 302; subjects of, 42, 48, 65, 79; synocha, 15, 44n.; synochus, 15, 20; typhine, 102; typhoid, 4, 16n., 19, 38, 43, 60, 94n., 102, 181, 183-4, 206, 248, 249, 250-1, 256, 258, 265ff., 269, 275, 276, 281-5, 286, 288-9, 291-3, 296, 300, 301, 302n.; typhus, 4, 15, 18-19, 20, 21, 23, 24, 28, 37, 47-8, 55n., 56, 61, 62, 64, 65, 76, 94, 98, 102, 165, 183n., 281ff., 287, 288, 292, 302n.; yellow, 18, 19, 22n., 23, 24, 27ff., 38, 56, 64, 68, 73, 80, 94, 102, 105, 251, 258, 302. *See also* Budd, W.; London Fever Hospital; plague; scarlet fever
Flourens, Marie-Jean-Pierre, 269

Forbes, John, 86, 111
Fordyce, George, 238
Fowke, Francis, 305
Fox, Edward Long (snr.), 189, 192, 201n.
Fox, Edward Long (jnr.), 189n.
Fox, Henry Hawes, 189n.
France, 12, 13, 15-16, 30ff., 43, 69, 77, 86, 88, 89, 94, 95, 134n., 185, 199, 239, 250, 266, 269n., 281, 298, 299
fungi, fungous theories, mycology, 148, 149, 151, 154, 165n., 169-70, 182, 186, 188-9, 190-1, 195n., 196ff., 199-201, 213, 259, 262, 277, 295. Cholera-fungus theory, the, 146, 148, 151, 156, 157, 163ff., 167-78, 180-9, 193-4, 197, 199, 200, 207, 208, 216, 217, 234n., 240, 245, 264, 278, 279, 304, 305ff. *See also* plants; uredos.

Garrod, Alfred Baring, 215
gases, 37, 59-60, 84, 91, 106-7, 122, 141, 217, 221, 228
Gaspard, Marie H. Bernard, 38n., 116n.
Gavin, Hector, 231
Gay-Lussac, Joseph Louis, 85, 126
Geoffroy Saint-Hilaire, Étienne, 85
geology, 154, 157, 198, 254, 287
germ theory, 1, 162n., 189, 197, 203, 207, 214, 229, 255n., 256, 260, 264, 285-6, 289, 295, 299, 303
Germany, 3n., 95, 126ff., 134n., 152, 153, 193n., 199, 230, 236, 257, 286, 295, 298
Giessen, 105, 126
glanders, 192, 238
Glasgow, 14n., 105, 128, 192, 219, 282n.
gluten, 122ff.
Gooch, Robert, 27
Good, John Mason, 92
Gotschlich, Felix, 3n.
Graham, Robert, 267
Graham, Thomas, 107-8, 142, 196, 221
Grainger, Edward, 26
Grainger, Richard, 58n., 60, 155
Grant, William, 19
Green, Joseph Henry, 230
Greenhow, Thomas Michael, 114
Greenwich, 71, 176
Gregory, William, 128

Griffith, John William, 177n., 183ff., 231
Grove, John, 189, 190, 192, 197-8, 214, 250, 264
growth, processes of, 1, 124, 135, 260, 262, 289
Gull, William Withey, 178, 179, 180-1, 182ff., 218, 226, 227, 304
Guy, William, 119n., 178

Hall, Sir Benjamin, 222
Hall, Marshall, 269
Hallier, Ernst, 195n., 295
Hampstead, 224
Hancock, Thomas, 56
Harvey, William, 213
Hassall, Arthur Hill, 175, 220-1, 223, 225, 234, 305
Hawkins, Francis Bisset, 82n.
Haygarth, John, 65
Health of Towns Association, 8, 34, 230
Health of Towns Commission, 34, 46n.
Heidelberg, 181n., 193n.
Henle, Jacob, 3, 73, 87-8, 104, 134, 135, 140, 189, 190, 192, 193-4, 195, 198-9, 200, 201, 207, 233, 243, 250, 257-60, 285
Henry, William, 238-9
Herapath, Thornton, 161n., 165n.
Herapath, William, 161n.
Herapath, William Bird, 161n., 186n., 197
heredity, 210-13
Herschel, John, 192
Heysham, John, 92
Hippocrates, 88, 95n., 102n., 104, 142
Hobhouse, John Cam, 28
Hodgson, Joseph, 51n.
Hoffmann, Christoph Ludwig, 136
Hofmann, August von, 128, 220, 221, 244, 245
Holland, Henry, 95n., 189, 190, 192-3, 195, 198, 199, 201, 217n., 253n., 269, 271, 274
hospitals, 10, 13, 31, 43, 69, 100, 164, 178, 179, 192, 215, 230, 268, 276, 289-90. Bath General, 148n.; Bristol General, 160n., 161; Bristol Infirmary, 158, 159n., 160n., 161, 189n., 265n.; City

Cholera (Edinburgh), 242; convalescent homes, 8; Dorset County, 195; *Dreadnought*, 174n., 176, 178, 265n.; Edinburgh Infirmary, 267n.; fever, in Edinburgh, 267n.; Guy's, 142n., 160n., 180n.; Jews', 9; King's College, 229n.; London Fever, 9-10, 13, 25, 26, 37, 95n., 281, 287, 289-90; Middlesex, 271; Murray's Royal Institution for the Insane, 241n.; St. Bartholomew's, 223, 264; St. Peter's (Bristol), 161, 186n., 265n.; St. Thomas's, 60, 155, 229n., 230; Shrewsbury Infirmary, 85; Smallpox (London), 115n.; temporary, for cholera, 163; University College, 183, 230; Westminster, 215
house-to-house visitation, 51-2
housing, 8, 18, 24, 34, 37, 78, 84, 138
Humboldt, Alexander von, 126, 210
Hume, Joseph, 20
humoral pathology, 14, 16, 20-1, 53, 55, 78, 88, 102, 103, 115-16, 118, 124-5, 130, 131, 136-40, 142, 144, 145, 148, 163, 179, 183-4, 196, 205-6, 208, 215-16, 223, 233, 234n., 237, 241, 244, 259, 267, 269, 270-1, 272, 273, 280, 306
Hunt, Robert, 149-50
Hunter, John, 115-16, 137, 238
Huxham, John, 136
Huxley, Thomas Henry, 255n.
hydrogen peroxide, 122, 150n.
hydrophobia, 101n., 103
hygiene, 70n., 84n., 85, 86, 181

immunity, 17, 22, 119, 124, 125, 193n., 252, 259, 290, 305
India, 1, 24, 27n., 48, 50, 51, 61, 69, 70, 71, 110, 149, 287
inductivism, 20, 82, 153
infection, 24, 65, 103, 106, 107, 115, 218, 224, 234, 243, 275
inflammation, 14-15, 21, 25, 54, 92, 94, 136, 233, 248n., 259, 260
influenza, 47, 48, 55, 56, 64, 67, 73, 95n., 101n., 150, 163, 258
infusoria, 199, 259
inoculation, 17, 77, 90, 103, 106, 238, 259
insects, 190, 193, 217, 277. Flies, 217;

insects (*cont.*)
   silkworms, 191, 198, 233
iodine, 118
Ireland, 45
Italy, 86, 242, 287

Jenner, Edward, 63, 238
Jenner, William, 9n., 183, 184, 281,
   283, 288, 292
Johnson, James, 25n.

Kay(-Shuttleworth), James Phillips, 6,
   12, 31, 32n., 35, 36, 38, 41, 42,
   70n., 222n., 280
King's College, London, 128n., 163n.,
   179n., 230, 271
Kircher, Athanasius, 190
Koch, Robert, 3, 173, 214, 286,
   295, 305
'Koch's postulates', 3, 243, 286n.
Kützing, Friedrich Traugott, 122

Laennec, René Théophile Hyacinthe,
   95n., 96
Lancet, The, 13n., 26, 27, 30, 77,
   84n., 105n., 111, 129–30, 133,
   143, 147, 167, 168, 172, 173,
   177, 178, 184–5, 197. 198n , 199,
   220, 283
Lancisi, Giovanni Maria, 115
Lankester, Edwin, 175, 176, 203,
   208, 209, 211
de La Place, Pierre Simon, 121, 208
laryngitis, 96
Latham, Peter Mere, 88n., 178, 181n
Latham, Robert Gordon, 53n.
Lawrence, William, 13, 222
Ledoyen, M., 58
Leeds, 40
Leeson, Henry, 58n., 60
Letheby, Henry, 231
liberalism, 28, 299, 301
Liebig, Justus, 86, 120–45, 193, 214,
   304. Biog. details of, 125–9, 244,
   271. *Animal Chemistry*, 126, 129,
   130, 133, 142n., 149, 194, 200.
   269; on decay, 102, 120, 121, 133,
   270; on disease, 103, 104, 120,
   122–5, 127, 130–1, 133, 138, 140,
   141–2, 190, 194, 196, 198n., 201,
   212, 233, 244–5, 257, 283, 286,
   299, 303; exciters as postulated by.
   102, 105–6, 108, 123, 125, 141–2,

143; and Farr, 84, 87, 94, 95n., 96,
   101ff., 104–5, 141–3, 229; on
   fermentation, 101, 103–4, 108,
   120ff., 133, 134–6, 138. 196,
   201, 233, 244, 270. 286. 303;
   influence of, 78, 104, 108, 126–34,
   137ff., 141–5, 207–8, 210, 212,
   234, 245, 261, 269–70, 280, 303;
   methodology of, 104, 125, 129,
   133–4, 135, 213; *Organic Chemistry*,
   126, 129, 133, 135, 141, 196, 200,
   270; on physiology, 104n., 124ff.,
   129, 130, 133, 137, 269–70; pupils
   of, 105, 127ff., 244; on putrefaction, 102, 103, 107, 120ff., 133,
   137–41, 199, 201, 221, 244, 270,
   286, 303; and sanitarianism, 107,
   137–41, 143–4, 220. *See also* contagious molecular action; zymosis
Lindley, John, 196
Lindsay, William Lauder, 240, 241–2
Linnaeus, 190
Lisfranc, Jacques, 84, 265, 266
Lister, Joseph, 155n., 236n., 295
Lister, Joseph Jackson, 152, 155n.
Liverpool, 126, 175, 230
localism, 15–16, 19, 21, 94, 206
London, 2, 4, 24–5, 26, 32, 34, 36,
   48, 54, 70, 71, 91, 93, 146n., 157,
   159n., 160n., 161n., 166–7, 168,
   215, 218, 229, 230, 236, 277
London Medical Gazette, 26, 58, 61,
   77, 147, 166ff., 172, 179, 185,
   200, 224
London Medical Society of Observation,
   289
Louis, Pierre Charles Alexandre, 16, 84,
   95n., 96, 102, 265, 266, 281, 287,
   289
lunacy, 160n., 162, 189n.

MacCann, Francis, 51n.
Maclean, Charles, 9, 19, 23n., 27–8, 29.
   30, 80, 298
McCulloch, John Ramsay, 85, 87
McGrigor, James, 178n.
MacMichael, William, 27
Magendie, François, 116n., 118
magnetism, 67, 79
malaria. *See* fever, intermittent
malignant pustule. *See* anthrax
Malthus, Thomas, 111
Manchester, 70n., 128, 138n., 158, 219

maps, 32, 39, 40, 109

marsh ague. *See* fever, intermittent

Marshall, John, 183, 184, 187, 188, 240-1, 246

Mayhew, Henry, 168

Mayo, Thomas, 135, 178n.

Mead, Richard, 35, 37

measles, 4, 60, 101n., 248, 253

medical education, 4-5, 9, 12ff., 28, 31, 69, 70n., 86, 97, 111, 130, 155, 158, 161, 192, 268. Blenheim St. medical school, 105; Bristol, 156n., 158, 159n., 160n., 161, 162n., 265n., 268, 281; Public or Carey St., 9n.; Webb St., 26, 60; Windmill St., 215

medical officers of health, 142n., 183n., 229n., 230-1, 254-5, 273n.

medical profession, the, 8, 35-6, 81, 83, 88, 104, 110-12, 114, 119, 131, 146-7, 148, 156, 161, 168-9, 172-3, 177-8, 188-9, 192, 215, 223, 231-2, 255-6, 268, 281, 284-5, 292, 295-6, 299-301, 308-10. Army and navy, 12, 36, 69, 70n., 86, 97; in Bristol, 157-62, 189n.; Chadwick on, 12-13, 31, 40, 41, 52, 111; and chemistry, 103, 111, 130, 131-3, 156, 163, 219, 227; in factories, 41; and the General Board of Health, 7, 52, 64, 69-70, 72, 74-80, 114, 139, 178, 179, 232, 300-1, 302ff., 309; influence of Liebig on, 108, 129-34, 138-45, 245, 270, 303; and microscopy, 153ff., 155-6, 162; numbers of, 4-5, 98, 161n.; physicians, 4, 72n., 111, 155, 299; and poor law, 12, 36-7, 59, 98, 112, 197n., 238, 264; and public health, 13, 35, 40-1, 52, 57, 111, 168, 222 231-2, 238; qualifications of, 4-5, 161; and registration, 81-2, 93ff., 96ff.; and sanitarianism, 7, 35-6, 52, 57, 58, 62, 74-5, 79, 111, 113, 147, 232; surgeons, 41, 48, 59, 72n.

medical reform, 13, 41, 111, 130, 169 178, 238

Medical Times and Gazette, 245

medical topography, 215, 239

mercury, 192, 273

mesmerism, 189n.

meteorology, 67, 79, 142n., 190, 223

Metropolitan Sanitary Commission, 7, 34, 46-51, 55-6, 58n., 59ff., 66, 74, 78

Mevagissey, 52

miasmatic theory, 59, 62-3, 84, 99, 107-8, 141, 193, 217, 258-9, 284, 297, 299, 300, 305, 307

Microscopical Society of London, 153-4, 156, 157, 174ff., 184n.

microscopy, 146, 151-6, 157, 162ff., 170, 173-4, 175ff., 181, 183, 191, 194n., 197ff., 206, 220, 273, 306

midwifery, 160n., 162

Mill, James, 11n.

Mill, John Stuart, 129n., 133-4

Miller, William Allen, 221

Milne, Joshua, 92

Milroy, Gavin, 72n.

Mitchell, John Kearsley, 189, 190-1, 195, 198, 201

Moffatt, T., 150

Monthly Journal of Medical Science, 61, 75, 77, 198

Monthyon prize, 267n.

morbidity, 2

Morning Chronicle, 143, 164, 168, 169, 172-3, 178, 184, 188, 195

Morton, Richard, 103, 142

Müller, Johannes, 134, 193n., 273

Mulder, Gerardus, 132

Munich, 127, 220, 235, 236n., 244, 245, 286

Murchison, Charles, 9n., 10, 259, 275, 287-91, 292, 293, 300

Murchison, Roderick, 287

Murray, James, 149

muscardine, 191, 198, 201, 233, 250, 258, 260

natural history, 20, 26, 54, 75, 94-5, 154, 191, 197, 209, 213, 253, 245, 260, 263-4, 301

Naturphilosophie, 149n., 212n.

Neild, John Cash, 159-60

nervous system, the, 8, 14, 15, 20-1, 53, 116, 118, 149, 189n., 248n., 259n., 267, 269-70, 271

neuralgia, 194n.

Newcastle, 114, 214, 215, 218n.

Newtonianism, 125, 131, 134

nitric acid, 220

non-naturals, the, 21

North Tawton, 265, 267, 292
Norwich, 268
nosology, 14, 30, 46, 92-4, 95n., 96-7, 105-6, 258. *See also* Farr
Nuisances Removal Act, 56-7
nutrition, diet, famine, food, 18, 21, 39, 45, 48, 78, 95n., 105, 110, 116, 120, 123, 127, 132, 133, 136, 137-8, 140, 149, 204, 228, 244, 248, 262, 270

odours, 59-60
ophthalmology, 161, 194n.
Orfila, Mathieu, 84, 116, 265
Oundle, 195
Owen, Richard, 10n., 34, 46, 154, 155, 157, 212, 222, 231, 247
Oxford, 5n., 161n., 175, 246
Ozanam, J. A. F., 95n.
ozone, 148, 149-51, 178n.

Pacini, Filippo, 3
Paget, James, 156n., 268
pangenesis, 256n.
parasitism, 140, 141, 171, 189, 191, 194, 196ff., 213, 233, 234, 247, 253-5, 258, 273, 286, 295, 305. Tapeworm, 207; worms, 99, 208.
Paris, 84-5, 96, 126, 159n., 160n., 161n., 181n., 236n., 264, 265-6, 287
Paris, John Ayrton, 178, 179, 222
Parker, Nicholas, 201
Parkes, Edmund, 16, 35, 70-4, 75, 76, 83, 112, 114, 175, 183n., 215, 216, 225, 226-7, 235, 240, 241, 274
Parkes, Joseph, 70
Parliament, 5, 8, 28, 36, 81
Parliamentary Candidate Society, 7
parthenogenesis, 212
Pasteur, Louis, 1, 3, 136, 189n., 229, 256n., 260, 262, 263, 295, 304
pathological anatomy, 10, 14, 15-16, 20, 26, 71, 75, 85, 94, 114, 162, 179, 223, 301
Pathological Society of London, 154, 214n.
Percival, Thomas, 43
petroleum, 148
Pettenkofer, Max von, 127, 235, 244ff., 283-4, 286-7, 293, 295, 302n.

phrenology, 266
phthisis. *See* tuberculosis
physiology, 1, 8, 15-16, 37n., 38, 85, 104, 111, 116, 124ff., 129, 130, 132ff., 148, 149n., 156, 181, 194, 198n., 204n., 205, 210, 211, 215, 263, 266ff., 269-70, 282, 306, 307
Piedvache, Joseph, 266
pig typhoid, 256
Pinel, Philippe, 21
Place, Francis, 7
plague, 4, 18-19, 21, 23, 24, 27ff., 37, 48, 56, 64, 65, 68, 76, 79n., 94, 213
plants, 107, 120, 174, 176, 254. Blight, 190, 198, 200; bran, 176, 187; diseases of, 196, 242; geographical distribution of, 198, 253; rice, 295; smut, 176, 177; wheat, husk of, 176. *See also* fungi; potato disease; uredos
Platonism, 212n.
Playfair, Lyon, 60, 128
Plomley, Francis, 209
pneumonia, 93, 100
poisons, viruses, 21, 22, 30, 36-8, 43-4, 46, 53, 62, 65, 66, 73, 74, 78, 102-3, 105-6, 108, 113-20, 123, 125, 139, 141, 143, 144, 148, 150, 161n., 181n., 205, 209, 228, 232ff., 244, 247, 248, 252, 260, 270, 271n., 272, 280, 288, 290. Arsenic, 102, 116; irritants, 208, 209; morbid, 115-16, 120, 124-5, 232, 233, 238, 260, 270, 271n., 285; paludal, 115, 233; venoms, 115, 116
police, 31, 32. *See also* State medicine
pollen, 107
poor, the, 2, 5, 9ff., 24, 31-2, 39, 41-2, 48, 59, 79, 283
poor law, 44, 46. New, 11, 41-2, 82, 112, 238; Scottish, 41-2. *See also* medical profession
Poor Law Commission, 6, 35, 38, 39n., 45
population, laws of, 10-11, 39, 40-1, 79, 83, 111, 128. Density of, 90-1, 106-8
potassium iodide, 117n., 270
potato disease, the, 149, 154, 163, 200, 262n.
Potter, Nathaniel, 22n., 38n.
press, the lay, 5, 74, 164, 167-9,

press (*cont.*)
184, 231, 245
Prichard, Augustin, 157, 159ff.
Prichard, James Cowles, 158, 160n., 189n., 198, 254
Pringle, John, 21, 37, 50, 136
prisons, 7, 181. Hulks, 71; Millbank, 181
Privy Council, 229n., 231, 237ff., 291
Provincial Medical and Surgical Association, 82, 158, 162-3, 179, 194-5, 218, 238, 239, 264, 281n. *See also* British Medical Association (2)
Public Health Acts, 34, 39, 42, 230
puerperal fever. *See* fever.
putrefaction, 18, 19, 21, 23, 24, 37-8, 53, 58ff., 62, 65, 78, 104, 107-8, 115, 116-17, 136-41, 143, 148, 150, 181n., 192, 208, 213, 219-20, 223-4, 234n., 235, 243-4, 248n., 258-9, 261, 271, 280, 288-9, 301. Animal, 21, 38, 288; antiseptics, 136-7, 140, 148, 245; of excretions, 224, 246, 247-8, 283, 284, 288; Liebig on, 102, 103, 107, 120ff., 133, 137-41, 199, 201, 244, 270, 286; vegetable, 17, 21, 38, 288
pyaemia, 137. Pus, 273, 289

quackery, 58, 133
quarantine, 10n., 24, 26-30, 47, 49, 55, 57, 61, 63, 66-7, 75, 83, 284, 296, 298
Quekett, Edwin, 153
Quekett, John, 153-4, 155, 166-7, 175
Quetelet, Lambert-Adolphe-Jacques, 150
quinsy, 96

Radcliffe, J. Netten, 203
Rainey, George, 155, 223
red snow (Pseudomonas nivalis), 190
Redi, Francesco, 262
reductionism, 190, 303, 304
Registrar-General's Office, 39, 81ff., 86, 99
registration, 81-3, 87, 93, 96-8, 292. Registration Acts, 81-2, 97, 98
Reid, John, 267
Richardson, Benjamin Ward, 53, 143, 197, 203, 207, 214-15, 243, 281
Robertson, W., 186n.

Roupell, George, 178
Royal College of Physicians, 5n., 27, 28, 69, 99, 135n., 147, 158, 163, 170, 178-80, 222, 223, 264, 271n., 300, 310. Cholera Committee of, 178-80, 184, 222; Report on Cholera (1849) of, 173n., 176n., 177, 181, 182-8, 227, 304; *Reports on Cholera* (1854), 180-1, 226-8, 310. *See also* Baly; Gull
Royal College of Physicians of Edinburgh, 96, 101
Royal College of Surgeons, 155, 158, 222, 223, 229n.
Royal Institution, 192
Royal Medical and Chirurgical Society, 117n., 129, 174n., 197n., 214n.
Royal Society of London, 128, 274
Russia, 46, 50n., 51, 52
Rymer, J., 53

Sanderson, John Burdon, 236, 237, 240, 243, 248n., 256n., 286n., 289
Sandgate, 175n.
sanitarianism, 6-7, 11, 16, 21, 22, 30-3, 35, 38, 39-40, 45-6, 52, 56-61, 63, 74-5, 79, 83-4, 86, 91, 93, 105, 106-8, 110ff., 113, 137-41, 144-5, 147, 167-8, 178, 180, 181, 184, 200, 221, 231-2, 248, 276, 280-1, 282-3, 292, 295-7, 300-1, 303, 305, 307
scabies, 192, 201
scarlet fever, scarlatina, 4, 60, 64, 76, 98, 101n., 296
Schleiden, Matthias Jacob, 134n., 152, 211, 213
Schönbein, Christian Friedrich, 150
Schwann, Theodor, 104, 134-6, 193, 196, 257, 273
Scotland, 41-3, 44, 68, 96, 161n.
scrofula. *See* tuberculosis
scurvy, 18, 95n., 99, 136
Semmelweis, Ignaz, 162n., 280
septicaemia, 78. *See also* humoral pathology
sheep-pox, 256, 265
Shrewsbury, 84, 85
Simon, Johann Franz, 196
Simon, John, 36, 83, 84, 89, 119, 221, 222, 226, 229-37, 246, 288n., 291-3, 295-6, 302n.. Biog. details

Simon, John (*cont.*)
of, 155, 229-31. On analysis, 155, 219n.; and Budd, 248, 273n., 274, 291-3, 295; on chemistry in medicine, 232-3; on cholera, 204, 229, 233-6, 242-3, 248-9; on contagion, 73, 232-4, 248, 263-4, 284-5, 292-3, 300; and Liebig, 233-4; sanitarianism of, 231-2, 248, 292-3, 295-6; and Snow, 204, 229, 234-5, 236, 247-9

skin diseases, 161, 181n., 272

smallpox, 4, 17-18, 22, 23, 45, 53, 60, 62, 67, 76, 88, 90-1, 93, 99ff., 114, 116ff., 141, 142, 148, 189, 206-7, 209, 213, 238, 248-53, 256, 258, 263ff., 272, 275, 278, 282, 293, 296, 307. Varioline, 102, 238. *See also* inoculation

Smee, Alfred, 231, 262

Smith, John, 28

Smith, Robert Angus, 60, 65, 219, 221n.

Smith, Thomas Southwood, 6-10, 18-26, 28ff., 34, 36, 37-9, 40, 46-53, 64, 82, 83, 110-11, 222n., 300, 301, 309. Biog. details of, 7-9, 70. And Armstrong, 9, 19, 26, 54; and Budd, 18, 23, 284, 309; and Chadwick, 7, 10, 12, 13, 31, 45; on cholera, 29, 31-2, 46-51, 54-8, 68, 78-9, 178; on contagion, 18, 22-4, 29, 30, 38, 58, 65, 66, 69-70, 76, 79, 105, 213, 284, 302; and disinfection, 58n., 61; on epidemic diseases, 18, 22-3, 30, 47-9, 54-5, 62, 64-5, 66-7, 68, 75-6, 80, 90, 100, 101, 302, 307; experiments by, 37-8, 62, 137n.; on fever, 6-7, 9, 10, 13, 18-25, 31, 41-4, 54, 66, 68, 95n., 302; and Maclean, 9, 19, 28, 30; on the medical profession, 13n., 28-9, 64; methodology of, 13, 20-3, 38, 66; on poisons, 21, 22, 37-8, 44, 62, 65, 114; and Sydenham, 53, 54-5, 56, 62, 68, 104; on zymosis, 143-4. *See also* Board of Health, General; Metropolitan Sanitary Commission

Snow, John, 1, 176, 202-49, 264, 291, 297, 300, 303. Biog. details of, 214-15, 267n., 274-5. On aerial transmission, 217, 221, 228, 277; and Baly, 180, 218, 227-8, 240; and Budd, 171, 207, 213, 215ff., 247, 249ff., 265, 268, 272n., 274-81; on communicability, 205, 206, 212-13, 218, 240, 247, 275, 277-8; on disease agents, 204ff., 212ff., 216-17, 229, 247, 307; on epidemiology of cholera, 71n., 203-4, 207, 218-19, 224-6, 228, 235-6, 246, 265, 275, 277-8, 290; and Farr, 109, 110, 203, 218, 228-9; and the General Board of Health, 71n.; and Liebig, 142, 207-8, 210, 212, 214, 280; measures urged by, 109, 279; and Parkes, 71n., 215, 216, 240; on pathology, 204, 205-7, 208, 216, 218, 224ff., 240, 242, 246, 248, 264n., 277-9, 280ff., 307, 309-10; and Simon, 204, 229, 234-5, 236, 247-9; on spontaneous generation, 105n., 213, 284; on water transmission, 171, 180, 203, 204, 206, 208, 216, 217-19, 276

Society for . . . Bettering the Condition of the Poor, 9n.

Society for the Diffusion of Useful Knowledge, 54, 230

South London Medical Society, 167

specificity, 20, 68, 73-4, 75-6, 79, 94ff., 100, 101, 105, 110, 111, 114, 125, 141, 191, 197, 206, 211ff., 229, 232, 244, 248, 253, 254, 256, 257, 262, 284, 286, 290, 301. *See also* natural history

spontaneous generation, 23, 30, 78, 105, 110, 190, 213, 253, 255, 257, 261-4, 273, 277, 282, 284, 288, 291

Spooner, Edward Oke, 175, 209, 251, 264-5

Spooner, William Charles, 264

Sprengel, Kurt, 95n.

Stahl, Georg Ernst, 133n.

starch, 176

Starr, Thomas, 198, 199n.

State medicine, medical police, 30n., 35-6, 40-1, 43, 83, 100, 222

Statistical Society of London, 81, 93

statistics, 2, 20, 39, 57, 79, 81-3, 86, 88, 92, 95n., 108-9, 111n., 112, 140, 163, 167, 218, 223, 225, 235, 252, 256, 279, 289-90, 307.

statistics (*cont.*)
International Statistical Congress, 99; life tables, 83, 92; numerical method, 223n., 289. *See also* Farr
Steenstrup, Japetus, 247
Stephens, Henry Oxley, 186, 188
Stevens, William, 16
Stewart, Alexander Patrick, 287
Stewart, Dugald, 41, 192
sugar, 122ff., 197
sulphur, 149, 192
Sunderland, 32
Sutherland, John, 35, 66, 78, 144, 162, 225–6
Swayne, John Champeny, 158, 160, 161, 162n.
Swayne, Joseph Griffiths, 157ff., 161–2, 163, 164, 166, 167, 169, 170, 172, 174ff., 183, 185, 186–8, 216, 264, 308, 309
sweating sickness, 79n.
Sweden, 50
Sydenham, Thomas, 19, 43, 53–6, 62, 68, 76, 87ff., 95, 100, 103, 104, 111, 139, 142, 213
Sydenham Society, 53, 195, 196
Symonds, John Addington (snr.), 159ff., 254–5
syphilis, 99, 101n., 258, 272

telluric theory, 148
Thenard, Louis Jacques, 85
therapeutics, 13, 14, 21, 25, 50–1, 53, 78, 100, 103, 132, 133, 146–7, 148, 151, 163, 167, 168–9, 179, 181, 191–2, 193, 194n., 222, 223, 269, 270, 279, 302
Thiersch, Karl, 127, 236–7, 240, 242–4, 245, 246–7, 248, 283, 286, 288, 293
Thom, Alexander, 79n.
Thomson, Anthony Todd, 71
Thomson, Robert Dundas, 95n., 105, 219–20, 221n., 223, 246–7
Thomson, Thomas, 105, 126
thrush, 191n.
Thwaites, George, 156, 157
Times, The, 31n., 167–8, 170ff., 184, 245
tinea favosa, 198
Tripe, John William, 142n.
Trousseau, Armand, 284

tuberculosis, 4, 5, 60, 86, 236, 258, 274, 289. Consumption, 92; phthisis, 95n., 163, 286; scrofula, 36, 43, 95n.
Tunstall, James, 148
Tweedie, Alexander, 9n., 25–6, 222, 309
typhoid, typhus. *See* fever

Unitarianism, 8–9, 70
University College, London, 5n., 70, 85, 86, 95n., 154n., 181n., 183, 184n., 194, 215, 230, 264, 268, 271n.
uredos, 176, 177, 185, 186n., 188

vaccination, 17, 35n., 63, 90, 163, 238
ventilation, 24–5, 43ff., 65, 107, 291
vibriones, 234
Vienna, 160n., 236n.
Villemin, Jean-Antoine, 236, 237, 248n.
Villermé, Louis René, 95n., 96
Virchow, Rudolf, 257, 260
vitalism, 41, 120, 121, 125, 130, 131–2, 137, 149, 190, 198, 210–11, 213, 214, 304

Wakley, Thomas, 13, 36, 73, 111
Ward, Nathaniel, 222
Wardrop, James, 13n.
Warsaw, 239
Warwick, 70
water supply, 32, 89, 91, 99, 109, 110, 144, 171, 172, 175n., 218–19, 229, 235–6, 241, 246, 248, 275, 276, 283, 288, 290, 293, 296. Analysis of, 105, 166, 176, 180, 182, 184, 187, 217, 219–21, 223, 225, 235; drinking, 1, 78, 138, 204, 206, 216, 217–18, 224–6, 227–8, 235, 276; filtration, 235; water-companies, 220, 225, 234–5, 236, 296; watercourses, 48, 109
Watson, Thomas, 119n., 142, 178, 231, 271–2, 274, 292n.
Webster, G., 85n., 87n.
Webster, George, 85n.
Western Literary Institution, 216
Westminster Medical Society (Medical Society of London), 167, 176, 214ff., 218

Westminster Review, The, 7, 11, 28
Westmoreland, 100
Whitechapel, 100
Whitehead, Henry, 203, 224n.
whooping cough, 101n., 265
Wilkinson, J. Stuart, 200
Willan, Robert, 42n.
Williams, Charles James Blasius, 95n., 178n.
Williams, P. H., 218
Williams, Robert, 117–20, 270
Willis, Thomas, 103, 133n., 142
Windsor, 291–2
Wöhler, Friedrich, 126, 244
Wollaston, William Hyde, 192

Woolwich, 71
Worcester, 158

yeast, 121–3, 134–6, 193, 196, 197, 200, 210, 233, 261. *See also* fermentation
yellow fever. *See* fever
York, 214, 239n.

Zurich, 193n.
zymosis, zymotics, 53, 66, 90, 99, 101–8, 109–10, 138–9, 143–4, 148, 208n., 224, 234, 248, 259. *See also* fermentation

NS.